PSYCHIATRY
CLERKSHIP GUIDE

PSYCHIATRY
CLERKSHIP GUIDE

SECOND EDITION

Myrl R. S. Manley, MD

Associate Professor of Psychiatry
Director of Medical Student Education in Psychiatry
New York University School of Medicine
New York, New York

Lindsay Maddocks is credited for the following illustrations:

Chapter 18, Figure 1
Chapter 23, Figures 1 and 2
Chapter 26, Figures 1 and 2
Chapter 27, Figures 1A, 1B, and 2
Chapter 29, Figure 1
Chapter 30, Figure 2

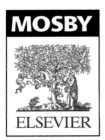

MOSBY

ELSEVIER

MOSBY
ELSEVIER

**WM
141
P9743
2007**

1600 John F. Kennedy Blvd.
Ste 1800
Philadelphia, PA 19103–2899

PSYCHIATRY CLERKSHIP GUIDE   ISBN: ⟨
Copyright © 2007, 2003 by Mosby, Inc., an affiliate of Elsevier Inc.

Notice

Knowledge and best practice in this field are constantly changing. As new research and experience broaden our knowledge, changes in practice, treatment and drug therapy may become necessary or appropriate. Readers are advised to check the most current information provided (i) on procedures featured or (ii) by the manufacturer of each product to be administered, to verify the recommended dose or formula, the method and duration of administration, and contraindications. It is the responsibility of the practitioner, relying on their own experience and knowledge of the patient, to make diagnoses, to determine dosages and the best treatment for each individual patient, and to take all appropriate safety precautions. To the fullest extent of the law, neither the Publisher nor the Authors assumes any liability for any injury and/or damage to persons or property arising out or related to any use of the material contained in this book.

The Publisher

Library of Congress Cataloging-in-Publication Data
Psychiatry clerkship guide / [edited by] Myrl R. S. Manley. — 2nd ed.
    p. ; cm.
    Includes index.
    ISBN 1-4160-3132-4
1. Psychiatry.   2. Clinical clerkship. I. Manley, Myrl R. S.
[DNLM: 1. Mental Disorders—diagnosis.   2. Clinical Clerkship.   3. Psychiatry—education. WM 141 P9743 2008]
RC480.5.P725 2008
616.89—dc22   2007001651

Acquisitions Editor: James Merritt
Developmental Editor: Nicole DiCicco
Publishing Services Manager: Linda Van Pelt
Project Manager: Francisco Morales
Design Direction: Louis Forgione

Printed in USA
Last digit is the print number: 9 8 7 6 5 4 3 2 1

Contributors

Carmen M. Alonso, MD
Clinical Assistant Professor of Psychiatry
Director of Pediatric Psychiatry Emergency Services & HBCI
New York University School of Medicine-Bellevue Hospital Center
New York, New York

Michael Dulchin, MD
Assistant Clinical Professor of Psychiatry
Unit Chief, Inpatient Psychiatry
Tisch Hospital/NYU Medical Centers
New York, New York

Dillon Euler, MD
Teaching Assistant in Psychiatry
Staff Psychiatrist
Project for Psychiatric Outreach to the Homeless
New York, New York

Nancy Forman, MD
Attending Psychiatrist
New York Harbor Healthcare System
Department of Veterans Affairs
New York, New York

Natalie Gluck, MD
Clinical Instructor in Psychiatry
Assistant Director of Medical Student Education in Psychiatry
Department of Psychiatry
New York University School of Medicine
New York, New York

Joel Gold, MD
Clinical Associate Professor of Psychiatry
Director, Psychiatric Emergency Services (CPEP)
New York University School of Medicine
New York, New York

Gary Gosselin, MD
Clinical Associate Professor of Psychiatry
Chief, Adolescent Inpatient Unit
Bellevue Hospital Center
New York, New York

Marianne T. Guschwann, MD
Clinical Assistant Professor of Psychiatry
New York University School of Medicine
New York, New York

Glenn Heiss, PhD
Clinical Assistant Professor of Psychiatry
New York University School of Medicine
General Track Coordinator
New York University-Bellevue Clinical Psychology Internship Program
New York, New York

Michelle Izmerly, DO
Clinical Instructor of Psychiatry
New York University School of Medicine
Associate Director of Ambulatory and Community Psychiatry
Bellevue Hospital
New York, New York

Ze'ev Levin, MD
Associate Clinical Professor of Psychiatry
New York University School of Medicine
Associate Director of Residency Training
New York, New York

Heather Lewerenz, MD
Assistant Clinical Professor of Psychiatry
New York University School of Medicine
Attending Psychiatrist, Bellevue Hospital
Comprehensive Psychiatric Emergency Program
New York, New York

Myrl R. S. Manley, MD
Associate Professor of Psychiatry
Director of Medical Student Education in Psychiatry
New York University School of Medicine
New York, New York

Raphael Morris, MD
Clinical Assistant Professor of Psychiatry
New York University School of Medicine
New York, New York

Heather Morse, MD
Clinical Instructor of Psychiatry
Unit Chief, Psychiatric Evaluation Service
Bellevue Hospital
New York, New York

Anand Pandya, MD
Clinical Assistant Professor of Psychiatry
New York University School of Medicine
Director of Ambulatory and Community Psychiatry
Bellevue Hospital
New York, New York

Molly E. Poag, MD
Assistant Clinical Professor of Psychiatry
New York University School of Medicine
Acting Chairman
Department of Psychiatry
Lenox Hill Hospital
New York, New York

Michelle Rottenstein, MD
Clinical Assistant Professor of Psychiatry
New York University School of Medicine
Department of Psychiatry
Lenox Hill Hospital
New York, New York

Arthur Sinkman, MD
Associate Clinical Professor of Psychiatry
Training Coordinator, Inpatient Psychiatry
New York VA Medical Center
New York, New York

Eric Teitel, MD
Clinical Assistant Professor
Assistant Unit Chief
Adolescent Inpatient Unit
Bellevue Hospital Center
New York, New York

Serena Yuan Volpp, MD, MPH
Unit Chief
Residency Training Unit
Bellevue Hospital
New York, New York

Van Yu, MD
Clinical Assistant Professor
New York University School of Medicine
Director, Project for Psychiatric Outreach to the Homeless
Medical Director
Center for Urban Community Services
New York, New York

Preface

Three years in clinical medicine is a long time and this is especially true of psychiatry. Since the first edition of the *Psychiatry Clerkship Guide* appeared four years ago a lot has changed. Many new medications have been approved for use in psychiatric disorders. At the same time, some drugs that were widely used are now recognized to pose greater risk than once thought. In addition, novel nonpharmacologic treatments are being pioneered, such as vagal nerve stimulation for the treatment of depression. The field continues to evolve, and our patients will benefit. Students of psychiatry, however, may feel they are trying to aim at a moving target. The "facts" of clinical psychiatry learned in the second year may be questioned by the time of the clerkship and outdated by the time of graduation. This new edition of the *Clerkship Guide* is our effort to keep pace with a rapidly changing discipline. All chapters from the first edition have been updated and most have been substantially rewritten. Four new chapters have been added. We have included in the appendix a table of current psychiatric medications listing mechanisms, indications, side effects, and dangers. The self-assessment examination has been completely rewritten in the style and format of the USMLE Step 1 exam. Despite these extensive changes, our goals remain the same. We want our students to share in the excitement, fun, and satisfaction of working with psychiatric patients, to recognize that psychiatric disorders can be understood medically and rationally diagnosed, and most of all to learn firsthand that these disorders can be treated—that even the most severely disturbed patients can be restored to reason and function, and brought back into the world.

I would like to thank Joseph P. Merlino, Christine E. Desmond, Lawrence Jacobsberg, Hillery Bosworth, Petros Levounis, and Aaron Metricken for their contributions in the first edition of *Psychiatry Clerkship Guide*.

Myrl R. S. Manley, MD

Contents

Orientation to the Psychiatry Clerkship

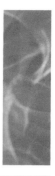

1

The Patient's Day on the Inpatient Unit

JOEL GOLD

 INVOLUNTARY TREATMENT

Why Are Most Psychiatric Units Locked?

Psychiatric disorders frequently affect a patient's ability to understand what is wrong with him or her. In psychiatry, this is referred to as *poor insight*. Even when psychiatric patients do understand what is wrong, some disorders prevent patients from aligning their behavior with their understanding. For example, a manic patient may be aware of the need for treatment but feel too agitated to remain in the hospital. If the patient is admitted involuntarily, this means that one or more physicians have filled out legal papers confining the patient to a hospital for a defined period of time. When this happens, the patient is legally not allowed to leave the hospital without a discharge order written by a physician.

What Are the Criteria for Involuntary Treatment?

Although it is necessary to have a psychiatric disorder to be admitted involuntarily, this is not all that is necessary. To override a patient's right to refuse treatment, every state in the United States and most of the provinces in Canada require that a person with mental illness be at some risk for harming himself or others as a result of his illness. In some states, such as New York, this danger is summarized as a "substantial risk of harm to self or others." In other states, such as California, a physician can commit a patient to involuntary treatment if the patient is "gravely disabled." It is important to remember that individuals cannot be hospitalized involuntarily because of psychosis alone. Many individuals have hallucinations and delusions and still live in the community. It is only when these symptoms threaten to cause harm to the individual or others that involuntary hospitalization is required. Nevertheless, some individuals with psychiatric symptoms are at an increased risk for harm to themselves or others when they are acutely ill. Table 1-1 presents a list of indications for psychiatric hospitalization.

Table 1-1

Some Indications for Psychiatric Hospitalization

Suicidal ideas

Homicidal ideas

Ideas of engaging in behavior that may evoke violence (e.g., planning to sneak into the White House to advise the President)

Command auditory hallucinations to hurt oneself or to hurt others

Command auditory hallucinations to engage in behavior that may evoke violence from other (e.g., the voice of God orders the patient to kiss everyone he or she meets)

Severe weight loss (e.g., as occurs in anorexia nervosa)

Repeated induction of vomiting, resulting in electrolyte imbalance (e.g., as occurs in bulimia nervosa)

Self-cutting or other self-harming behavior that, although not intended to kill, is potentially more dangerous than the patient realizes

Disorganized behavior that can hurt oneself or others (e.g., trying to dry one's hair with a lighter)

Forgetful behavior that can hurt oneself or others (e.g., forgetting to turn off the stove because of dementia)

Behavior deemed intolerable to the community (e.g., walking naked in the streets shouting obscenities)

VOLUNTARY TREATMENT

What Are the Criteria for Voluntary Treatment?

In a strictly legal sense, a patient can be hospitalized for almost any condition that requires psychiatric or medical attention. There is no law that prevents a psychiatrist and a patient from arranging a weekend in a hospital for the treatment of relatively mild anxiety, just as there is no law that prevents a surgeon from performing plastic surgery on a patient with relatively minor blemishes. However, in practice, most individuals have their psychiatric care paid for by third-party payers such as Medicaid, Medicare, the Bureau of Veterans Affairs, or a private insurance company. These third-party payers pay for inpatient treatment only for conditions that cannot be safely treated on an outpatient basis. Thus, most patients who are admitted to an inpatient psychiatric service meet one of the following criteria: (1) they are a danger to themselves because of their mental illness, (2) they are a danger to others because of their mental illness, (3) they have a medical condition that cannot be adequately treated on an outpatient basis because of their mental illness, (4) they engage in behavior that is intolerable to society, or (5) they cannot adequately attend to the basic necessities of living.

An example of behavior that is intolerable to society is that of an individual with schizophrenia who is so disorganized that he defecates on himself in public. Such an individual may not necessarily pose a threat to himself or to others but probably meets the criteria for a voluntary admission in most settings. When patients meeting the preceding criteria are able and willing to sign in voluntarily, they should be allowed to do so. If however, they are unable to do so, they can and should be admitted involuntarily.

Where Do Patients on the Inpatient Unit Come From?

Patients may have walked into an emergency room by themselves or with family or have been brought to an emergency department by police or emergency services. After being found appropriate for admission, they are transferred to the unit. In some hospitals, patients may be admitted directly to a unit by an outpatient physician who has admitting privileges at that hospital. Those patients may be observed by their outpatient physician while in the hospital, or their care may be transferred to attending physicians and house staff who work in the hospital. Still other patients may be admitted from medical and surgical inpatient units by a consultation-liaison psychiatrist.

All patients should be aware of their legal status and their rights as patients in the hospital, including access to mental hygiene attorneys. In addition, patients should be informed of the rules on the unit and should be introduced to the members of their treatment team.

 RULES AND REGULATIONS

Why Are There So Many Rules on Psychiatric Inpatient Units?

Inpatient psychiatric units often have a long list of contraband items, a long list of restricted behaviors, and a system of privilege levels. Patients often complain that they are not allowed to do things that they did every day before admission. Medical students can find themselves defending rules and regulations that they do not understand.

The reason for most rules and regulations is safety. Most items that are contraband on inpatient units are things that could be used to hurt people. Even simple things such as shampoo and headphones may be banned because suicidal patients have been known to drink shampoo and homicidal patients have tried to strangle someone with the wire from headphones.

Many hospitals no longer allow smoking. Patients with psychiatric illnesses are more likely to be smokers than the general public. Although patients often complain about not being able to smoke, nonsmoking facilities feel strongly that smoking is a public health danger and also a fire hazard. On units with smoking bans, patients should be offered alternatives such as nicotine gum or a patch or perhaps bupropion, an antidepressant used to dull nicotine craving.

Why Do Staff Interfere with Relationships between Patients?

Aside from the risk of violence, inpatient psychiatry is very concerned about the risk of patients engaging in sexual behavior. Although sex is

The Patient's Day

a normal part of life, there often is a universal ban on intimate behavior on acute inpatient units. First, patients may not be able to consent to sexual behavior when they are acutely ill. When people are hospitalized in a psychiatric unit, there is a good chance that their mental illness is so severe that they cannot make rational decisions. It is the responsibility of the staff to ensure that they do not engage in behavior that they might later regret.

Enforcing rules about sexual behavior is sometimes hard for medical students and younger staff. Often, medical students identify with patients and have trouble seeing the harm in a hug or a kiss. However, experience has shown that without a strict boundary, it is often difficult to prevent individuals from progressing to more risky behavior. Even if a particularly healthy pair of patients appears to have a "harmless" intimate relationship, other, sicker patients may see this behavior and not understand why they get in trouble when they attempt the same thing.

MILIEU THERAPY, GROUP THERAPY, ART THERAPY, AND ACTIVITY THERAPY

What Is Milieu Therapy?

Milieu therapy (or the *therapeutic ward milieu*) refers to the positive effect of the inpatient unit environment, achieved through appropriate manipulation of the environment by the staff for the benefit of the patients. The inpatient unit can be thought of as a microcosm of the "outside" world, a place where patients can practice social skills with peers, work on maintaining good impulse control and safety, and prepare for a return to the community. Staff should be flexible in building a therapeutic milieu that addresses the specific needs of the community: schooling on child and adolescent units; age-appropriate activities on geriatric units; culturally sensitive programming, including staff who speak patients' languages. Homeless patients may be reassured of having a bed for the night. Other patients feel safe in the hospital, believing that the staff will take care of their physical and psychiatric problems.

Despite this, most patients are ambivalent about being in the hospital. They may express only part of this ambivalence. Some express only gratitude for being hospitalized, whereas others express only fears and regrets about being hospitalized. It is important to remember that some patients benefit from the milieu of the hospital despite their expressed preference for being out of the hospital.

What Is the Difference between Group Therapy and Individual Therapy?

There are significant differences between group therapy and individual therapy. Instead of focusing on the problems of one individual, *group therapy* attempts to provide a positive therapeutic effect on several people at once. This means that the leader of the group needs to balance the needs of different individuals. No one member should dominate a group, but that does not mean that everyone in the group has to participate equally. Inevitably, some patients are more talkative than others. The problems of one individual may be the focus for some period of time as long as the group leader is aware of how that benefits the rest of the group.

Depending on the makeup of a group, its structure and focus vary. Groups with lower functioning patients may be more psychoeducational, focusing on symptom recognition, medication indications and side effects, or current events. Groups with higher functioning patients are often *process* groups that focus on interactions between group members (including the group leader) as the group is happening.

Doesn't Group Therapy Violate Patients' Confidentiality?

The violation of patients' confidentiality is a potential problem that must be taken seriously. The group leader must not reveal confidential information about any particular patient unless the patient brings it up himself. Most groups begin by stressing confidentiality: after the group session, members should not discuss anything that was revealed with anyone who was not a part of the group.

What Do I Do if I'm Asked to Lead a Group?

One of the biggest differences between conducting an individual session with a patient and leading a group is the experience of being outnumbered. In an individual session, you have much more control over what is being said. Fortunately, the group leader is not expected to control what develops in the group. You should resist the urge to answer every question that is raised. Even if the group begins to focus on what is good or bad about the hospital, it is not your job to fix the problem. Instead, the group leader maintains the structure of the group. The group leader may also help the members of the group to help each other and to find answers and solutions for themselves. Although it is important to have a flexible approach when running groups, it is equally important to set the structure and inform members of the rules for the particular group.

If the Group Leader Is Not Supposed to Solve Every Problem and Answer Every Question, How Does Group Therapy Work?

Table 1-2 lists several therapeutic factors that occur in group therapy. A group leader may be able to steer the discussion in such a way that some of these therapeutic factors are present. However, because the group process is so complex, the group leader is unlikely to be completely aware of all of the therapeutic factors as they occur.

What Are Activity Therapy and Art Therapy?

Activity therapy is based on the observation that mastering simple skills such as an exercise routine or planting a garden has a therapeutic effect. Many psychiatric patients have impaired concentration, an impaired ability to initiate actions, cognitive deficits, and movement disorders.

Table 1-2

Therapeutic Factors in Group Therapy

Factor	Definition	Example
Altruism	The patient has the experience of helping others.	A depressed patient is able to feel a sense of mastery and control when she can give advice to help another patient.
Corrective familial	The experience of the group parallels the experience of the patient's family but without the pathologic features.	A patient with obsessive-compulsive personality disorder has brothers who mocked him when he cried, but in group other members respect his feelings.
Modeling	A patient learns skills by imitating others in the group.	By imitating the behavior of others in the group, a schizophrenic patient learns to wait until others stop speaking before she begins talking.
Instillation of hope	Positive motivation and optimism are increased.	A more depressed patient feels better when he hears that a less depressed patient is now ready for discharge.
Universalization	That others have similar experiences is recognized.	A patient who feels ashamed about his alcoholism can finally admit it after hearing others speak about their problem.
Cohesion	The patient has the experience of oneness or of working toward a common goal.	A group of depressed patients feels less lonely and depressed after they unite to make a suggestion box for the unit.
Education	The patient learns about a disease and its treatment, increasing his ability to cope with his illness.	A bipolar patient hears from another bipolar patient about the importance of medication, even when feeling well.
Reality testing	Reality is confirmed and distortions corrected.	A schizophrenic patient with persecutory delusions hears other patients also complain about the quality of the food but without feeling they are being poisoned.
Ventilation	Feelings or thoughts are expressed, giving a sense of relief.	An alcohol-dependent patient overcomes her embarrassment after she admits in a group that she is an alcoholic.

Activity therapy helps patients with simple activities that may be very practical (e.g., learning activities of daily living such as grooming) or less directly relevant to life outside the hospital (e.g., learning a folk dance). Because some psychiatric medications cause sedation, obesity, and even diabetes mellitus, psychiatric patients are at increased risk for cardiac disease. Activity therapy that includes aerobic exercise is especially important in this population.

Art therapy is based on a similar observation about the positive effect of artistic expression on patients. Artistic expression reflects what is important for the patient. It may convey everything from the concrete concerns to the emotional experience of an individual. Often, patients create art that refers indirectly to ideas and feelings that are too charged to express directly to their physician. In addition, the production of a work of art may give a patient confidence and a sense of mastery that is therapeutic.

Because activity therapy and art therapy are usually conducted in a group format in the inpatient setting, the therapeutic factors of groups (see Table 1-2) may also contribute to the positive effect of these therapies.

In addition to the therapeutic benefit provided by art and activity therapies, these groups help shed light on the patient's current functioning motivation, ability to concentrate, energy level, degree of organization, and ability to work with others. This information helps you and the staff evaluate the effect of medication and assess the need for continued hospitalization or readiness for discharge.

 ## COMMUNITY MEETING

Who Should Attend Community Meeting?

Theoretically, *community meeting* should include all of the staff and all of the patients of an inpatient unit. In practice, there are always some patients who choose not to attend community meeting, and on some units, patients may be excluded from community meeting because of disruptive behavior. Thus, some staff must also be excluded from community meeting to take care of the patients who do not attend.

What Is the Purpose of Community Meeting?

Community meeting is a form of group therapy that fosters cohesion and increases communication among the staff and the patients. It may also serve as an opportunity for many of the other therapeutic factors listed in Table 1-2.

How Is Community Meeting Different from Other Groups?

More staff and more patients attend community meetings than most other group activities. This larger forum usually requires a different set of rules to maintain order. For example, individuals may be asked to raise hands before speaking. One of the main jobs of the leader of this group is to keep the focus on "community issues." This means that individual issues, such as when an individual patient is leaving, are not usually allowed. Inevitably, some patients have difficulty understanding what a community issue is and raise questions that pertain to their personal treatment, such as "Why am I on this medication?"

Because most staff attend community meeting, it is a rare opportunity for patients to speak to the whole treatment team involved in their care. Patients often express their many frustrations, concerns, and demands during this meeting. It is common for less experienced staff to see this as a negative atmosphere; it is important to remember that it may be therapeutic.

OBSERVATION, SECLUSION, AND RESTRAINTS

What Is Observation?

All patients on inpatient units are monitored regularly by members of the staff, usually by nurses or psychiatric technicians. As patients might be a danger to themselves or others, all patients are checked at regular intervals, both day and night, often every 30 minutes. If staff members are more concerned about a particular patient, that patient may be checked more frequently, perhaps every 15 minutes. A patient who is in imminent danger (e.g., who is actively suicidal or assaultive) or an elopement risk may require one-to-one observation. In such cases, a member of the staff watches the patient at all times.

What Is Seclusion?

Seclusion is the placement of an individual in a room separate from the rest of the patients and staff to protect him, other patients, and the staff. The patient cannot leave the room either because the door is locked or because staff members block his exit. Seclusion differs from involuntary hospitalization because in seclusion, a patient is limited to one room, without access to the rest of the psychiatric unit. Seclusion also differs from placing a person in isolation. The purpose of isolation is to prevent the spread of infectious disease. The purpose of seclusion is to minimize psychiatric morbidity and mortality.

What Are Restraints?

Restraints are mechanical devices such as a straitjacket, straps, or a net that physically prevent an individual from moving. The restraints used in modern psychiatric settings are designed to minimize harm and discomfort to the patient. The use of restraints varies considerably from facility to facility. The types of restraints used for a given purpose may also vary.

What Are Pharmacologic Restraints?

The term *pharmacologic restraints* has different meanings. It is sometimes used to describe any medication that is given as needed (pro re nata [PRN]) to decrease the acute risk of violence. In other settings, it is used only to describe medications used for that purpose that are not part of the usual psychiatric armamentarium, such as anesthetics. The term pharmacologic restraint is itself controversial in psychiatry; it implies that medication is being administered to restrain the activities of a patient. Although medication may be administered to decrease the risk of violence, it is not used to restrain the patient but rather to help the patient to control himself. When psychiatric medication is administered to a patient who is at risk for violence, the goal is usually to decrease agitation, decrease anxiety, and decrease irritability or explosive rage. In general, it is best to avoid the term pharmacologic restraint and instead to describe the specific medications that are being used and the specific purpose of each medication.

When Does Someone Need Seclusion?

Seclusion is indicated when the risk of danger from an agitated or violent patient outweighs the negative effects of seclusion. Predictions of dangerousness are based on the totality of clinical information. Often, the risk of danger is demonstrated when a patient has already engaged in violence or threatened to engage in violence. At other times, staff must conclude that a patient is at a substantial risk for imminent danger when the patient is increasingly agitated and has a history of violence or when an agitated patient is unable to follow the rules of the unit and is unable to respond to verbal redirection by the staff.

Balanced against the dangerousness are the negative effects of seclusion. Being secluded is often traumatic. Patients who have been secluded may report feeling that they were treated like an "animal" or an "object." Patients may report feeling humiliated and scared. Some patients develop symptoms of post-traumatic stress disorder after experiencing seclusion. At the very least, seclusion may severely strain or disrupt the alliance between the patient and the treatment team. Both the patient and the treatment team may feel profoundly uncomfortable about what happened and may avoid talking about it. At the same time, a lack of trust between the patient and the team may undermine the rest of the treatment. For all of these reasons, seclusion must be used judiciously.

When Does Someone Need Restraints?

Because restraints are more restrictive than seclusion, they are more effective at preventing violence. Patients generally experience restraints as more traumatizing, so restraints are used only when a patient is so agitated that it is unsafe to keep him secluded in a room. A patient who bangs his head against the wall of the seclusion room or who punches or kicks the door to get the attention of individuals outside the room may require restraints.

When Should Seclusion or Restraints Not Be Used?

Seclusion should not be used if a patient may hurt herself in the seclusion room. Suicidal patients should not be placed in seclusion unless they can be continuously observed and supervised.

In addition, it is dangerous to keep patients in restraints or seclusion if they are acutely intoxicated or medically unstable. Intoxicated individuals may aspirate vomitus while in restraints because they are unable to turn onto their side. Individuals who are intoxicated with phenylcyclidine (PCP) or who are delirious may become more psychotic if they are restrained. The use of seclusion and restraints usually leads to decreased verbal and visual stimuli, and individuals who are intoxicated with PCP or who are delirious may become more agitated and psychotic. Although they are sometimes necessary, restraints can be dangerous both for the patient and for the staff placing the patient in restraints. As such, they should be used as a last resort when other less restrictive measures have failed.

Finally, it is important that seclusion and restraints are never used for the convenience of the staff or to punish a patient. If you believe that a patient is being secluded or restrained for punishment or for the convenience of the staff, it is important that you speak to your supervisor to clarify the purpose of these serious interventions.

What Needs to Be Done When a Patient Is Placed in Seclusion or Restraints?

After a patient is secluded or restrained, the first job of the medical staff is to assess the patient. Was the patient physically hurt in the process of being placed in seclusion or restraints? Does the patient require medication to help him calm down? Is the patient safe in seclusion, or does he need restraints? Are the restraints placed properly, or can the patient wiggle into a position where he can (accidentally or intentionally) strangle himself? The staff should offer to contact the patient's family to inform them about the incident as soon as possible.

The next responsibility is to document what has occurred. All uses of seclusion and restraints require an order from a physician specifying how long the individual is to be kept secluded or restrained. In addition, it is important to write a note in the progress notes explaining why a person was put in seclusion or restraints. Although these are often chaotic situations, it is important to think carefully about how to document them. A complete note concerning seclusion or restraints should mention the time of the incident, the date, what behavior the patient demonstrated during the incident, what may have precipitated the incident, and why the incident could not be handled with a less restrictive measure. A sample note is provided in Box 1-1.

The medical staff must periodically reassess the need for seclusion or restraints. It is never acceptable to renew an order for seclusion or restraints without reevaluating the patient. When the patient is ready to be released, it is important to talk to the patient about his or her experience. Allow the patient to express negative feelings about what was experienced. If the patient feels that he was wronged, it is important not to get into an argument. Respectfully disagree and emphasize that the staff wants to continue to work with the patient on the problems that led to the hospitalization. However, if the patient cannot see anything wrong with his previous actions and indicates that he intends to complete a plan

The Patient's Day

BOX 1-1

A SAMPLE NOTE DOCUMENTING SECLUSION

7/1/2001 Medical Student Note 3:30 PM

The patient became agitated after speaking on the telephone with his mother about a half-hour ago. The medication nurse attempted to calm him down and offered him medication to help him calm down, but he refused and began to scream threats. The patient was then so agitated that he was a clear and substantial risk of imminent violence toward the medication nurse and therefore he was placed in the seclusion room. The patient accepted Haldol 5 mg PO and Ativan 2 mg PO at that time and is now somewhat calmer but still visibly angry. The resident offered to call the patient's family, but the patient refused. The patient was secluded at 3:20 PM for a maximum of 2 hours but can be released earlier if he is calm and able to verbalize that he will not try to hurt anyone.

of hurting himself, staff, or other patients, it may be unsafe to release this patient into the community, and alternatives such as continuous observation by staff must be considered.

Can a Patient Be Forced to Take Medications?

A patient may receive medications emergently—usually intramuscularly—if she is an acute danger to herself or others, often in the context of severe agitation. Otherwise, patients have the right to refuse medication. If a patient is refusing medication and the medical staff believes that such medication is required, the hospital may apply to the court to have the patient receive medication over her objection. If a judge signs such an order and the patient continues to refuse oral medication, the staff may proceed to give the medication intramuscularly when such a preparation exists (e.g., intramuscular haloperidol.)

KEY POINTS

- ◆ Psychosis alone does not justify involuntary hospitalization.
- ◆ Art and activity therapies, in addition to being a part of treatment, are used to assess the patient's abilities to perform complex tasks and to interact with others.
- ◆ Seclusion or restraints must never be used for staff convenience or to punish patients.

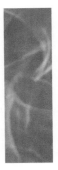

2

The Medical Student's Role on the Inpatient Service

JOEL GOLD

THE STUDENT AS A MEMBER OF AN INTERDISCIPLINARY TREATMENT TEAM

What Is an Interdisciplinary Team?

Most psychiatric inpatient units use an *interdisciplinary team model*. The team includes the medical staff, the nurses, the social workers, and staff from other disciplines who provide clinical care, such as activity therapists, art therapists, psychologists, and case managers. The team makes decisions concerning the care of the patient with input from members of all the disciplines. These decisions may include determining when a patient is ready for additional privileges, when a patient is ready for discharge, and what kind of follow-up is necessary after discharge. Table 2-1 describes the activities of some members of the multidisciplinary team.

Why Does Psychiatry Use an Interdisciplinary Team?

Patients may report different symptoms to different members of the staff for a variety of reasons. A patient may trust physicians more than she trusts nurses, or she may feel more comfortable admitting symptoms to individuals of the same sex or of a similar background. A patient may be invested in convincing a physician that she is healthy so that she can be discharged. On the other hand, some patients want to convince a social worker that they are helpless so that they can receive additional services after discharge. This process of appearing different to different people is usually done unconsciously; discrepancies do not necessarily mean that the patient is lying. In addition, the illness may manifest differently at different times of the day or in different situations. A patient with major depressive disorder with melancholic features may appear more depressed to the medical staff in the morning and less depressed to the nursing staff in the evening. Finally, because members of different disciplines have different training, they observe different aspects of the same patient. An activity therapist who watches a patient complete complex tasks may be impressed by how healthy the patient appears to be, whereas

Table 2-1

Responsibilities of Members of the Multidisciplinary Team

Profession	Responsibilities in Inpatient Psychiatry
Psychiatrist	Psychotherapy, psychoeducation, medication management*; certification for involuntary hospitalization*; writing orders for restraints,* seclusion,* and discharges*; conducting group therapies including community meeting, disposition planning, and family meetings
Nurse	Dispensing medication, psychoeducation, implementing most physician orders and ward rules, conducting group therapies including community meeting, providing daily assessments of patients' progress
Social worker	Discharge planning (including application for entitlements and outpatient services), conducting family meetings, psychoeducation to families, conducting group therapies including community meeting
Psychologist	Psychological testing (including neuropsychiatric testing and intelligence testing), psychotherapy, and psychoeducation
Occupational therapist	Conducting group activities, systematically evaluating patients' ability to engage in activities of daily living, training patients to engage in activities of daily living and in other simple skills
Recreational therapist	Conducting group activities, helping patients develop a healthy leisure lifestyle
Creative arts therapist	Conducting group activities, using creative arts such as music, drama, dance, and art as a means of self-expression that can foster self-awareness

*These functions are the exclusive responsibility of physicians.

a nurse who needs to exhort the same patient to take each dose of medication may be struck by how ill the patient appears to be. Before you make important decisions about your patient, you need to hear the perspectives of members of the different disciplines.

What Is the Medical Student's Role in an Interdisciplinary Team?

The medical student functions in the role of the physician; the level of responsibility varies from school to school. During team meetings, a medical student is often asked to report on the patient's psychiatric and general medical conditions. This includes a brief summary of the patient's symptoms and signs, any effect or side effects from the medication, and a summary of the patient's current treatment. Commonly, the medical student has 3 minutes or less to summarize the case. Members of other disciplines report their perceptions of the patient before or after the medical student reports her perceptions. Often, contradictory perceptions of the patient are presented, but it is not the job of the medical student to defend her point of view. Medical students are perceived as better clinicians if they can incorporate the different reports into a more complex view of the patient.

When Will I Meet with My Patient?

Initially, a new patient will probably be evaluated with members of the treatment team including the attending psychiatrist, the resident psychiatrist, a social worker, a nurse, and perhaps a member from other disciplines, such as an activity therapist. For the first several sessions, you may feel more comfortable meeting the patient with another member of the treatment team, but soon you will be meeting the patient by yourself. Although this may be a stressful experience at first, meeting one on one is often the best way to forge a strong therapeutic alliance. Over the course of your time on the unit, you are likely to be observed by other members of the team. Both watching others interview patients and interviewing a patient while being observed are valuable experiences.

Who Makes the Final Decisions in an Interdisciplinary Team?

Because different individuals have different experiences with the patient, it is common for there to be disagreements about clinical decisions. However, only a physician can sign an order to start, stop, or change medications. All discharges require an order by a physician, and most states require a physician to certify when a patient needs to be involuntarily hospitalized. Thus, the physician must agree with the ultimate decision.

CHART ROUNDS AND WALK ROUNDS

What Do I Need to Know about My Patients for Rounds?

Most inpatient units have daily rounds; these may include *chart rounds* (rounds held in a conference room), *walk rounds* (where the team as a whole goes to see the patient while discussing the case), or both. Table 2-2 provides a list of information that medical students should have for each of their patients.

Table 2-2
Patient Information for Daily Rounds
Name
Age
Race/ethnicity
Marital status
Psychiatric diagnoses
Medical diagnoses
Current medications
Medication history (during this hospitalization and before admission)
Most recent mental status examination, including the most recent cognitive examination

PROGRESS NOTES

What Is the Form of Psychiatric Progress Notes?

Most psychiatric inpatient units use the SOAP (subjective reports, objective findings, assessment, and plan) format for progress notes (Box 2-1). You may note that the mental status examination includes subjective elements such as the patient's report of his or her mood or perceptual disturbances. Because these are standard parts of the mental status examination, it is conventional to include them in the "O" section. You can also include some of this in the "S" section as long as your note does not become too long or redundant.

What Should I Say in the Assessment Section of the Progress Note?

In addition to having the right format, it is important to have the right content. When writing in the "A" section, keep three things in mind. First and

---

BOX 2-1

PSYCHIATRIC PROGRESS NOTE FORMAT

Date, Time

Type of Note (Medical Student Progress Note)

S = Subjective Report.

Include the patient's report of symptoms, change in reported symptoms since the last note or overall change since admission, new complaints, and side effects. In addition, it is common here to report on the patient's activities, such as the patient's experience while out on a pass.

O = Objective Observation.

In psychiatry, this usually consists of a mental status examination, but if the patient has medical comorbidity or if she reports somatic complaints, it is important also to document an appropriate physical examination here. Also document test results in this section.

A = Assessment.

This section includes a list of all of the patient's diagnoses with a comment on how the patient is progressing. A "problem list" is also useful.

P = Plan.

This section should include a complete biopsychosocial plan. (See Table 2-3 for details.)

    Signature (leave room for your supervisor to countersign your note)

foremost, you must accurately convey the change in your patient. Writing the identical assessment day after day does not convey much to the reader. The changes in psychiatry may be subtle compared with those that occur in other areas of medicine, but if you are not observing any changes for several consecutive days on an acute inpatient unit, you may want to ask for additional supervision before writing the same assessment again.

Second, it is important to comment on any new problems that are mentioned earlier in the note. For example, if you report in the "S" section that the patient has a somatic complaint, it is important to comment on whether this may be a dangerous medical development. If you do not intend to treat or to evaluate further a problem identified in the "S" or "O" section, it is important to explain why in the "A" section.

The third consideration for this section is to resist the urge to paint too bright a picture. If a patient is described as "stable" each day, he probably does not need to be in an inpatient unit. Your assessment should reflect why the patient still needs to be in the hospital.

What Is a Biopsychosocial Plan?

The biopsychosocial model described by George Engel in 1977 remains a major working model in clinical psychiatry. It proposes that psychiatric disorders are influenced by biologic, psychological, and social factors. A biopsychosocial plan acknowledges each of these three factors (Table 2-3).

The *biologic* evaluation should include an evaluation of possible biologic causes for the patient's psychiatric condition as well as an assessment of the patient's general health. Biologic causes for psychiatric symptoms, such as intoxication, head injury, or infection, are usually evaluated with the use of laboratory tests, physical examinations, or radiologic tests. A complete biologic evaluation should also include a review of past biologic treatments for the psychiatric symptoms. Obtaining old records and reviewing previous medication trials are tedious but crucial parts of good psychiatric practice.

A *psychological* evaluation may include formal psychological testing, but the most important psychological evaluation involves talking with your patient. You can identify areas for further discussion, and you must find out what psychological treatments have been tried in the past and how well they worked. If they worked poorly, what were the reasons?

A *social* evaluation usually includes gathering information about the stresses at home, work, or school that may have contributed to the patient's illness. In addition, it is important to assess the social supports that are available to the patient after discharge. Are there friends or family who can help the patient? Regardless of how a patient does on an inpatient unit, it is impossible to plan a successful discharge unless you evaluate what will be available after discharge. Can the patient return to a home, or will she be homeless?

How Is This Model Used to Prepare an Actual Comprehensive Treatment Plan?

Consider the case of a 21-year-old man with bipolar I disorder who is admitted with a manic episode. He is so agitated and hypersexual at

Table 2-3

Factors in the Biopsychosocial Model

	Past	Present
Biologic	Significant family history History of heavy alcohol or drug use History of head trauma History of central nervous system (CNS) illness History of systemic illness that may affect the CNS	Current alcohol/drug use Toxic/metabolic abnormalities Current CNS illness Current illness that may affect the CNS Recent head trauma Adherence or nonadherence to medication Side effects of medication
Psychological	Content of past symptoms Early family dynamics Important past relationships and friendships	Content of present symptoms Meaning to patient of current stressors Psychological strengths (e.g., intelligence, social skills, frustration tolerance) Nature of current friendships and relationships Self-esteem and sense of self
Social	Early home environment Past social matrix (family/friends) Past living arrangements Past employment Past cultural/religious/political environment	 Current social matrix Current living situation Current employment Current cultural/religious/political environment

the time of the admission that he cannot provide a coherent history during the initial interview. He is supposed to be taking lithium prescribed by an outpatient psychiatrist. Recommendations 1 through 6 of the plan in Box 2-2 correspond to the biologic evaluation. Recommendations 7 through 9 represent a psychological evaluation. Recommendation 10 represents a social evaluation. Recommendations 11 and 12 are biologic treatments. Recommendations 13 and 14 are psychological treatments. Recommendations 15 and 16 are social treatments or interventions. There is a great deal of overlap among these different areas. For example, the family meeting may accomplish recommendations 10 and 15. Also, some interventions do not fit neatly into one category or another. For example, group therapy can be a psychological and a social treatment. Nevertheless, keeping Table 2-3 in mind can help you to develop a complete plan like the one shown in Box 2-2.

Biologic treatments for psychiatric conditions include medications and electroconvulsive therapy. Psychological treatments for psychiatric

BOX 2-2

SAMPLE INPATIENT PLAN FOR A PATIENT ADMITTED DURING A MANIC EPISODE

1. Urine toxicology tests to rule out intoxication as a cause of the current symptoms
2. Electroencephalogram to rule out temporal lobe epilepsy as a cause of the current symptoms
3. Thyroid function tests to rule out hyperthyroidism as a cause of the current symptoms and to rule out hypothyroidism secondary to previous lithium treatment
4. Lithium level to assess medication compliance before admission and to assess the risk of lithium toxicity
5. Electrocardiogram and renal function tests to assess the safety of continuing lithium in this patient
6. Discussion with the patient's outpatient psychiatrist to review past medication trials and the reason for stopping previous medications
7. Discussion with the patient's outpatient psychiatrist to review past psychotherapy trials and the effects of psychotherapy on the patient's course and overall functioning
8. Neuropsychological testing to assess the patient's cognitive capacity to benefit from psychotherapy and to assess whether the patient is likely to have the capacity to manage medications and other responsibilities independently after discharge
9. A complete sexual history to assess the risk of the patient's having acquired a sexually transmitted disease during this or previous mood episodes
10. A family meeting to identify any stressors that may have precipitated the current manic episode; this meeting also assesses the level of family support and whether the family can engage in specific interventions such as monitoring the patient's compliance with medication after discharge
11. Lithium 600 mg PO twice a day
12. Clonazepam 1.5 mg PO twice a day
13. Psychoeducation to teach the patient about behavior that may increase his risk of relapse after discharge
14. Psychotherapy to help the patient accept his diagnosis and help him to adapt to this diagnosis without self-destructive behavior such as stopping his medication
15. Family meeting to plan a more structured environment for the patient after discharge
16. Group therapies to help the patient learn appropriate interpersonal behavior

conditions include psychotherapies and psychoeducation. Social treatments include family therapy, couples therapy, group therapy, and therapies that improve social skills. In the acute inpatient setting, there is usually insufficient time to provide ongoing family or couples therapy, and briefer interventions are used, such as family meetings.

FOLLOWING INPATIENTS: "PSYCHOTHERAPY" AND MEDICATION MANAGEMENT

What Should I Talk about with My Patients?

You can think of your interviews with patients as having two parts: *evaluation* and *treatment*. You evaluate changes in your patient's psychiatric condition by performing regular mental status examinations, although it may not be necessary to repeat the complete mental status examination at every interview. For example, if the patient does not have any history of cognitive impairment and the cognitive section of the mental status examination has been documented during the current admission, you may be able to skip this section (unless there is an acute change in the patient).

Although the assessment part of speaking with a patient is relatively straightforward, many medical students struggle with the treatment part of speaking with the patient. After assessing the symptoms, medical students often feel at a loss for words and feel uncertain about how to fill the time that they are expected to spend with the patient. It is important to remember that the process of learning about the patient is itself therapeutic. Patients can feel tremendous relief when they are given an opportunity to speak and when others take an interest in them. You can speak about whatever interests the patient or, if the patient has difficulty with sitting and talking, you can engage in activities together. Playing a game together may be especially valuable with children or psychotic patients.

Aside from offering the patient your ear, there are active parts to this "speaking treatment." This active part can be broken down into two categories: psychoeducation and psychotherapy.

What Is Psychoeducation?

Psychoeducation teaches patients about psychiatric disorders and treatments. It helps them understand their symptoms as aspects of a psychiatric disorder, and they learn the benefits and limitations of treatment and the need for compliance. Through psychoeducation, patients recognize the cause of their disorder and may be able to identify initial emerging symptoms before they require hospitalization.

What Is Psychotherapy?

Psychotherapy is the process of helping people to overcome problems by talking about them. Psychoeducation is important, but it does not solve the whole problem. Although some individuals with alcohol dependence are able to stop drinking when they are taught about the adverse effects of alcohol, many more alcoholics already know that alcohol is bad for them but are unable to stop drinking. Psychotherapy may help. It is not possible to learn how to conduct psychotherapy during the few weeks of a psychiatric clerkship. You can, however, develop an understanding of psychotherapy and of how talking with patients can be therapeutic, even if it is not formal psychotherapy.

Is It Dangerous to Talk to Patients?

Although violence on inpatient units is rare, it does happen. You should be aware of the environment and take precautions. Patients should not be seen in their rooms. When interviewing patients, you should stay between the patient and the exit in case the patient becomes agitated. Boundaries are important. You should not hold hands with or hug patients. You should maintain an appropriate and respectful distance from patients, neither too close, making you or the patient uncomfortable, nor too far, giving the impression that you are afraid or disgusted. You should never hesitate to end an interview or step away from a patient if he feels unsafe. In those circumstances, you should report the episode of agitation to other members of the staff. If you are unfamiliar with the patient or if the person has a history of violence, conduct meetings in open areas in view of other staff. If you sense that particular topics are unduly upsetting, do not press the patient to talk more. Finally, if you see an episode of violence between patients, do not attempt to intervene physically. Call for help. There are members of staff who are trained to work with agitated or violent patients.

What Should I Do if I Feel Uncomfortable or Confused about My Feelings?

Patients can engender feelings in seasoned clinicians and students alike. Sometimes this is due to overt behavior on the part of the patient and sometimes it is due to unconscious processes within the mind of the person working with the patient. Broadly, these feelings are termed *countertransference*. Finding yourself surprised by feelings of anger, attraction, or identification is not in and of itself harmful. The feelings become problematic only when not examined or if they are acted upon. If you find yourself having such reactions, it is important to receive appropriate supervision so that those feelings do not interfere with the patient's treatment.

In fact, countertransference can be quite helpful in providing useful information about your patient. A patient may make you uncomfortable by telling you something and asking that it not be shared with the rest of the team. Another patient may express affectionate or romantic feelings for you. Yet another may share information that you find overwhelming. In all of these situations, ask your supervisors for guidance.

▌ FAMILY MEETINGS

What Should I Learn in a Family Meeting?

Family meetings are intended as a two-way exchange of information. The information that you obtain from family meetings includes collateral information about the patient's history, such as a history of dangerousness, past treatment efforts, and recent signs of mental illness that the patient may not have reported. It is important to ask the family about barriers they see to the patient's discharge.

In addition to verbal information, family meetings are an opportunity to gather other data. Observing the way that the family interacts may shape your treatment. What is the quality of the relationships in the family? If the family is angry at the patient for being sick or if the patient is angry at the family for having him hospitalized, this needs to be addressed, especially if the family is going to be active in the patient's discharge plans. Is the patient extremely obedient to his family, or does he threaten them? If the patient defers to his family for all decisions, psychoeducation of the family is crucial to the patient's well-being after discharge. Does the patient look and feel healthier or sicker when she is with her family? If the patient is returning to live with her family, her mental status with her family may be more important than the way she appears when surrounded by hospital staff. On the other hand, the patient's ability to minimize pathology may mislead the family. If the family does not appear to be aware of the seriousness of the patient's illness, you may need to educate them further.

To gather this valuable nonverbal data, it is important to start with open-ended questions. Allow the family to talk and interact with each other. Notice who speaks for the family and who, if anyone, is allowed to contradict the family spokesperson. Although time is at a premium in all of medicine, resist the urge to make every family meeting a brief meeting with a strict agenda.

However, if a family meeting begins to devolve into a shouting match, it is appropriate to interrupt and try to reframe the meeting in a more productive way. It may even be necessary to end the meeting if the patient or a member of her family becomes uncontrollably upset. If a particular family member routinely agitates the patient, it may be appropriate to exclude that person from family meetings. This restriction may also apply to visitation. The patient should be informed why someone is restricted or excluded.

What Should I Convey in a Family Meeting?

Family meetings are your chance to engage the family in tasks necessary for your patient's recovery. Before a family meeting, you should have some ideas about how the family can help. Will they be monitoring the patient's medication after discharge? Will they be responsible for getting the patient to the follow-up appointments? Should the family relieve their ill relative of all responsibilities? Should they push the patient to get back into a productive routine as quickly as possible?

Aside from giving the family concrete instructions on how to care for their ill relative, you often need to educate the family about the illness. This psychoeducation is similar to the psychoeducation described earlier in this chapter, but the focus is often slightly different. Many families feel they are responsible for their relative's illness. On the other hand, some families blame the sick relative, harboring the belief that the patient could consciously control his symptoms or that the illness reflects some kind of moral failing. These beliefs about the cause of disorders can impair the family's ability to care for the patient. Emphasizing the "no-fault" biologic model for psychiatric disorders may help a family accept the patient's illness without judgment.

DISCHARGE PLANNING

What Is Included in Discharge Planning from a Psychiatric Inpatient Unit?

The biopsychosocial model is useful in discharge planning: a complete discharge plan considers the medical and psychological follow-up as well as the environment in which the patient is going to live.

In general, the medical student is involved in the process of arranging how and where the patient is going to obtain treatment after discharge. Will the patient need to go to a clinic once a month, once a week, or every day? Will he require brief psychopharmacology appointments, psychotherapy, or a day treatment program? Chapter 3 will help you understand the different options that are available after discharge. It is important that a medical student understand the expectations of a particular outpatient treatment program before calling up to make an appointment. For example, some outpatient physicians and some clinics are prepared to provide treatment only for patients who are medically stable or who are at low risk for violence. Knowing this before you make a call will help you to provide relevant history. Although it may be tempting to distort information so that your patient can obtain an outpatient appointment, it is unethical and unwise to do this; you or your inpatient unit will probably have to discharge other patients to the same outpatient providers in the future.

Generally, when calling to make a follow-up appointment for a patient, you need to provide the following: the patient's address and telephone number, the patient's insurance information, and the patient's clinical information, including his current medications and his diagnoses.

Social workers usually help to ensure that the patient has food, money, transportation, and shelter after discharge, but it is often the medical student's responsibility to identify the patient's needs. Aside from scheduling follow-up appointments, you must consider the social environment of your patients. Will the patient need a referral to a support group such as Alcoholics Anonymous or the National Alliance for the Mentally Ill? Does the patient even have a home, or will she be going to a homeless shelter? Is the patient sufficiently mobile to get home and to get to follow-up appointments, or will she require an ambulance?

KEY POINTS

◆ The most important psychological assessment is talking with your patient.

◆ Most psychiatry inpatient services use a multidisciplinary team approach.

◆ Talking with patients is often therapeutic, even if it is not psychotherapy.

◆ A patient's mental status with his or her family can be more important than the mental status with the staff in assessing readiness for discharge.

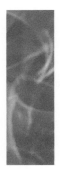

3

The Medical Student in the Outpatient Clinic

ANAND PANDYA AND HEATHER MORSE

 ORIENTATION TO THE CLINIC

How Are Outpatient Services Different from Other Psychiatric Services?

Most simply, the patients in clinics are not currently hospitalized, although they may have recently been hospitalized or may soon be hospitalized.

There are other differences as well. During your inpatient psychiatry experience, you will notice the intensity of care provided on a day-to-day basis. It quickly becomes apparent that the hospitalized patient is much sicker than patients treated on an outpatient basis. The inpatient unit provides around-the-clock protective support and treatment; outpatient care offers more autonomy and consequently less protective oversight. Patients treated on an outpatient basis may still be quite ill; however, they are not assessed as being dangerous to themselves or other people and they have reasonable supports to be cared for safely out of the constant protective supervision of the hospital.

Because outpatients have the liberty to come and go, the treatment inevitably must allow greater autonomy and engagement of the patients, and their own goals become far more important than in inpatient settings. Because of the relatively brief length of stay in inpatient settings, the focus remains primarily on acute symptomatology. But in outpatient settings one must address other issues that do not fit as neatly into a disease model. These include long-standing patterns of behaviors that may not lead to dangerousness but that greatly affect the person's functioning or distress, such as vocational and relationship issues.

Are Outpatients Similar to Patients Seen on the Inpatient Unit?

Yes and no. Certainly, every diagnosed form of mental illness you encounter on the inpatient wards is also found in the outpatient clinic. However, there are individuals with some psychiatric diagnoses that typically are not seen on your inpatient service. Because only individuals with the most severe forms of mental illness are hospitalized these days, many people treated in the outpatient setting have less serious psychiatric disorders, including anxiety disorders, adjustment disorders, mild depression, and several types of personality disorders. Although all of these diagnoses bring with them suffering and impairment, typically the affected individual is able to function well enough to remain out of the hospital. Some people function extremely well but still experience problems in living, for which outpatient treatment can be helpful.

The inpatient and outpatient divisions often work in concert in the treatment of patients. Because patients cannot live on the inpatient unit forever (although this did occur prior to the deinstitutionalization movement of the 1960s), sooner or later they become outpatients. When illness episodes result in unsafe behavior, the hospital inpatient unit provides the necessary respite care and secure setting until the patient can return to the community once again. Many forms of mental illness (e.g., schizophrenia and bipolar disorder) are marked by exacerbations and periods of stability.

Is the Psychiatric Outpatient Clinic like Other Outpatient Clinics?

In some ways they are similar, but there are some important differences. Most outpatient clinics treat patients for one or a few visits per illness episode. Psychiatric outpatient treatment, even brief therapies, usually requires the patients' regular follow-up for 3 or more months. Many patients come to the clinic for regular weekly visits for several months or years, especially when psychotherapy is a major component of treatment. Another major difference is that most psychiatric clinics work on a schedule in which patients' visits are arranged for a defined period of time, often 30 or 45 minutes. The schedule is usually more rigidly adhered to than the schedule in a medical clinic in order to ensure consistency and predictability in treatments that can involve intense emotions. Finally, because of the stigma of mental illness and the intensely private material that can be discussed in psychiatry, patients and clinicians may have a heightened awareness of the importance of confidentiality.

How Does a Patient Get to Be an Outpatient?

There are several paths to the outpatient clinic. Many individuals simply walk in, recognizing that there is something troubling them for which they seek assistance. Other people are referred from other parts of the health care system including inpatient units (upon discharge), the emergency room, or other hospital clinics. Community agencies, including religious organizations, also refer patients to outpatient treatment, as do employers. Of course, family members and friends also make such referrals. Knowing how the patients came can tell you much about them, such as what supports they have and whether or not they have insight and motivation for treatment.

What Is the Structure of the Typical Outpatient Psychiatric Clinic?

The structure varies from program to program, but many clinics include a walk-in service for patients who come without an appointment. This enables clinicians to see patients who cannot tolerate the delay waiting for an appointment or who have difficulty scheduling their lives to make an appointment in advance.

Other patients are able to make a scheduled appointment for an intake evaluation. In this session, background information and a summary of the problem are documented. From that point, clinics differ in the procedures used to determine whether a patient is appropriate for treatment and what treatment modalities are appropriate.

Who Is in the Outpatient Treatment Team?

In addition to the psychiatrists, typical outpatient clinics employ the expertise of psychologists, social workers, case managers, and psychiatric nurses. Other kinds of therapists usually seen on the inpatient unit (e.g., music or art therapists, vocational therapists, and aides) are less often found in the outpatient setting.

What Do the Team Members Do?

Psychologists assist in the psychological assessment and evaluation of patients through testing assessment, and they participate in several different modalities of therapy. Social workers help with environmental and social problems (e.g., housing, medical insurance, entitlements, food). Social workers are often called upon to address domestic violence and child abuse concerns. They also provide ongoing psychotherapy.

Psychiatric nurses educate about medication and illness, assess vital signs and medical history, act as a liaison with other medical health care providers, and provide ongoing treatment. Many decanoate clinics—in which long-acting medication is administered by injection—are run by nurses.

What Does the Psychiatrist Do in the Clinic?

A psychiatrist manages medication and may provide psychotherapy. Psychiatrists typically provide the overall leadership for the clinical operation of the outpatient service. Determining whether any medical, neurologic, or substance-related issues are involved in the patient's condition is the singular responsibility of the psychiatrist, although in some settings preliminary screenings are done by other clinicians. In addition, the psychiatrist is responsible for the coordination of the medical and psychiatric care and may be responsible for the education and supervision of other staff.

Will I Get to Do Psychotherapy in the Clinic?

Given the length of your clinical clerkship (usually 6 to 8 weeks), it is unlikely that you will perform psychotherapy, which typically lasts months to years. Moreover, because of the intensely personal nature of psychotherapy, it is difficult for a student to sit in on an ongoing therapy without disrupting treatment. In some settings, observation of therapy is possible through one-way mirrors or with videotaped demonstrations.

The Outpatient Clinic

If I Don't Do Therapy in the Clinic, What Will I Do?

Because of the limitations of time and experience, students typically work in one of three outpatient services: triage, evaluation, and medication management.

 TRIAGE SERVICE

What Does Triage Mean?

Triage is a quick initial assessment that ensures that the sickest and most at-risk patients are treated first. Patients with emergencies are referred to the emergency department or are treated on the spot; other patients who can tolerate the delay are assessed for future treatment.

How Do I Do a Triage Assessment?

Patients are screened in different ways in different clinics. At some clinics, patients are first seen by a clinician in a walk-in clinic. Other places may screen patients over the telephone or in the emergency room. Wherever the screening takes place, the most important information to obtain is a safety assessment and a medical assessment.

How Do I Assess Safety?

Is the patient suicidal or homicidal? Is he able to attend to his basic needs such as clothing, food, and shelter? Answers to these questions help you decide whether the patient requires immediate hospitalization. Patients who have suicidal thoughts may require hospitalization. Factors that are used to determine whether a suicidal patient can safely leave the clinic include having a suicide plan, having a history of attempts, being able to commit convincingly to not attempting suicide until the next appointment (sometimes referred to as "contracting for safety"), and being able to describe a convincing plan of action if suicidal thoughts return or become worse. Similarly, if the patient has thoughts of hurting someone else or appears violent or impulsive, hospitalization should again be considered and parallel factors should be evaluated. (See Chapters 17 and 18 for a more detailed discussion of assessment of suicide and violence.) A final form of the safety assessment is evaluating whether a person can care for himself or herself. For example, has the patient been living on the street and refusing clothing or shelter in freezing weather? It is important that these issues are discussed in a straightforward manner—even if they cause some discomfort.

Why Do I Need to Do a Medical Assessment?

Some psychiatric symptoms are caused by underlying medical conditions. Failure to detect the medical condition can result in morbidity and mortality. Patients who present with an acute mental status change or who are disoriented may have a delirium, a syndrome akin to "brain failure."

This is caused by an underlying medical or drug condition and poses a great risk. The mortality rate for delirium is about 10% (some studies report rates as high as 20%). Patients with a possible delirium must be assessed immediately in a medical emergency room or other acute setting. Other patients may have a condition that is appropriate for outpatient psychiatric treatment but simultaneously present with a medical problem that needs immediate attention; for example, an asthma exacerbation. In this case, you need to decide what level of care the patient requires. A medical problem may also be less acute and may need to be followed by the treating psychiatrist, or the medication you start during your screening may have side effects that need to be monitored (e.g., venlafaxine and hypertension). Does the patient need an appointment in the medical clinic or do the psychiatrists monitor this themselves? For these reasons, it is important to learn how each clinic functions. Specific areas that need to be addressed are present medical complaints, past medical and surgical history, allergies, and medications.

What Should I Know about the Clinic's Population of Patients for Triage?

Patients' economic, social, and cultural backgrounds all give you clues to what may be important to them and to what you may need to do to help them on their first visit. For example, is the patient homeless? Does the patient have insurance? If so, does your clinic accept that insurance? Does the patient live in the area that your clinic serves? Are there programs at your hospital or neighboring hospitals that provide specialized services to a specific cultural group? Unlike inpatient treatment, outpatient treatment is usually continued for an extended period of time. These questions help the clinician attend to the patients' needs more effectively and therefore may increase a patient's compliance with and motivation for treatment.

What Do I Do if My Patient Doesn't Speak English?

The temptation to use family members to translate is very real in busy clinics where interpreters may be scarce; however, this should not be done. Information obtained in a psychiatric interview is extremely personal. The patient may not feel comfortable being honest if his or her mother or husband is the interpreter. You also are not aware of the nature of the relationship. A battered woman most likely will not be honest about violence in the home with her partner taking part in the interview.

Find out whether your clinic has an on-site interpreting service. It is always best to use a trained interpreter if one is available. If all else fails, check with the clinic staff to see if you can use an interpreting service by telephone. There are many such services, but their use may be restricted because of expense. Remember, when you are using the services of an interpreter it is important to maintain eye contact with your patient and address questions directly to her.

How Do I Know if a Patient Is Appropriate for Treatment in the Clinic?

Clinics vary in their eligibility criteria. Language, insurance, current substance abuse, and where the person lives may all be factors. Many public hospitals and clinics serve only a certain geographic area, referred to as the "catchment area." An important question is whether the patient would do better with a day treatment program instead of the less structured and less frequent visits to the outpatient clinic. Patients who are heavy drug or alcohol users have to be assessed for the need for inpatient detoxification before beginning outpatient treatment. Often, substance abuse services are provided separately from other mental health services. Information on the frequency and extent of use, history of previous withdrawal symptoms, and present signs and symptoms helps in that assessment.

When Should I Get a Social Work Assessment?

Whenever additional services cannot be provided in the clinic, consider consulting a social worker. This includes financial, vocational, housing, medical, or family issues. Another important reason for urgent social work intervention is abuse—child, elder, or domestic. All clinicians are required by law to report suspected child abuse; however, social workers are very often experienced in this process and should be consulted.

EVALUATION

How Do I Prepare to Do an Evaluation?

If you were not the clinician who participated in the screening process, now is the time to review the data already collected and generate questions for the interview. Make sure all the necessary points were covered in triage. If referrals were made, contact those departments. It is also a good idea to review any laboratory tests that were ordered. If the patient was referred from another area of the hospital, you should attempt to obtain a copy of the discharge summary or the chart itself. Contact the referring physician and learn what her concerns were. Gathering this information before the interview allows you to use your time with the patient more effectively. Remember, you cannot speak with outside collateral sources (family, friends, outside doctors) without first obtaining the patient's verbal or written consent.

How Is Outpatient Assessment Different from Inpatient Assessment?

The interview itself may differ because the patient is more stable and most likely more able to tolerate a longer interview. Many initial interviews are scheduled for 45 to 90 minutes. When patients are admitted to the hospital, they can usually tolerate only brief interactions, especially at the beginning of their stay. The longer interview may allow you to gather more details of their family history, social support system, past level of functioning, developmental history, and other areas. Because the patient is less acutely ill, on review of symptoms you may discover concerns aside from the primary diagnosis that will contribute to the patient's recovery and general well-being. These concerns may not fit well into a diagnostic category. For example, in outpatient settings, a relationship problem or problem with procrastination at school may become the focus of an initial interview and subsequent treatment, although it may not have an obvious connection to any psychiatric diagnosis.

How Do I Make a Treatment Plan?

After you have formed your differential diagnosis, the treatment plan naturally follows. What do you need to know in order to rule in or out any of these diagnoses—more laboratory tests, a medical examination, imaging studies, neuropsychological testing, or collateral information? Once you have a working diagnosis, it helps you decide on the appropriate treatment: medication, some form of therapy, or both. Because outpatient treatment is usually voluntary and less coercive, the patient's preference becomes far more important than in inpatient psychiatry. In the case of some higher functioning patients, because the patient's motivation and participation is such a critical factor in certain forms of treatment, it may appear that the patient completely dictates whether the treatment includes medication or psychotherapy and even what type of psychotherapy is used. The outpatient treatment plan must also address social issues such as housing and benefit applications.

How Do I Know Which Therapy Is Best for Which Patient?

There is a growing body of outcome studies that offer empirical data on the effectiveness of different kinds of psychotherapy in treating various disorders. You certainly want to make a treatment decision based on the available evidence, but that is seldom sufficient. Also important are any previous experiences in psychotherapy. With this information, you may determine that a particular form of therapy is not suitable for a particular patient. For example, some patients become too uncomfortable—or even psychotic—if their therapist is less active in the treatment. At the very least, information about prior treatments can give you some idea about what does and does not work for that patient. Other factors to consider are the patient's preferences and the clinic's available resources. A list of common modalities of therapy, along with indications and contraindications, is given in Table 3-1. Table 3-2 describes some additional factors to consider when prescribing psychotherapy.

What Do I Include in My Oral Presentation or Written Evaluation?

The evaluation follows the standard format for clinical case reports, as discussed in Chapter 8. After the differential diagnosis (i.e., a list of all possible diagnoses from most likely to least likely), you are expected to present your reasons for your choice of presumptive diagnosis. Following this are the treatment course and discussion sections. Briefly summarize any treatment

Table 3-1

Some Modalities of Psychotherapy and Their Uses

Therapy	Techniques	Goals	Indications	Contraindications
Psychodynamic psychotherapy (also called "exploratory," "insight oriented")	Free association Dream exploration Discussion of childhood antecedents Recognition of transference and resistance	Bringing unconscious thoughts and impulses into conscious awareness	Adjustment disorders Problems in living (V code on DSM-IV) Dysthymia	Psychotic symptoms Paranoid symptoms Mental retardation or dementia Antisocial personality disorders
Supportive	Surveys past coping strategies in order to support and strengthen existing adaptive capacities and minimize maladaptive tendencies	Symptom reduction through insight Improved functioning	Generalized anxiety disorder Some somatoform disorders Some personality disorders (e.g., histrionic, dependent, borderline) Chronic psychotic disorders such as schizophrenia Patients with limited intelligence or cognitive impairment Some personality disorders (e.g., schizoid, schizotypal)	Conditions for which the effectiveness of other therapies is well established (e.g., specific phobias) None
Behavioral	Prescription of specific activities or exercises Little or no use of remote antecedents or unconscious processes	Symptom removal	*Treatment of choice for* Specific phobias Obsessive-compulsive disorder Panic disorder Many sexual dysfunctions	No absolute contraindications, but less useful for chronic disorders without clearly demarcated pathologic behaviors

(Continued)

The Outpatient Clinic

Table 3-1

Some Modalities of Psychotherapy and Their Uses (Continued)

Therapy	Techniques	Goals	Indications	Contraindications
Cognitive	Identify and eliminate cognitive distortions (mistakes in assessing novel situations and one's own capacities)	Symptom reduction	Major depressive disorder Dysthymia Anxiety states Somatoform disorders	Psychotic symptoms Cognitive impairment
Dialectical-behavioral therapy (DBT)	Combines individual with group therapy focusing on specific, defined maladaptive behaviors. Suicide prevention is given priority	Improved functioning and symptom reduction	Borderline personality disorder	The use of DBT for other conditions has not been widely implemented or studied

Note:
Many therapists use an eclectic mix of techniques from a variety of therapeutic models. An individual's therapy is unlikely to be purely one modality to the exclusion of all others.

The indications for a particular therapy are overlapping and nonabsolute. The choice for a given patient may be guided as much by the patient's preference and available resources as by theoretical considerations.

Contraindications are relative, not absolute. Exceptions may be warranted for individual patients.

Table 3-2	
Psychological, Personality, and Cognitive Factors to Consider in Prescribing Therapy	

Psychodynamic Psychotherapy
Mild to moderate symptoms
Psychologically minded, introspective, intelligent, highly motivated, good frustration tolerance
Financial resources (this modality is not always reimbursed by third-party payers)

Supportive Psychotherapy
Less able to consider explicit discussion of psychological issues

Cognitive-Behavioral Therapy
Mild to moderate symptoms
Absence of cognitive incapacity such as mental retardation or dementia
Specific well-delineated behaviors or specific distorted assumptions or ways of thinking

Group Therapy
Problem areas compatible with the goals of the available groups
Able to tolerate attention focused on others for long periods of time
Ability to perform group tasks, motivation for change

Family Therapy
Relationship difficulties/conflict in the family or couple
Distress, problems communicating, motivation for change
Willingness of family members to participate

to date and present your suggestions for future treatment. You may wish to support your suggestions with a discussion of the course and prognosis of illness or knowledge of treatment outcome studies.

 MEDICATION MANAGEMENT

What Experience in Medication Management Will I Get in the Outpatient Clinic?

In both the triage and assessment phases, you may have the experience of starting or continuing medications with patients. In addition, some teaching clinics have opportunities for students to participate in ongoing medication management of patients who may or may not be in psychotherapy.

What Is Different about Outpatient Medication Management Compared with Inpatient Medication Management?

Because of the length of time in outpatient treatment (months or years compared with weeks or days), you will be able to assess more subtle side effects than are often possible to detect in an inpatient setting, where the main concern is rapid stabilization. For example, many people taking selective serotonin reuptake inhibitors report sexual side effects such as delayed orgasm and decreased libido, and increased vividness of dreams. These side effects are unlikely to be of major importance during a short hospitalization but may be of considerable importance in managing medication over a long period. Unpleasant and disturbing side effects are a common reason for stopping medication.

Also, tapering and discontinuing medication are more typical of outpatient than of inpatient management. All aspects of medication management are more likely to involve negotiations between the physician and the patient. The physician tries to work with the patient to devise the most agreeable medication plan, taking into account cost, dosing schedules, side effects, and personal issues. This is less an issue on inpatient units, where treatment may be urgent, involuntary, or court ordered. In addition, because of the high cost of inpatient treatment, medications are often increased rapidly to stabilize the patient as soon as possible. Once stabilized and engaged in outpatient treatment, the patient may be able to be maintained on a lower dose, which may be more comfortable and carry a lower risk of long-term side effects.

Is Cost a Factor in Prescribing Outpatient Medications?

Yes, it should be, although it is often not discussed. It is important for physicians to know how much their patients are paying for medication. Cost may make the difference in whether a patient fills a prescription and whether it is taken as prescribed. Some patients who are prescribed expensive antidepressants, for example, attempt to ration them to the few times during the week when they feel most depressed—an unsatisfactory strategy because the drugs work only if taken regularly for extended periods of time.

In many circumstances, a less expensive but equally effective drug is available. When the Food and Drug Administration approves a new drug, the pharmaceutical company that developed the drug is given a patent for its exclusive manufacture and distribution for a period of 17 years. During the period of monopoly, the pharmaceutical company attempts to establish its brand name and market share and to recoup research and development costs. At the end of the patent, generic forms of the drug can be marketed to compete with the brand name. These pharmacologic equivalents are almost always cheaper—sometimes dramatically so—than brand-name medications. Some drug cost comparisons are presented in Table 3-3. What people actually pay for their prescriptions depends on their medical coverage. Many private insurance policies pay a substantial portion of the cost of prescriptions, often requiring the patient to make a co-payment. The co-payment may be higher for brand-name drugs than for generics. Medicaid includes outpatient prescription coverage; Medicare traditionally did not cover outpatient medications, but a new voluntary program, Medicare Part D, allows Medicare recipients to purchase private insurance to cover much of their pharmacy costs.

The Outpatient Clinic

Table 3-3

Costs of a One-Month Supply of Some Psychiatric Medications

Brand	Medication Generic	Dosage (mg/tablet)	No. of Tablets	Retail Price
	Lithium carbonate	300	90	$19.04
Depakote		500	60	$123.99
	Valproic acid	250	120	$55.96
Prozac		20	30	$121.42
	Fluoxetine	20	30	$15.99
Celexa		20	30	$72.99
	Citalopram	20	30	$39.99
Zoloft		50	30	$75.99
Effexor XR		75	30	$89.99
Wellbutrin		150	60	$115.99
	Bupropion	100	90	$66.99
Zyprexa		20	30	$519.99
Risperdal		4	30	$250.69
Seroquel		300	60	$459.54
Abilify		30	30	$417.97
	Haloperidol	5	90	$15.80
Risperdal Consta		25	2	$533.00
Clozaril		100	90	$401.89
	Clozapine	100	120	$312.00
Ativan		2	30	$63.99
	Lorazepam	2	30	$21.99

The Outpatient Clinic

What Is the Difference between Medicare and Medicaid?

Medicare is a federal program begun in 1966 to provide medical care benefits for older people participating in the Social Security program. In 1972, the program was expanded to cover younger people with disabilities and older people not in the Social Security program but willing to pay a premium.

Medicare was designed to provide coverage for acute conditions, and services such as long-term care, preventative services, ongoing pharmaceuticals, or dental care are typically excluded. The traditional Medicare program has two parts, Part A being primarily hospital insurance (as well as some outpatient hospital care, including partial psychiatric hospitals) and Part B, a voluntary medical insurance program that requires a monthly premium.

Medicaid was enacted in 1965 to provide medical insurance for poor people. Funding for Medicaid comes from federal and state matching funds. States may impose limitations on the services they fund as well as the level of reimbursement. Medicaid pays for a substantial fraction of all psychiatric care in the United States.

KEY POINTS

◆ Psychiatric triage involves assessment of safety and a medical assessment.

◆ Psychotherapy is prescribed based on the evidence of outcome studies, the patient's preferences and capacities, and available resources.

◆ Family members should not be used as translators for patients who do not speak English.

◆ All clinicians are required by law to report suspected child abuse.

4

The Medical Student on the Psychiatry Consultation-Liaison (or Psychosomatic Medicine) Service

NANCY FORMAN

THE PSYCHIATRY CONSULTATION-LIAISON SERVICE

What Is Consultation-Liaison Psychiatry?

Consultation-liaison (C-L) psychiatry, now often referred to as psychosomatic medicine, is the branch of psychiatry that deals with psychiatry in the general hospital (as opposed to on the psychiatric units). The patients served are those on the medical, surgical, and obstetric units and, often, those in the medical and surgical emergency services. Increasingly, C-L services are expanding into outpatient areas as well, including general medical and specialty medical and surgical clinics. (There is usually a separate psychiatry C-L group that serves the pediatric population.) The *consultation* portion of the work generally refers to the direct care of patients, in which a clinician requests a psychiatric evaluation, usually by asking a specific question, for a particular patient.

What's the Liaison Part?

Liaison refers to the ongoing relationship that develops between the psychiatrist and any of the units in the hospital, allowing a deeper familiarity with the staff, the functioning of the unit, the types of patients, and the particular stresses of that unit. This sets the stage for a different kind of interaction in which the psychiatrist is able to work with the staff to facilitate a better working environment and to provide ongoing education about psychiatric issues that arise in a medical or surgical setting.

39

What Is the Relationship between Consultation-Liaison Psychiatry and Psychosomatic Medicine?

In 2003, as part of the process of becoming a recognized and accredited subspecialty within the field of psychiatry, C-L psychiatry underwent an official name change to psychosomatic medicine (PM). Some services changed their names to reflect this, but many did not. Whether you find yourself on a service that is referred to as C-L or PM, the substance is the same; the change in name is part of the historical development of a field that is in a period of rapid and exciting growth and development.

What Kind of Patients Will I See?

Because you will be seeing medical and surgical patients on the C-L psychiatric rotation, the patients will most likely fall into a few general groups, as summarized in Tables 4-1 and 4-2. Sometimes, you will be asked for assistance with the diagnosis, sometimes with proper medication use, sometimes to provide psychotherapy, and often for a combination of these.

Is C-L Psychiatry Just like Psychiatric Emergency Work?

There is a significant overlap between emergency psychiatry and C-L psychiatry. The main difference is that in C-L psychiatry, the patients have medical or surgical problems that require acute evaluation and treatment in addition to psychiatric issues. Also, you are an invited consultant who has been asked to provide expert specialty evaluation of someone else's

Psychosomatic Medicine

Table 4-1

Some Common Reasons for Psychiatric Consultations

To help manage patients with chronic persistent mental illness such as schizophrenia
To evaluate and help manage patients with new acute psychiatric symptoms
To evaluate and help manage patients with acute behavioral changes
To evaluate patients whose capacity to make treatment decisions on their own behalf is being questioned

Table 4-2

Some Common Diagnoses Seen in Psychiatric Consultation

Adjustment disorders with depressed or anxious mood
Major depressive disorder and dysthymia
Dementia
Delirium
Substance use disorders (intoxication, withdrawal, or long-term complications)
Personality disorders
Psychiatric symptoms secondary to an underlying general medical condition or to medication

patient. As such, you will be making recommendations, many of which are for the requesting physician to accept or reject. For this reason, consultants do not usually write orders.

RESPONSIBILITIES ON THE SERVICE

How Do I Start?

Usually, you will be assigned a consultation that a clinician has called in by telephone. You will be given limited data, which will include the patient's name and hospital location, and some clinical information, usually in the form of a question or problem statement that you are being asked to address. It is often helpful to call the requesting clinician before you see the patient and to clarify more specifically the perceived psychiatric issues. (Often, there are differences between the issues that are called in to the C-L psychiatric service and those that are told to you directly over the telephone.) Because of the persistent stigma of mental illness, it is important for the treating team to alert the patient to the psychiatric consultation and to put it into an appropriate therapeutic context, rather than for you to catch the patient off guard when you march in and announce that you came from psychiatry to see him.

What Do I Do When I Get to the Ward?

Once you know why the team has requested psychiatric evaluation for the patient, it is helpful to do several things before you see the patient. Always look through the chart; it will often help you to figure out the time course of events. Make sure that you write down the list of medications the patient is receiving and received before the hospitalization. Thoroughness requires not only checking what was ordered but also checking the nursing records to see what the patient actually takes. (Before you decide that the patient's symptoms are due to a medication that has been ordered, be certain that the patient has not been refusing to take the medication in question.) While you are looking at the chart, also look at the nurses' notes, which will tell you about the patient's behavior over time and on different shifts, and look at the social workers' notes, which not only are full of psychosocial information but also may have information from collateral sources. Scan the laboratory test results. You may find important abnormalities and might notice that additional tests may be needed. The medical and surgical services are not always cognizant of what laboratory tests are necessary to rule in or out the psychiatric disorders or symptoms that need to be addressed. However, do not tarry too long over the chart; you are just collecting information with which to proceed to the evaluation of the patient.

What if a Patient Is Agitated?

You should have sufficient information from speaking with the patient's primary clinician and from looking at the chart to have a first impression of whether you will feel comfortable going in to speak with the patient alone. Because the medical and surgical units generally are unable to tolerate the level of behavioral disturbances that occurs in a psychiatric emergency department, the patient may already be sedated or have someone sitting with him by the time you arrive. If you have any concern, however, you should find someone to accompany you to see a patient (although finding someone may not be as easy as in the psychiatric emergency unit). The safety issues are similar—make sure that you are near an open door and that you know the way out. Should the patient become agitated and you are unable to calm him down verbally, let the patient know that he appears to be upset, that it seems unwise to continue, and that you will return when things have calmed down. Then leave and immediately and inform either the unit staff or your supervisor. It is *not* your job to restrain physically someone who is agitated or to force someone to remain in the room with you while you complete your interview. All hospitals have professional police or security staff who are experienced in calming and restraining agitated patients, and should you encounter such a situation, your job is to alert the floor nursing staff of this situation immediately so that they can call for assistance. You will not be able to perform an adequate evaluation if you do not feel safe, so ensure that you do feel safe before proceeding.

How Should I Introduce Myself?

In most psychiatric settings, the patients know that they are being cared for by psychiatric staff. In the C-L psychiatric service, however, you are on someone else's turf. If you have prepared properly, you will already know whether the patient expects to be seen by someone from psychiatry. Because the patient may not remember having been told, it is usually best to start off by letting the patient know that you are from psychiatry and have been asked by the physician (whose name you will know and say to the patient) to help with the treatment. Although not telling the patient directly that you are from psychiatry may make the interview easier (at least for you) for the first few minutes, it will become obvious very quickly. Either the patient will ask why you are there or he will figure it out and realize that you were not being straight with him from the beginning. After seeing a certain number of patients you will find a comfortable way to introduce yourself.

How Is a C-L Psychiatric Evaluation Different from Other Psychiatric Evaluations?

Usually when you see a new patient for the first time, you will have been provided a question by the clinician seeking consultation. You have several tasks. You must ensure that the question is appropriate for a psychiatric consultant to be asked. Often, you will find that the question needs to be reshaped or reframed, and part of the task of the consultation is to assist the requesting service in doing that. For example, the question may be, "Does this patient have the decisional capacity to sign out against medical advice (AMA)?" This is not an unreasonable question, but the short answer—yes or no—is not always adequate to address the clinical issues at hand. There are often complicated issues that contribute to the patient's request to leave AMA, and it may be helpful for you to comment on as many of them as possible. In addition to addressing the referral question, you will need to conduct a general but brief screening psychiatric evaluation to look for signs and symptoms of psychopathology.

What Should I Look For?

One of the most important things to remember on the C-L psychiatric service is to "think organic." That is, you must maintain a high index of suspicion for medical or drug-related etiologies underlying the symptoms you see. Although not everything you see will have an organic cause, you will be seeing patients who are medically ill, receiving medications, undergoing procedures, sleep deprived, and otherwise physiologically stressed, and you will see a high prevalence of organic pathology. Clues to the presence of underlying organicity include a waxing and waning level of alertness (which may not be evident on a single, brief visit) and disorientation to time, place, or person.

Some form of cognitive screening evaluation should be a routine part of every evaluation. Use whichever tool your institution has available, but be sure to use one. All of the cognitive screening instruments include orientation to time and place. If it does not address orientation, your consultation will not be complete. As a general rule, patients with primary psychiatric (nonorganic) disorders—however disorganized, psychotic, or withdrawn they may be—are not disoriented. If, when writing up your consultation note, you realize that you forgot to address orientation, *do not* simply write "A & O × 3." Go back to the patient. Orientation is crucial; do not neglect it.

It is also important to check vital signs as a routine part of your consultation. You do not want to miss a fever or autonomic hyperactivity, which might significantly change your differential diagnosis. Do not accept other notes in the chart that say "VS WNL" and just copy that into your note. "WNL" is just as likely to mean "we never looked" as it is to mean "within normal limits." Look at the vital sign sheet yourself.

What Do I Do with All the Information I've Gathered?

Should the patient express to you suicidal or homicidal ideation, you may need to act immediately. If you have reason to believe that a life is in danger, either the patient's or someone else's, do not leave the patient alone. Contact the nursing staff on the floor so that someone can stay with the patient while arrangements are made in accordance with hospital policy to ensure everyone's safety. Once safety is ensured, it is useful to contact collateral sources for information about the patient. Ask the patient for a name and telephone number of someone who knows her well—a family member, a friend, a therapist, or the treating psychiatrist—and ask for permission to contact that person. Let the patient know that this is a routine part of the evaluation. If the patient refuses permission, you may be constrained by the local laws and statutes; check with your supervisor about what you legally can and cannot do.

What Do I Put in My Consultation Note?

Because you already went through the chart before you saw the patient, you have at least some sense of what the notes and consultation notes look like. Succinct, clearly written, and pertinent notes are good. Studies have shown that clinicians do not read long, wordy consultation notes but instead flip to the end section for impressions and recommendations. Box 4-1 provides the outline of a typical consultation note. Make your recommendations very clear; state exactly what needs to be done, when, and by whom. For example, if you write the recommendation "Contact private psychiatrist," it is unclear whether you are going to do it or are suggesting to the medical service that they do it. Be very specific about what you will do and what they should do. If you have contacted outside sources, include them in your written note with names and telephone numbers. You will probably be discussing your cases with a supervisor before you write specific recommendations, so make sure that you are clear about your *exact* recommendations, such as dosages of medications and intervals and parameters for the medications. Be sure to include when you will be seeing the patient again or whether the requesting service should call you if additional help is needed. Always include your name legibly printed and a contact telephone or beeper number in case questions arise.

If I've Written a Note, Do I Still Have to Talk to the Requesting Physician?

It is usually helpful to contact the referring clinician and share with her your diagnostic impressions and suggestions for treatment. This is particularly true if there are things you need her to know or do in a timely

Psychosomatic Medicine

BOX 4-1

SAMPLE OUTLINE FOR A PSYCHIATRIC CONSULTATION NOTE

 I. Reason for consultation
 II. Sources of information and your estimate of their reliability
 III. History of present illness, making brief reference to the medical or surgical issues and concentrating on the psychiatric issues
 IV. Past psychiatric history
 V. Past medical history
 VI. Social history (including drug or alcohol use and human immunodeficiency virus risk factors)
 VII. Medications (both current and before hospitalization if different)
 VIII. Medication allergies
 IX. Laboratory and vital sign review
 X. Complete mental status examination
 XI. Summary and formulation (or impression and plan), including a multiaxial diagnosis and clear recommendations, including plans for follow-up if indicated

manner, including one-on-one constant observation, issues of restraint, need for immediate medication, and urgent testing. However, just touching base with the referring clinician can be helpful. You can determine whether you have answered her questions and how you can be of continuing help.

How Often Should I See My Patients in Follow-Up?

This is not always an easy question to answer, and your supervisor will be able to help you. It depends in part on the clinical situation. If your patient was very agitated and required medication to calm down, you might want to go back in a couple of hours to see whether the medication worked. If the patient is depressed, you might want to schedule to see the patient regularly several times a week, perhaps for relatively brief periods. Work out a schedule that is acceptable to the patient and clinically reasonable, both for you and for the patient. If you are not sure when you can get back to see the patient, do not set a time and date. Patients often look forward to the visits and depend on them, and you are much better off not setting up a situation that can both hurt and disappoint the patient. In general, the services requesting consultations prefer that patients be seen on a somewhat regular basis until they are discharged from the medical or surgical service.

KEY POINTS

◆ Always make sure the patient knows a psychiatric consultation has been requested.

◆ Always consider organic etiologies in your differential diagnosis.

◆ Always check for orientation to person, place, and time, and check the patient's vital signs.

Psychosomatic Medicine

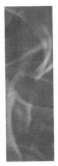

5

The Medical Student in the Psychiatric Emergency Room

VAN YU AND HEATHER LEWERENZ

What Will I See in the Psychiatric Emergency Room?

The psychiatric emergency room provides an opportunity to see a wide range of psychiatric patients with a variety of presenting problems and illnesses. You will evaluate and treat everyone from patients who present simply because a prescription ran out who are otherwise stable to patients who are agitated, assaultive, and psychotic. As the main gateway to mental health care, not only is the psychiatric emergency room a natural destination for people whose behavior or symptoms are most floridly abnormal, it is also a place where a patient's illness will not yet be ameliorated by treatment. Because of this, the psychiatric emergency room provides a unique opportunity to see severe pathology.

What Constitutes a Psychiatric Emergency?

A psychiatric emergency is any situation in which a person is in physical danger because of psychiatric illness or treatment. The person in danger is not always the one with the illness. Obvious examples are suicide attempts or assaults on others, but being too psychotic or depressed to attend to basic needs (taking insulin, wearing warm clothes when it's cold, feeding young children) can also be an emergency. As with any treatment, psychiatric medications may have side effects or toxicities that constitute emergencies: acute dystonic reactions, neuroleptic malignant syndrome, the sequelae of medication overdoses. Some common psychiatric emergencies are listed in Table 5-1.

What Happens in a Psychiatric Emergency Room?

A psychiatric emergency room has four functions: (1) to prevent suicide, homicide, and assault; (2) to evaluate and diagnose psychiatric illness (or to identify medical or neurologic illness as the cause of psychiatric symptoms); (3) to determine the appropriate level of psychiatric care; and (4) to treat psychiatric illness.

Table 5-1
Common Psychiatric Emergencies

Associated with Psychiatric Disorders
Suicidality
Threat of violence
Acute psychotic episode
Panic attack

Associated with Psychiatric Medication
Acute dystonic reaction
Akathisia
Lithium toxicity
Tricyclic antidepressant overdose
Neuroleptic malignant syndrome

Associated with Other Drug Use
Acute intoxication and withdrawal states
Disordered behavior because of drug use
Anticholinergic delirium

Medical Conditions
Delirium

How Does the Emergency Room Prevent Suicide and Assault?

This is accomplished in two ways. First, the psychiatric emergency room and its staff serve as physical barriers to violence directed at self or others. The level of containment and supervision required to accomplish this depends on how ill and determined a patient is. Some patients are effectively contained simply by being prevented from leaving, whereas others may require physical restraint or medication. The second intervention to prevent suicide, homicide, or assault is to initiate treatment for whatever psychiatric condition is causing the person to be suicidal, homicidal, or aggressive.

Can Patients Be Held Involuntarily?

Yes. Even the patient who walks into the emergency room on his own may end up being held against his will. Depriving a person of liberty is a serious infringement of a person's rights. The legal justification for doing so is that there are some instances in which the state's interest in protecting its citizens outweighs an individual's right of liberty. There have been many examples in history of governments quarantining people in an attempt to control the spread of infectious disease. Similarly, a state's interest in preventing a person from harming himself or other people resulted in laws allowing the involuntary commitment of dangerous persons. Because involuntary commitment laws are legislated at the state level, the exact wording of criteria varies with jurisdiction. In New York State, for example, a person can be involuntarily committed to a psychiatric facility if that person has "a mental illness for which immediate observation, care, and treatment in a hospital is appropriate and which is likely to result in serious harm to himself or herself or others." Serious harm is defined as "a substantial risk of physical harm to the person as manifested by threats of or attempts at suicide or serious bodily harm or other conduct demonstrating that the person is dangerous to himself or herself, or a substantial risk of physical harm to other persons as manifested by homicidal or other violent behavior by which others are placed in reasonable fear of serious physical harm." Patients should be referred to appropriate legal services for assistance if they wish to contest admission to the hospital, medications, or any part of their treatment.

Who Besides Patients Will I Find in a Psychiatric Emergency Room?

You can deduce this by remembering the tasks of a psychiatric emergency room. The first people you may encounter are those who bring patients in. These people are, of course, not regular emergency room staff and may include police, officers of other law enforcement agencies, emergency medical services, outreach workers, and staff of outpatient mental health facilities. The psychiatric evaluation is performed by psychiatrists, psychologists, nurses, nurse practitioners, social workers, or some combination of these. There are always nurses whose primary function is to give medication. Security officers and specially trained psychiatric technicians aid in the nonpharmacologic management of patients' behavior. In some large metropolitan emergency departments, security is provided by a division of the city police department. Social workers and sometimes addiction counselors handle disposition planning. Clerical staff help manage the creation and flow of patients' medical records. Staffing may vary depending on the size and location of the institution. Smaller or rural hospitals may not have a separate psychiatric emergency room and you may be evaluating psychiatric emergency patients in a general emergency department, whereas larger, urban or tertiary care facilities have fully staffed, freestanding psychiatric emergency departments.

Is It Dangerous to Work in a Psychiatric Emergency Room?

The potential for danger is there. Before evaluating any patient, you must be clear with yourself about how you, other staff, and patients will remain safe. In some ways, the psychiatric emergency room is the safest unit in the hospital because of design and procedures created with the potentially violent patient in mind. Many potential weapons that are common on medical units are absent in the psychiatric emergency room. There are few, if any, intravenous (IV) line poles to throw or swing at others, chairs and beds are bolted or built into the floor or wall, there are no IV lines to wrap around necks, and there are no needles with which to stab people. In most psychiatric emergency rooms, police and other law enforcement officers must unload their weapons or leave them behind before entering.

In addition, there are precautions for you to take. Familiarize yourself with where you may sit and talk with patients. Find the panic button and know your escape routes and lines of sight with other staff. If you talk with a patient in a room, sit close to the door and make sure it is open and unblocked. If a patient balks at this arrangement, by complaining about a lack of privacy, for example, be honest about your concern for safety and explain that the rules must apply to all patients fairly. If a patient refuses the seating arrangement you feel comfortable with, do not interview the patient. You may also ask other staff to accompany you. Don't be afraid to ask—most staff appreciate the danger and fear that can be associated with this work. Most important is vigilance: consider every patient to be dangerous. When staff injuries do occur, it is often due to a lapse of attention with a patient who is not obviously dangerous.

How Can I Identify Medical or Neurologic Illness as the Cause of Psychiatric Symptoms?

Medical screening must precede psychiatric assessment. Most acute medical problems cannot be adequately treated in a psychiatric emergency room. Two key screening assessments are vital signs and level of consciousness. Delirium is a descriptive term denoting an altered level of consciousness. Delirium is always caused by a medical or neurologic process. No psychiatric illness causes delirium; however, because delirium is a perturbation of the central nervous system, psychiatric symptoms may be the most prominent presentation of delirium. Most of the time you can rule out delirium clinically very quickly. A person who appears awake and alert, who engages in conversation, and who is oriented to person, place, time, and situation is most likely not delirious. Another very quick clinical test is to convince yourself that a person can register information. You can do this by simply asking a person to repeat a sentence that you utter. Even the most psychotic persons should be able to do this (provided they are willing and able to speak). On the other hand, a person who cannot do so needs closer medical scrutiny.

A word of caution is required about this kind of quick clinical assessment for delirium. The altered consciousness is often waxing and waning. A person can be awake, alert, and oriented at one moment and somnolent the next. Therefore, you must have both a longitudinal and initial assessment for each patient. The assessment and treatment of delirium are discussed more fully in Chapter 26.

What Happens to Patients after They Are Assessed in the Emergency Room?

A major function of the psychiatric emergency room is triage of patients to the appropriate level of care. The most intensive disposition is an involuntary admission for people who are determined to be an acute danger to self or others. This does not only include suicidality and homicidality but may also include people whose psychiatric symptoms impair the ability to care for basic needs, attend to medical illnesses, or interact appropriately with others. For example, an insulin-dependent person who believes insulin is poison may require an involuntary admission. Another example would be the person with disorganized schizophrenia who repeatedly masturbates in a train station waiting room. Voluntary inpatient admission may be offered to patients whose psychiatric condition would be more effectively managed in the intensive setting of an inpatient unit than in an outpatient setting. For example, a person suffering from an episode of major depression whose vegetative symptoms impair her ability to attend outpatient visits may benefit from inpatient treatment. A person whose psychopharmacologic intervention is very complicated because of refractory disease or comorbidity may be more safely treated—at least initially—on an inpatient unit.

What Do You Do with Patients Who Are Too Sick to Be Sent Home But Who Don't Need to Be Hospitalized?

Many psychiatric emergency rooms now have extended observation units. These units, often physically part of the emergency room itself, have beds where patients can be held up to 72 hours when they do not clearly need hospitalization but are too unstable to be sent home right away. Extended observation is a common disposition for people who are intoxicated with alcohol or other drugs because that influence usually abates over the course of 24 to 72 hours. For example, people often appear to be suffering from a major depressive episode for a short period following cocaine use. In addition, emotional crises caused by personality disorders or acute psychosocial stress are often effectively managed over the course of 24 to 72 hours. For example, a person with borderline personality traits is sometimes suicidal in the immediate aftermath of an interpersonal upset but may be able to recompensate quickly.

How Do I Decide When Simply to Send Somebody Home from the Emergency Room?

The appropriateness of this choice depends not only on the severity of psychiatric illness but also on the environment to which the patient is released. Even patients with relatively severe symptoms may be safely discharged if they can be released to a setting of adequate support such as a reliable family or a supervised residence.

What if There Is Not a Separate Psychiatric Emergency Room?

Most hospitals do not have a freestanding psychiatric emergency room, in which case a psychiatrist serves as consultant to the regular emergency staff. It is more dangerous to manage psychiatric patients in a general emergency room. Potential weapons such as needles and IV poles are readily available, and the staff of general emergency rooms are often not trained or experienced in dealing with potentially dangerous patients. The psychiatric consultant to the emergency department does not have as much flexibility as the psychiatrist working in a separate psychiatric emergency room. There are often no extended observation beds that can be supervised intensely enough for psychiatric patients, and usually there are no social workers who are trained or experienced in psychiatric discharge planning. You should familiarize yourself with the resources available at your hospital and utilize supervision by residents and attending psychiatrists.

The Emergency Room

What Is My Role in the Psychiatric Emergency Room?

One of the primary functions of the psychiatric emergency room is to evaluate and diagnose psychiatric illness. If you can take a relevant history and perform an accurate mental status examination, you can be a valuable member of the treatment team. On most other services in the hospital, unfamiliarity with treatment modalities and inexperience with a variety of procedures limit the activity of the average medical student. On the other hand, any third-year student should be able to engage patients in conversation, observe their behavior, review medical records, and contact others who know the patient. With information collected through these activities, the treatment team should be able to evaluate and diagnose the vast majority of people who arrive in the psychiatric emergency room.

KEY POINTS

◆ Medical screening precedes psychiatric screening in psychiatric emergencies.

◆ The psychiatric emergency room is your best chance to see unmedicated psychopathology.

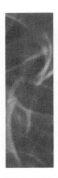

6

The Medical Student in the Forensic Psychiatry Setting

RAPHAEL MORRIS

What Is a Forensic Psychiatric Service?

A forensic service is a ward or hospital where the patients are facing criminal charges or have been acquitted of their charges by reason of mental disease or defect (the insanity defense). Dangerous violent patients are not automatically forensic patients until officially incarcerated and under the jurisdiction of a correctional system or the state mental health system. Although much of the work of forensic psychiatrists is done in the outpatient setting and there are opportunities for civil, non–criminal related, evaluations, most of a medical student's exposure is to inmates or hospitalized forensic patients involved in the criminal justice system at some level.

Where Do Forensic Patients Come From?

Forensic patients are generally brought to the forensic ward or hospital by police officers from the community or by correctional officers directly from jail. Some cases involve sending the patient directly from a court hearing, and some are transferred to the hospital from a police lockup (central booking). The agencies generally involved with forensic patients include the police, city and state department of corrections, criminal and supreme courts, the state forensic hospital system, legal aid society, and the mental hygiene legal service.

Why Are Forensic Patients Sent to the Hospital from Jail?

Forensic patients come to the hospital from jail when their high-risk behaviors are unmanageable in the jail setting despite their access to mental health professionals. Risk behaviors that may require emergency medication include threatening suicide or provoking altercations in the jail. In addition, the jail often requests a more thorough evaluation in order to better manage the patient/inmate. Some other forensic patients are sent to the hospital to facilitate the completion of a competence to stand trial evaluation where treatment is not the primary issue.

Do I Call the People I Work with Inmates or Patients?

This depends on your role. To the correctional officers, the forensic client is an inmate. To the treatment team, the client is a patient, and to the court-appointed forensic evaluator, he or she is a defendant.

What Is My Role on the Forensic Service?

The student on the forensic service is a member of the treatment team and—with supervision—is responsible for the management of a specified caseload. This includes clarifying diagnosis by gathering relevant history, conducting interviews with patients, and collaborating with other disciplines while recommending both pharmacologic and psychotherapeutic treatments and monitoring for treatment efficacy. The student takes into consideration the impact of substance abuse, comorbid medical conditions that may include physical trauma in the jail, criminal history, and the severe social stressors forensic patients are under during the formulation of cases and development of treatment plans.

What Evaluations Are Conducted on the Forensic Service?

The most common evaluations are of competence to stand trial that assess the individual's capacity to assist in his or her defense and to develop a rational appreciation of the individual's legal predicament. At times, a judge asks for an evaluation of the treatment needs of a particular forensic patient/defendant for the purpose of ordering a treatment alternative to incarceration.

What Is My Role in Determining Whether My Patient Is Competent to Refuse Treatment and How Is That Different from His Competence to Stand Trial?

Psychiatrists are often called upon to provide opinions concerning decision-making competence issues. As a student, you must consider whether a refusal by the patient is motivated by delusions, depression, or other psychiatric symptoms and whether or not the patient appreciates the consequences of his or her decision. Any physician can assess for competence to refuse treatment, but in most hospitals, psychiatrists are relied upon to provide consultation on competence issues. Competence assessments are task specific. In treatment refusal cases, the patient's ability to weigh the risks and benefits of refusing treatment or leaving against medical advice is considered. In criminal cases, the defendants' ability to consider the risks and benefits of following different legal strategies is considered and their ability to work with their attorney is at the forefront of the assessment. A judge is interested in whether or not the defendant can make a rational and reasoned decision when entering a plea or deciding to take his or her case to trial. The judge takes into consideration the defendant's appearance and demeanor in the courtroom, speech patterns, and interactions with the defense attorney.

Is Competence to Stand Trial the Same as the Insanity Defense?

No. An evaluation for "insanity" is the assessment of the role mental illness played in the commission of a crime, usually a violent crime. It is rarely invoked and is a retrospective evaluation based on all of the available data related to the nature of the crime, the defendant's history, and the events that led up to the alleged crime. Competence is not concerned as much with the crime itself but focuses on the current mental status of a defendant and his or her ability to assist in a legal defense. See Table 6-1.

How Do I Assess Depression? Wouldn't Anyone Be Depressed if They Were Facing a Long Prison Term?

The psychiatrist assesses mood changes, energy levels, appetite, and sleep patterns. The prison sentence is a contributing social stressor. Many forensic patients who do not meet criteria for major depressive disorder may meet criteria for adjustment disorder or suffer from reactive mood symptoms related to their personality disorder.

How Do I Assess Suicide Risk in a Forensic Patient Who Claims "I Will Kill Myself if I Have to Go Back to Jail"?

Just as in nonforensic settings, the psychiatrist must conduct a thorough suicide risk assessment considering acute and chronic risk factors. Acute risk factors would include the presence of panic symptoms, meeting criteria for major depression, and the presence of psychotic symptoms. Chronic risk factors could include prior suicide attempts or comorbid human immunodeficiency virus (HIV) infection. It is also essential to take into consideration some of the established high-risk periods for completed suicide among prison inmates. See Box 6-1.

Table 6-1

Competence versus Criminal Responsibility Assessments

Competence to Stand Trial Evaluations	Criminal Responsibility (Insanity) Evaluations
Here-and-now evaluation	A retrospective review of the mental state at the time of the crime
Relies on current mental status	Relies more on history
Evaluation is requested based on the defendant's mental state, not the nature of the alleged crime	Rarely requested outside violent felonies
Can be requested by the defense, the prosecutor, or the judge	Requested by the defense team

HIGH-RISK PERIODS FOR SUICIDE AMONG PRISON INMATES

The first 24 hours of lockup
Before and after court dates
The time right before transfer to state prison
After receiving a "Dear John" breakup letter

Don't Some Forensic Patients Exaggerate Their Symptoms to Avoid Jail?

Yes, many forensic patients exaggerate symptoms to avoid some aversive situation in the jail setting such as gang violence or being kept in punitive segregation following a violation of rules.

What Is Malingering and Do I Have to Be on the Alert for It in All of My Forensic Patients?

Malingering is the intentional production of false or grossly exaggerated physical or psychological symptoms motivated by external incentives. Although the psychiatrist in the forensic setting should keep it in mind, only a small percentage of patients meet criteria for malingering without any other psychopathology. Some of the circumstances that warrant suspicion of malingering are presented in Table 6-2.

How Do I Assess the Severity of an Alleged Suicide Attempt Prior to One That Led to Hospital Admission?

This differentiation is difficult, and the patient's account of events alone is inadequate to make a determination. Table 6-3 presents some useful guidelines.

Table 6-2

Circumstances Associated with Malingering

When should one suspect that a forensic patient could be feigning psychiatric symptoms?
1. Clear secondary gain can be established; for example, the patient is hoping to serve his sentence in a forensic hospital rather than in the jail setting.
2. There is no history of prior treatment.
3. The symptom onset is later than expected for that particular condition.
4. There are prior evaluations suggesting malingering.
5. There is no evidence of distress despite the report of hallucinations or delusions.
6. The patient behaves differently in the ward milieu than during direct interviewing.

Forensic Psychiatry

Table 6-3
Steps for Differentiating Suicide Attempts from Gestures in Forensic Settings
Look for physical signs, for example, marks on the neck.
Look for evidence of loss of consciousness.
Look for the presence of toxic blood levels of medications.
Did the patient require monitoring in a medical intensive care unit (ICU)?
Review past risk behaviors and risk factors for self-harm; patients with multiple superficial scars on their extremities may be at higher risk for making gestures consistent with their personality disorder and at lower risk for completed suicide.
What was the patient's awareness of the level or intensity of monitoring? For example, did the patient know that an officer or a nursing aide would be passing by in 1 minute or did he believe that no one would find him to cut him down from the hanging rope?

How Is a Forensic Service Similar to a General Civilian Psychiatric Unit?

Clinicians must abide by the same government-set regulations and standards regarding the use of emergency medications and the emergency use of seclusion or restraint. In New York State, prisoners are allowed to refuse medications that are not court ordered. Just as on general psychiatry units, treatment teams include psychiatrists, psychologists, social workers, nurses, and activity therapists. Forensic patients are not locked down or behind bars when they are hospitalized. Forensic wards are secured by correctional or safety officers and therapy aides. Access to the units is limited to a centralized gate controlled by officers who screen and search patients and their visitors. In some respects, the heightened attention to risk assessment by the staff and the presence of officers make the ward even more secure than a typical nonforensic unit where the staff are often less prepared for aggressive patients.

Do I Need to Be Concerned about Anything Besides Diagnosis in My Forensic Patient?

Yes. Patients on a forensic service receive treatment as well as diagnostic evaluations. In working with this population, the psychiatrist must appreciate the nature of the unique social stressors including facing long prison sentences, facing uncertain legal dispositions, and facing potential retribution from enemies in the jail setting. By virtue of their lifestyles, forensic patients are often unreliable. This leaves many clinicians reluctant to prescribe medication out of concern for abuse or failure to follow up. For this reason, many subtle mood symptoms may go undetected or undertreated or attributed to external factors in the forensic setting. Table 6-4 reviews some of the constraints to treatment.

Table 6-4
Some Constraints to Effective Treatment in Forensic Settings
Court-ordered transfers can be immediate and interrupt therapy and an established therapeutic alliance.
Court orders for medication over objection do not extend to the jail or prison in many jurisdictions.
Court appearances during inpatient admissions interfere with routine daytime clinical programming.
Many outpatient settings do not accept forensic patients.
Many forensic patients are homeless and are without established benefits.

Why Is It Important to Take a Comprehensive Criminal History?

First, the nature of the alleged crime can tell a great deal about the acuity of psychiatric symptoms or the level of functioning of that patient. Second, prior arrests may give relevant information about severity of substance abuse. Third, criminal history is relevant to enhancing the patient's risk assessment. The more violent the alleged crime, the more alert staff should be to the risk for aggressive behaviors on the unit. Important aspects of the criminal history are presented in Table 6-5.

How Do I Talk with My Patient about His Current Crime?

Unless otherwise instructed by the attending physician, it is fine for the student to discuss the current charges with the patient after reviewing the limits of confidentiality and reminding the patient that confessions are not required in this setting. You can simply ask, "What do the police say you did?"

Table 6-5
Information Relevant in the Social History of Forensic Patients
Juvenile record, including institutions and state hospitalizations
Past arrests/convictions
Felonies versus misdemeanors
What was the nature of past offenses? That is, were they disorganized, suggesting more psychopathology?
How many and how long were prison sentences?
Have there been any failed supervisions in the community, that is, violation of parole?
Has the patient sustained physical or psychological trauma while incarcerated?
Has the patient spent time in punitive segregation for infractions?
What are the circumstances surrounding the most recent legal charge, referred to as the instant offense?

What Happens if I Find Out That My Patient Has Committed an Unsolved Crime That I've Read about in the Newspaper?

All issues that might involve risk management services or hospital security would warrant immediately speaking directly to your supervising attending psychiatrist. Although there is no duty to report to the police on the past crimes of your patient, the psychiatrist must take that information into consideration when reviewing the discharge plan. Knowledge about a past crime may affect the assessment of the patient's level of dangerousness in the community and may necessitate further involuntary commitment to a hospital. It is important to clarify at the onset of treatment with the patient what constitutes the circle of confidentiality or, in other words, what members of the treatment team will have access to information divulged during sessions. Even for students, clarifying with patients the limits of confidentiality is important, as the medical records of forensic patients can find their way to court.

Aren't All Psychotic Patients Violent?

No, psychosis is certainly a risk factor that should be considered, but schizophrenia does not equate with violence. Substance abuse and psychopathy (a severe form of personality disorder) are greater risk factors. Should you combine psychosis with substance abuse, the risk rises substantially.

Where Do Forensic Patients Go after They Leave the Hospital Unit?

The majority of forensic patients are not discharged directly to the community. They are often transferred to forensic state hospitals for extended treatment. If their charges are dropped and they are released from custody, they are generally stepped down to a regular inpatient psychiatric service until they no longer pose a danger in the community. When still under correctional custody but stable enough to leave the hospital, they are generally housed in mental observation units in the jails. The chances of bumping into such a person are highly remote, and doing so would probably indicate that the person had been charged with a very minor nonviolent misdemeanor.

Is the Forensic Service Much More Dangerous Than a Regular Psychiatric Inpatient Unit?

No, on forensic units safety is addressed in the following ways:

- Correctional officers patrol the units.
- Frequent room and body searches are conducted for contraband.
- A risk assessment is completed for each patient upon admission.
- New-onset risk factors are communicated among members of a multidisciplinary treatment team.

If I Am Treating a Forensic Patient and Know His History, Am I Also Responsible for Providing Information to the Court Regarding Competence to Stand Trial?

The goal of a forensic evaluation is to provide an objective assessment that will assist the court. For this reason, it is important for the psychiatrist to avoid taking on the dual role of treating clinician and forensic evaluator. This is the concept of "dual agency." Whenever practical, a separate treating clinician is assigned to provide comprehensive medical treatments. This separation facilitates a more objective forensic evaluation and allows the treating clinician to develop a therapeutic alliance, which at times calls for a degree of advocating for the patient.

Do I Really Need to Obtain a Urine Toxicology Screen from the Patient if He Has Been in Jail for 2 Months?

Yes, despite the security provided, inmates can and do obtain drugs in jail, and they can develop substance-induced symptoms that lead to hospital admission. In fact, the patient may intentionally forgo treatment for withdrawal symptoms in order to avoid the potential consequences of admitting to drug use in the jail.

KEY POINTS

◆ Patients on a forensic psychiatry service are facing criminal charges or have been acquitted of their charges by reason of mental disease or defect ("insanity").

◆ Psychiatric diagnoses on a forensic service are made in the same way as diagnoses on a civilian service: based on signs, symptoms, and clinical course according to DSM-IV-TR criteria.

◆ Assessments for competence and insanity serve different purposes and are conducted in different ways.

◆ Forensic assessment and psychiatric treatment are best done by different people ("dual agency.")

Evaluating the Patient

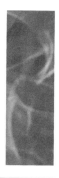

7

Using DSM-IV-TR

MYRL R. S. MANLEY

CLASSIFICATION OF PSYCHIATRIC DISORDERS

What Is DSM-IV-TR?

The *Diagnostic and Statistical Manual of Mental Disorders,* fourth edition (DSM-IV-TR), published by the American Psychiatric Association in 1994, classifies psychiatric disorders. For each disorder, DSM-IV-TR provides a set of diagnostic criteria accompanied by text that describes the essential features and the differential diagnosis of each disorder. DSM-IV-TR does not address treatments. TR indicates "text revision." DSM-IV-TR, published in 2000, updates DSM-IV-TR. The sets of diagnostic criteria are the same in the two volumes, but the accompanying text in DSM-IV-TR has been revised to incorporate more recent research data and epidemiologic surveys. The text has also been expanded to make DSM-IV-TR more broadly educational and not simply a handbook of diagnostic criteria.

Does DSM-IV-TR Provide a Definition of Mental Disorders?

Yes. Mental disorders are behavioral or psychological syndromes that cause *distress* or *disability.* If there is neither, the behavior is not considered a disorder. For example, depression can cause distress, mental retardation causes impaired functioning, and both are considered disorders in DSM-IV-TR. However, culturally sanctioned responses, deviant behavior, and conflicts with society are not in themselves mental disorders. For example, grieving the loss of a loved one, being gay, and being upset about higher taxes are not mental disorders.

Why Does Psychiatry Use a System of Formalized Diagnostic Criteria When Other Medical Specialties Do Not?

Because psychiatry is different. The greatest diagnostic difference is that psychiatry does not (yet) have external markers such as laboratory tests or imaging studies that can be used to establish the diagnosis. The absence of such markers leads inevitably to disagreement among clinicians about the correct diagnosis. DSM-IV-TR attempts to increase *diagnostic reliability* (i.e., agreement about the correct diagnosis) in two ways. First, it establishes criteria that are highly specific, leaving little room for individual interpretation. (The diagnosis of "anorexia," for example, requires the loss of at least 15% of normal body weight, not just "a lot of weight.") Second, DSM-IV-TR diagnostic criteria are based on descriptive phenomenology.

What Is Phenomenology?

Phenomenology is information known directly through the senses: what is seen, heard, felt, and so forth. DSM-IV-TR diagnoses are based on descriptions of observed phenomena: the clinical symptoms and the clinical course. The diagnoses make no use of interpretations or inferred intrapsychic processes. Observed data are always more reliable than inferred data.

USING DSM-IV-TR

Is DSM-IV-TR Used All Over the World?

DSM-IV-TR is widely used throughout the United States. In many other parts of the world, including member states of the World Health Organization, the 10th edition of the International Classification of Diseases (ICD-10) is preferred. In the United States, Medicare uses only ICD-10 codes.

What's the Difference between DSM-IV-TR and ICD-10?

DSM-IV-TR includes only psychiatric diagnoses; ICD-10 includes medical as well as psychiatric diagnoses. In addition, the two systems were designed for different purposes. ICD-10 codes are used for general epidemiologic and health management functions such as monitoring the incidence and prevalence of diseases and compiling national morbidity and mortality statistics.

DSM-IV-TR attempts to increase diagnostic reliability through the formulation of highly specific operationalized diagnostic criteria. ICD-10 contains only brief descriptions of the disorders

Over the years there has been increasing convergence between the two systems. Most (but not all) psychiatric disorders are now identified by the same numeric codes in ICD-10 as in DSM-IV-TR.

How Is DSM-IV-TR Organized?

The DSM-IV-TR classification system is multiaxial. The clinician is asked to assess five different aspects of a patient's life. These five aspects are called *axes* and are summarized in Table 7-1. A patient may have one, more than one, or no diagnosis or rating on each axis.

Table 7-1	
DSM-IV-TR Multiaxial System	
Axis I	Clinical disorders
	Conditions that are not mental disorders but that may be a focus of clinical attention
Axis II	Personality disorders
	Mental retardation
Axis III	General medical conditions
Axis IV	Psychosocial and environmental problems
Axis V	Global assessment of functioning

What's the Difference between Axis I and Axis II?

The formulators of DSM-III (the first DSM to use a multiaxial system) believed that there was a qualitative difference between personality disorders and other psychiatric disorders. Their thinking was influenced by Freud's distinction between "character neuroses" and "actual neuroses." Personality disorders were coded on Axis II, separate from the main group of disorders coded on Axis I. Although Axis I disorders tend to be episodic and *state* dependent and Axis II disorders tend to be chronic and *trait* dependent, there are numerous exceptions. The difference now is really one of definition: personality disorders (and traits) and mental retardation constitute Axis II disorders; everything else is an Axis I disorder. Axis I and Axis II disorders can coexist in a patient.

What Kinds of Problems Should I Put on Axis IV?

Psychosocial and environmental problems are reported on Axis IV. Table 7-2 lists the major classes of such problems. Remember that both good and bad things can cause stress. In fact, any major change in a person's life is most likely to be stressful. For example, both matching to the residency of one's dreams and not matching at all can cause significant psychological stress.

Table 7-2
Psychosocial and Environmental Problems (Axis IV)
Problems with primary support group (e.g., family conflicts)
Problems related to the social environment (e.g., retirement)
Educational problems (e.g., illiteracy)
Occupational problems (e.g., discord with boss or coworker)
Housing problems (e.g., homelessness)
Economic problems (e.g., insufficient welfare support)
Problems with access to health care (e.g., inadequate health insurance)
Legal problems (e.g., incarceration)
Other problems (e.g., exposure to disasters, war, or other hostilities)

How Do I Assess Functioning for Axis V?

Axis V is the Global Assessment of Functioning (GAF), a numeric score from 1 to 100 that reflects a person's overall functioning. Lower scores reflect greater impairment and higher scores less impairment. Given adequate information (inadequate information is coded as GAF = 0), a GAF rating can be estimated on the basis of psychological, social, and occupational functioning.

How Do I Estimate a GAF?

Think of the 1-to-100 GAF scale as divided by the numbers 20, 50, and 80 (Table 7-3). After you decide which one of the four ranges is most appropriate, consider how the particular individual is functioning compared with other individuals within the range. Remember that after a suicide attempt, a person cannot be given a GAF score higher than 20.

Where Do I Report Mental Disorders with Drug-Related or Medical Causes?

These are reported on both Axis I and Axis II. Several primary psychiatric disorders include both drug-related and medical causes in their differential diagnosis. Regardless of the cause of the disorder, the diagnosis is reported under Axis I or II. For example, "Cocaine-Induced Psychotic Disorder" and "Dementia Due to HIV Infection" are Axis I diagnoses. When a medical condition is the direct cause of symptoms, the medical condition is also reported on Axis III. For example, if the depression develops in a patient as a direct result of a brain tumor, the diagnosis of "Mood Disorder Due to Brain Tumor, With Depressive Features" should be coded on Axis I and "Brain Tumor" should be coded on Axis III.

What Is NOS, and How Do I Use It?

NOS indicates "not otherwise specified." It is used to indicate that the patient fits a general class of disorders but that a more specific diagnosis cannot be made, either because the clinician lacks sufficient information or because the patient's cluster of symptoms do not meet formal criteria. For example, a patient may be given the diagnosis "Mood Disorder NOS" if she presents with an episode of major depression and it is not clear whether she has ever had an episode of mania or hypomania. As more

Table 7-3

Gross Estimate of the Global Assessment of Functioning (GAF)

Score	Level of Functioning
81–100	No problems
51–80	Holds a job, likely an outpatient
21–50	Has no job, likely an inpatient
1–20	In serious danger of hurting self or others

information becomes available, the diagnosis might be revised, for example, to "Bipolar II Disorder." Try to avoid using NOS as an excuse for not getting sufficient clinical information to make a specific diagnosis from the start.

Is "Neurotic" a DSM-IV-TR Term?

No. The term "neurotic" is derived from psychoanalytic theory and was intended to describe people who had psychiatric symptoms related to unconscious intrapsychic conflicts but whose capacity to "test reality" was unimpaired (as opposed to "psychotic"). These concepts are highly interpretive and nonphenomenologic. They were explicitly excluded from earlier editions of DSM. The term psychotic is retained but as an adjective to describe certain symptoms, not individuals. (The term neurotic is preserved in ICD-10 but with specific mention that it is not intended to imply etiology.)

Do I Need to Memorize DSM-IV-TR Diagnostic Criteria?

No. It is much more important to have a general conceptualization of the presentation of a disorder than to have memorized specific, detailed diagnostic criteria. Many patients who fail to meet full criteria are nevertheless given a presumptive diagnosis. Moreover, the formal criteria will certainly change in the future as understanding of psychiatric disorders improves. You should use DSM-IV-TR as a reference, not as a textbook of psychopathology.

Are There Any Disadvantages to Using DSM-IV-TR?

Having a checklist of signs and symptoms risks leaving the actual person out of the picture. In search of clarity and reliability, DSM-IV-TR may have lessened an appreciation for the uniqueness of each patient. In addition, clinicians sometimes focus on DSM-IV-TR–driven questioning, which does little to help develop an effective patient-physician relationship. The physician should use DSM-IV-TR but should also learn about the patient's life, establish rapport, and create a supportive and caring environment for the patient.

KEY POINTS

◆ Axis I and Axis II disorders are not mutually exclusive and often coexist.

◆ The DSM-IV-TR method of determining a diagnosis is phenomenologic-descriptive; it specifically avoids interpretation or inference.

◆ Psychosocial stressors (Axis V) include positive as well as negative life events.

◆ Most hospitalized patients have a GAF score between 20 and 50.

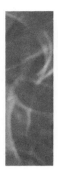

8

The Psychiatric History and Mental Status Examination

MYRL R. S. MANLEY

 THE PSYCHIATRIC HISTORY

Is History-Taking as Important in Psychiatry as in Medicine?

Absolutely! Because there are no external markers or laboratory tests in psychiatry, the only way to make a diagnosis is on the basis of symptoms and course. A careful history elicits the major symptoms (including some symptoms that the patient may not think important enough to report) and how they have evolved over time. An outline for the psychiatric history is presented in Table 8-1.

How Do I Take a History?

A history is taken as much by listening as it is by asking questions. Start with an open-ended question ("What brings you here today?"). Allowing the patient to talk uninterrupted for a while is more likely to reveal formal thought disorders or delusional beliefs than is posing a series of specific questions. Use the patient's responses as a guide for follow-up questions. Know the outline for the psychiatric history, but be flexible in addressing material as it arises in the interview rather than sticking to a rigid mental outline. For example, if you are getting a history of prior medication treatments and the patient mentions current suicidal thoughts, you should immediately switch to a suicide assessment. At other times, if the patient raises an issue that seems minor and unrelated to what you are asking, you can say, "Let me set that aside for a moment if you don't mind. I'd like to finish the list of drugs you have taken in the past."

Why Should I Put the Chief Complaint in the Patient's Own Words if It Doesn't Make Sense?

The use of the patient's own words tells a great deal about the patient's thinking, understanding, and insight. If the chief complaint is given in incoherent gibberish, for example, that is valuable information to record. In the history of the present illness, you can clarify the reasons and sequence of events leading to admission.

Table 8-1

Outline for the Psychiatric History

I. Identifying data (always age and sex; ethnicity, occupation, and marital status when significant)

II. Chief complaint (in the patient's own words)

III. History of the present illness

A. When did the current episode begin? What were presenting symptoms? How have symptoms progressed?

B. Is the patient receiving treatment? If so, what? Effectiveness? Side effects? Compliance?

C. Pertinent negatives

IV. Past psychiatric history

A. When was the first-ever onset of symptoms (whether treated or not)? Have there been recurrences? If so, what frequency and length of episodes? Changes in symptom pattern?

B. All prior treatments in detail

1. For medications: Dose, length of treatment, side effects, therapeutic response, patient's compliance

2. For psychotherapy: Modality, length of treatment, perceived benefits, patient's involvement or noninvolvement

V. Medical history (especially current medical problems, current prescription medications, drug allergies)

VI. Family history (Who is in the family? Who else has had psychiatric symptoms or treatment?)

VII. Personal history

A. Relate the significant events of a patient's life, and create a picture of functioning over time. Some important elements: early friendships, academic record, job experiences, romantic relationships, sexual experiences, military experience, incarceration experience, drug and alcohol use, recreational pastimes

VIII. Mental status examination

IX. Physical examination

X. Laboratory findings

XI. Differential diagnosis

Do I Really Need to Be Specific about Past Treatments if They Haven't Worked?

Yes; you must be specific about past treatments especially if they haven't worked. One of the most valuable services you can perform for your patient is to dig through old records, talk to prior treating clinicians, and document precisely what has been tried, what has worked, and what has not worked. The best predictor of future treatment response is past treatment response. However, without documenting the medication dose, the length of time taken, and the patient's compliance, it is impossible to distinguish a therapeutic nonresponse from a subtherapeutic drug trial (e.g., too low a dose or too short a course of medication).

What Are "Pertinent Negatives"?

As the history unfolds, some diagnoses will begin to seem more likely than others, and you will expect to hear about symptoms that commonly occur with those disorders. A pertinent negative is the absence of an expected sign or symptom. For example, in a patient who has depression, you would expect to find sleep and appetite disturbances. When the expected does not exist, it should be mentioned explicitly and not ignored. Its absence may have diagnostic implications.

Is the Medical History Really Necessary if My Patient Has Only a Psychiatric Condition?

Yes. You may not know that the condition is only psychiatric until you have taken a careful medical history, review of systems, and performed an attentive physical examination. Many medical conditions include psychiatric symptoms, and your patient's presenting symptoms may be the manifestation of a previously undiagnosed medical problem. In addition, medical conditions affect a person's overall sense of health and well-being and may complicate treatment. Cardiac conduction defects, for example, may limit the use of tricyclic antidepressants.

Will the Family History Help Establish My Patient's Diagnosis?

Most often not. Although many psychiatric disorders run in families (and probably have a genetically transmitted vulnerability), your patient's diagnosis will be based only on her signs, symptoms, and clinical course, not on the diagnosis of someone else in the family. Several recent studies have suggested that the vulnerability transmitted through families is not to a particular diagnosis but rather to a spectrum of disorders. Some families, for example, may have a predisposition to psychotic disorders that in some family members is expressed as schizophrenia and in other members as schizoaffective disorder or a psychotic mood disorder.

A positive family history should alert you to possibilities, however. A history of alcoholism in the family means that the individual is at greater risk for alcohol-related disorders. A family history of suicide substantially increases the risk for suicide in your patient regardless of the diagnosis.

What Should I Put in the Personal History?

Rather than including everything you ever heard about your patient, try to be selective. You should include major life events (e.g., army service, marriage), but you also want the personal history to trace the trajectory of an individual's life, describing the capacity for independent functioning over time. Aim to include information that is directly relevant to the diagnosis, treatment, and management; leave out all else. For example, developmental milestones of childhood (e.g., walking, talking, toilet training) are rarely of use in working with adult patients and need not be routinely mentioned.

It is essential, however, to enquire about drug and alcohol use. Which are currently used? How much and how often? When was the most recent drink or drug use? What has been the use in the past?

For patients with significant substance use or abuse, it may be preferable to include a "substance use history" separate from the personal history. (See Chapter 26.)

Should I Take a Sexual History of My Patient?

Sexual histories are important components of comprehensive evaluations for all patients—medical as well as psychiatric. Sex is such an important part of life for most people, so much a part of one's sense of identity, and such a useful barometer of physical and emotional well-being that to leave this topic out is to do your patient a disservice. At a minimum, you want to know whether your patient is currently sexually active, preferred partner or partners (sexual orientation), and any recent changes or concerns. Some changes have diagnostic implications: increased libido is common in manic states, decreased libido in depression. In addition, many psychiatric medications have sexual side effects. Selective serotonin reuptake inhibitor (SSRI) antidepressants, for example, often cause decreased libido and delayed orgasm. It is more difficult to assess these changes without a broad understanding of baseline sexual functioning. As with drug and alcohol use, it is sometimes useful to summarize this information in a separate section on "sexual history." (See Chapter 31.)

MENTAL STATUS EXAMINATION

What Is a Mental Status Examination?

The mental status examination (MSE) is analogous to the physical examination in physical medicine. It is a format for organizing your observations about your patient's thoughts, feelings, and behavior and for documenting specific abnormalities. Your direct observations of the patient are very likely to include findings that are not mentioned in the history (e.g., blunted emotional expression or a formal thought disorder). Taken together, the history and MSE provide the data from which a differential diagnosis is derived. The MSE should include only the findings that are present at the time you interview the patient. If, for example, your patient has a history of auditory hallucinations but is not hallucinating when you talk to her, hallucinations would not be included in the MSE. In addition, your MSE observations must be as descriptive and noninferential as possible. Describe only what you see, not what you think is the situation. For example, state that "The patient had tears in her eyes," not "The patient was feeling upset over the breakup with her boyfriend." An outline for the MSE is given in Table 8-2.

Do I Need to Ask Specific Tests to Describe the Cognitive Functions under "Sensorium"?

Very often you do not. In fact, your descriptions of the patient's cognitive capacities will be more valid and reliable if they are drawn from the whole of the interview and not from one or two isolated tests. Just by engaging the

---

Table 8-2

Outline of the Mental Status Examination

I. Appearance: Oddities of dress or demeanor, signs of physical illness, behavior with the examiner

II. Speech: The physical production of speech (not the ideas): slurred, monotone, soft, pressured, etc.

III. Emotional expression: Consider the range of emotions, the intensity, lability, and appropriateness to the topics being discussed
   A. Subjective: How the patient feels
   B. Objective: How the patient looks

IV. Thinking and perception
   A. Content: Delusions, obsessions, preoccupations, suicidal or homicidal thoughts
   B. Form: Logical and goal directed versus presence of a formal thought disorder
   C. Perceptions: Hallucinations, illusions

V. Sensorium (cognitive functions)
   A. Alertness
   B. Orientation
   C. Concentration
   D. Memory
      1. Immediate recall
      2. Short-term (or recent) recall
      3. Long-term memory
   E. Calculations
   F. Fund of knowledge
   G. Abstract reasoning

VI. Insight and judgment

---

patient in an extended conversation, you will usually be able to describe something about the patient's concentration, fund of knowledge, memory, and other functions. For example, can the patient focus on your questions? Answer without being distracted? Remember what was discussed earlier? If a particular area needs greater clarification, specific tests can be used; some of these are listed in Table 8-3.

What Is "Fund of Knowledge" Supposed to Assess?

Does the person know what is going on in the world around him? Are major events registering in the person's mind in the way you would expect them to for any sentient person. Fund of knowledge is not intended to be a measure of education or intelligence, although it is certainly affected by them. (You will need to keep this in mind so that you can tailor your questions to the appropriate educational and intellectual level of your individual patient.)

One of the most time honored—and least reliable—ways of evaluating fund of knowledge is to ask the patient to name presidents of the United States backward, starting with the current president and going back as far

Table 8-3

Some Ways to Test Cognitive Functions for the Mental Status Examination

Always use the whole examination in forming your observations. These tests may help clarify deficits and the degree of abnormality. In many instances, formal tests will not be necessary because sufficient information was obtained just by talking with the patient.

Concentration
"Count backward from 100 by 7." (Note that this is not intended to be a test of calculation. What matters is the patient's ability to sustain focus on the task, not whether she gets all the right answers.)
"Spell 'world' backward."
"Say the letters of the alphabet backward."

Calculations
"How many quarters are in $3.75?"
"If you buy something that costs $1.60 and pay with a $5 bill, how much change should you get back?"

Memory
Immediate: Ask the patient to repeat a series of five to seven digits after you.
Give the patient three objects to remember and then immediately ask what they are.
Recent recall: Ask the patient to repeat three objects after 5 minutes.
"What did you have for breakfast this morning?"
"How did you come in to the hospital this afternoon?"
Long term: "What grade school did you attend?" (Note that asking a patient her birthday does not test long-term memory; she is not "remembering" being born but rather is reciting information learned by rote.)
"Who was your fifth grade teacher?"
"Where did you first learn to drive?"

Fund of Knowledge
"What is a major news story that's on TV or in the newspapers these days? Tell me about it."
"Tell me about a recent movie (or book)."
"What countries border the United States?"
"What countries border France?"

Abstract Reasoning
"Which object doesn't belong in this group: fish, tree, rock? Why?"
"How are an apple and an orange alike?" (Note that abstract reasoning cannot be assessed by asking differences because the only plausible answers are concrete.)
"What does it mean when people say 'A stitch in time saves nine'?"

as possible. This is a poor test because it tests several cognitive functions simultaneously—fund of knowledge, but also memory and concentration. Political events are more important to some people than others. Moreover, recent immigrants to the United States might be able to give you detailed histories of their home countries and not know the names of more than one or two recent U.S. presidents. Table 8-3 suggests some alternatives.

How Do I Test for "Abstract Reasoning"?

Students are often taught to evaluate abstract reasoning by asking for interpretations of proverbs, but this is problematic. Most of us learn the meaning of proverbs the same way we learn all language—through day-to-day use. When you ask a patient to "interpret" a proverb, you are really asking her to recite the meaning learned over years of use, not to demonstrate abstract reasoning at the moment. Interpreting unfamiliar proverbs can be difficult, even for intelligent and highly educated individuals. (Test yourself with this East African proverb: You can't throw a canvas cloth over a horned animal. The traditional meaning: You can't cover up evil deeds forever.) An alternative is to ask about similarities or to ask which object doesn't belong in a group of three. Keep in mind, however, that abstract reasoning can often be assessed just by talking with the patient, without having to resort to specific tests.

How Can I Assess Abstract Reasoning without Formal Testing?

Patients reveal a capacity for abstract thinking in a variety of ways, such as through the use of jokes, metaphors, and proverbs. One patient, speaking of the psychiatrist who had treated her psychotic disorder, said, "I was blind. He gave me back my sight." The use of the word "blindness" to describe psychosis is a powerful metaphor and reveals the woman's ability to think in abstract terms.

What Am I Looking for in "Insight and Judgment"?

These closely related capacities help you to understand the patient's ability to cooperate with treatment and to behave in ways that will not get her into trouble. Insight describes the recognition of having a disorder, the symptoms related to the disorder, and the need for treatment. Judgment describes the ability to contain the more disruptive symptoms of a disorder and behave in socially accepted ways and to comply with necessary treatment.

How Can I Assess Insight and Judgment?

Much information can be observed in the course of the general interview. Does the patient behave with you in socially appropriate ways? Does she acknowledge having a disorder and needing treatment? Students are sometimes taught to "test" judgment by posing hypothetical problems, such as "What would you do if you found a stamped, addressed, and sealed envelope lying on the sidewalk?" These questions almost never yield useful information. The intended answer seems obvious to most people and may have nothing to do with how the patient would actually behave. It is much better to ask questions based on the patient's real-life circumstances: "What would you do if you ran out of medication?" "What would you do if the electricity in your apartment were turned off?" At all events, make your assessment in the context of the whole interview. The manic patient who has just given away his car, his wedding ring, and $10,000 in cash to strangers and who still thinks that was a good thing to do is demonstrating poor judgment.

KEY POINTS

◆ In taking a psychiatric history, you must include some open-ended questions to detect thought disorders and delusional beliefs.

◆ The chief complaint should be in the patient's own words, even if it does not make sense.

◆ Limit the observations in the personal history to information that will help with diagnosis, treatment, and management.

◆ The mental status examination records only the findings that are present at the time of the interview.

◆ The assessment of cognitive functions should be based on the totality of the interview and not on isolated "tests."

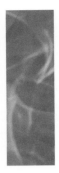

9

The Medical Evaluation in Psychiatry

ARTHUR SINKMAN

Why Is a Medical Evaluation Important in the Assessment of a Psychiatric Patient?

There are several reasons why it is essential for you to perform a medical evaluation of the psychiatric patient:

1. Psychiatric signs and symptoms can be part of the initial presentation of a medical illness. For instance, anxiety and irritability can be part of the presenting complaints of hyperthyroidism. What looks like a psychiatric illness may turn out to be a medical condition.
2. Psychiatric medications can have significant medical consequences. A medical work-up is essential before you start treatment. For instance, signs of liver disease may steer you clear of using divalproex (Depakote) for mania.
3. Having a medical illness can have a significant emotional impact and be the root cause of the patient's emotional troubles.
4. Conversely, having a psychiatric illness can severely affect the patient's medical illness. For instance, depression often makes it very difficult for diabetic patients to care for themselves.

What Physical Illnesses Present with Psychiatric Symptoms?

Many illnesses can masquerade as psychiatric conditions. The list is very long, including conditions as diverse as brain tumors and hyperparathyroidism. Some of the medical conditions that are more likely to cause psychiatric symptoms are listed in Table 9-1. Unfortunately, there is no direct correlation between a particular medical illness and a specific pattern of psychiatric symptoms. Psychotic symptoms, anxiety, depression, and confusion can each occur in various medical conditions. Keep in mind that it is not just medical illnesses that can cause psychiatric symptoms. Medications and substance abuse can have psychiatric side effects. Make sure to keep an eye open for these important factors.

Table 9-1

Some Medical Illnesses Associated with Psychiatric Symptoms

Infections	Encephalitis (particularly herpes), human immunodeficiency virus, tertiary syphilis, Lyme disease, pneumonia, Creutzfeldt-Jakob disease
Tumors	Brain (primary and metastatic), pancreas, paraneoplastic syndrome
Inflammatory	Systemic lupus erythematosus
Seizures	Postictal, psychomotor
Neurologic	Alzheimer's disease, Wilson's disease, Huntington's disease, subdural hematoma, traumatic brain injury
Metabolic	Hypercalcemia, hyponatremia, hyper- and hypothyroidism, Cushing's disease, Addison's disease, pernicious anemia, chronic renal failure, hepatic encephalopathy, acute intermittent porphyria

Note: This list is not exhaustive, but illustrative.

How Do I Conduct a Medical Evaluation on a Psychiatric Patient?

The short answer is, in the same thorough way that you would perform a medical evaluation on any other patient. The key components are well known to you: history, review of systems, physical examination, and laboratory studies.

How Do You Use Physical Signs in Psychiatry?

There are no direct physical signs of psychiatric illness. However, a good clinician may discover signs of a medical illness that explain the psychiatric symptoms. Some of these are listed in Table 9-2.

Should I Do a Physical Examination on All My Psychiatric Patients?

Examinations should be performed for inpatients because on an inpatient psychiatric service the psychiatrist is the responsible physician. Outpatients can be referred to a consulting internist as long as the resulting assessments (even if the finding is of no abnormalities) are sent to the psychiatrist and appropriately recorded in the patient's record.

Which Parts of the Physical Examination Are Important?

In the end, the important part of the examination will be the part that revealed abnormalities. It can be a grievous error to prejudge and to assume what will be important and what will not be. Do not proceed by rote, but train yourself to think about the examination as you are doing it and be alert for unanticipated findings.

What Should I Do if My Patient Is a Healthy Adult with a Negative Review of Systems?

Even when there is no reason to suspect that your patient has a medical problem, it is crucial to make sure the physical examination is completed

Table 9-2

Use of Physical Signs in Psychiatry

Patient's Appearance	Symptoms	Diagnosis
Sad	Jerky movements of arms and legs	Huntington's chorea
	Butterfly rash on cheeks	Systemic lupus erythematosus
Hyperactive and anxious	Dilated pupils, muscle wasting	Stimulant abuse
Confused and irritable	Wet pants, blood on lips	Postictal states
Emotions are blunted	Stooped posture, pill-rolling tremor	Parkinson's disease
Anxious	Rapid pulse, tremor	Hyperthyroidism
Excited	Round face, truncal obesity	Cushing's disease
Short tempered	Muscle-bound body builder	Anabolic steroid abuse
Apathetic	Dry skin, pale conjunctiva	Chronic renal failure
Visual hallucinations	Tremors, sweating	Alcohol withdrawal
Mood swings, demanding	Wheelchair bound	Traumatic brain injury

and considered in formulating the patient's diagnosis and treatment. Although invasive examinations such as rectal or pelvic exams may be deferred or referred to a consultant, they must always be done when there is a medical indication, such as a male patient complaining of symptoms of prostatism. Whatever you do, do not lie and say that your patient "refused" a rectal examination if you never attempted one.

My Supervisor Says I Shouldn't Do a Physical Examination on My Patient because It Will Contaminate the Transference. What Does That Mean?

Transference refers to the tendency of a patient to have feelings toward his doctor and ideas about him. These are often not realistic responses but are based on automatic (unconscious) patterns of relating to others that had their origins in childhood. In psychodynamic psychotherapy, the work of discovering these patterns is an important part of the healing process. However, patients can develop transference responses toward any of their caregivers, not just psychiatrists. All physicians need to be aware of this possibility as it can significantly affect treatment. Think of the rebellious teenage diabetic angrily challenging the authority of his physician and refusing to do finger sticks. For the psychiatrist doing psychodynamic psychotherapy, performing a physical examination herself on the patient would complicate the task of trying to explore the transference and it would be best to refer the patient to a consultant for the examination. However, on an inpatient psychiatric unit the situation is different and it is essential that you conduct a thorough physical examination on your patient. Being aware of transference may guide you in dealing with the patient. For instance, with a seductive patient it is important to have someone else present during your examination.

What Does PERRLA Mean?

PERRLA is a commonly used acronym for describing normal pupils: *p*upils are *e*qual in size, *r*ound, and *r*eactive to *l*ight and *a*ccommodation. It is important to recognize what the acronym does not tell you. It says nothing about pupil size, which can be one of the most important physical signs in identifying drug- and alcohol-related disorders. For example, pupils are very constricted ("pinpoint") in opiate intoxication and dilated in stimulant intoxication.

Is There a Standard Battery of Laboratory Tests That Should Be Ordered for All Patients?

No, but there are tests that are useful for medical screening in most patients. These are listed in Table 9-3.

When Should I Suspect That My Patient's Psychiatric Symptoms Are Caused by an Underlying Medical Condition?

There are particular clinical situations that should heighten your suspicion that a nonpsychiatric condition is at work. These are outlined in Table 9-4. Even when one of the factors listed is not present, keep an open mind and assume that an underlying physical illness, medication side effect, or substance abuse can be a factor causing psychiatric symptoms.

Are Laboratory Studies Useful in Monitoring Treatment?

Laboratory studies and structural neuroimaging investigations do not necessarily correlate with symptom progression or resolution. However,

Table 9-3

Some Laboratory Tests Useful for Screening Medical Conditions in Psychiatric Patients

Complete blood count
Electrolytes (Na, K, Cl, CO_2)
Glucose
Calcium
Renal function tests (blood urea nitrogen, creatinine)
Liver function tests (alanine aminotransferase, aspartate aminotransferase, gamma-glutamyl transpeptidase)
Rapid plasma reagin
Thyroid function tests (free thyroxine, thyroid-stimulating hormone)
Vitamin B_{12} level
Urine drug screen

Table 9-4

Factors Suggesting a Medical Cause for Psychiatric Symptoms

An elderly patient develops psychiatric symptoms for the first time in his life, or the pattern of his chronic psychiatric symptoms changes in a dramatic way.

Urinary or fecal incontinence is present. (In the severely and chronically mentally ill, this rule may not apply.)

The patient is confused or forgetful.

The patient has tremors, difficulties with movement, or other movement abnormalities.

The patient has a chronic medical illness and is taking various medications.

There is a history of a recent head injury.

the blood levels of some medications such as lithium and anticonvulsant mood stabilizers need to be monitored to ensure that the levels are within an established therapeutic range. Excessively high levels can lead to potentially dangerous toxicity.

What Does It Mean when the Laboratory Reports a Result as "Abnormal"?

Test results are reported as abnormal if they fall outside a "reference range," customarily set at the 95% confidence interval. Such a confidence interval means that if the test were repeated the result would fall within the range 95 out of 100 times. Thus, a "normal" result would fall outside this range on the basis of random statistical fluctuation 5 of 100 times. Therefore, if a panel of 20 tests is performed, it is expected that one of them will be outside the 95% confidence interval and will be reported as abnormal yet not represent any pathology. It is the degree of the abnormality of the laboratory result that is crucial. Also, it is essential to put the abnormal laboratory result in the context of the patient's clinical situation.

How Does the Presence of an Underlying Physical Illness Affect Treatment?

Treatment of the underlying physical illness is primary. If the medical illness is causing psychiatric symptoms, these symptoms should disappear when the illness is treated. In the interim, treatment of these secondary psychiatric symptoms is usually indicated, as they will make the patient more comfortable and increase compliance.

The Medical Evaluation

KEY POINTS

◆ There are no direct physical signs of psychiatric illness.

◆ Medical illnesses can masquerade as psychiatric conditions.

◆ Skipping components of the physical examination risks missing crucial underlying medical causes of psychiatric symptoms.

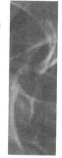

10

Guide to Psychological Testing and Psychiatric Rating Scales

GLENN HEISS AND MYRL R. S. MANLEY

PSYCHOLOGICAL TESTING

What Is Psychological Testing?

Psychological testing is an umbrella term for various interventions intended to formalize observations about patients. Unlike the usual clinical assessment in which a physician interviews a patient to collect data for diagnosis and treatment, psychological testing is more rigorous about establishing standardization, reliability, and validity (Box 10-1). Psychological tests address one of three general areas: intelligence and aptitude, personality makeup, and cognitive impairment caused by brain damage (neuropsychological assessment). Common tests used for each of these areas are listed in Table 10-1.

Can I Use Psychological Tests to Make a Diagnosis for My Patient?

No. Psychiatric diagnoses are made only on the basis of descriptions of signs, symptoms, and clinical course. Psychological testing cannot provide a psychiatric diagnosis. However, data yielded by such tests can aid in the diagnostic process by revealing issues that had not previously been apparent in routine clinical assessment. For example, testing may raise the possibility that the patient has an undetected delusional system, has a disorder of logical reasoning, or is lying. In such instances, you would then reevaluate the patient while keeping in mind the new information.

Can I Administer Psychological Tests Myself?

Generally not. Psychological testing is usually done by licensed psychologists who have formal training in psychological assessment. The proper administration and interpretation of tests require considerable experience and cannot meaningfully be accomplished by a novice.

BOX 10-1

PRINCIPLES OF PSYCHOLOGICAL TESTING

Standardization

Tests are administered in a *uniform* and *replicable* manner. Test results are compared for both clinical and nonclinical populations who have taken the test under similar conditions.

Reliability

Test results are *consistent* and *reproducible*. Tests taken at different times by the same patient or administered to the patient by different examiners tend to yield the same results.

Validity

The test truly measures what it purports to measure. A valid intelligence test, for example, measures intelligence and not socioeconomic status.

Should Psychological Testing Be Done for All of My Patients?

Psychological testing is not a routine part of the assessment of psychiatric patients. It is expensive and time consuming, and in many instances it does not yield any compelling information beyond that gathered in the original assessment. Formal testing is reserved for special situations.

When Should I Refer a Patient for Psychological Testing?

The psychologist who performs the testing will want a specific referral question in order to choose appropriate test instruments. Common reasons

---

Table 10-1

Some Psychological Tests in Common Use

Intelligence and Aptitude
Wechsler Adult Intelligence Scale (WAIS)
Wechsler Intelligence Scale for Children (WISC)

Personality
Personality Assessment Inventory (PAI)
Minnesota Multiphasic Personality Inventory (MMPI)
Rorschach inkblot test
Thematic Apperception Test (TAT)

Neuropsychological
Halstead-Reitan Neuropsychological Test Battery
Luria-Nebraska Neuropsychological Test Battery
Repeatable Battery for the Assessment of Neuropsychological Status (RBANS)

for referral include to assess intelligence and aptitude, to help with discharge planning, to clarify personality issues in guarded patients, to clarify vague and nonspecific symptoms when the diagnosis remains unclear, and to assess for brain damage in patients with cognitive deficits. Psychological testing is commonly included in forensic evaluations. When you request testing, you should be able to articulate a specific question you want answered. It is not appropriate to send your patient for testing with the question, "What is the diagnosis?" Table 10-2 lists some common reasons for obtaining psychological testing.

PSYCHIATRIC RATING SCALES

Are Psychiatric Rating Scales Different from Other Forms of Psychological Testing?

In many respects, they are substantially different. Rating scales present a series of questions that focus on a particular aspect of psychopathology, such as psychotic symptoms or symptoms of depression. Patients are asked to rate themselves for the presence and severity of specific symptoms. Each response is given a point score, and the sum of all scores forms an overall numeric rating. The scales thus provide a *quantitative* assessment of symptom severity. They are particularly useful (and were originally designed) as outcome measures in studies of the effectiveness of drugs or psychotherapy. Psychiatric rating scales are easy and quick to administer and do not require special training or extensive experience. Some widely used rating scales are listed in Table 10-3.

Table 10-2

Common Reasons for Psychological Testing

Intelligence and Aptitude
To help with discharge planning
To establish a diagnosis of mental retardation

Personality Testing
To help clarify symptom patterns when the diagnosis is unclear
To help detect malingering
To identify issues for consideration in psychotherapy
To help uncover additional information about aspirations, fears, conflicts, and self-perception, particularly in reticent or guarded patients

Neuropsychological Testing
To distinguish between brain-damaged and neurologically intact psychiatric patients
To identify specific neurologic problems such as dyslexia
To localize brain damage

Table 10-3
Some Commonly Used Psychiatric Rating Scales

Scale for the Assessment of Positive Symptoms (SAPS)
Measures psychotic symptoms

Scale for the Assessment of Negative Symptoms (SANS)
Measures negative symptoms typically seen in schizophrenia such as social withdrawal and decreased motivation

Hamilton Rating Scale for Depression
Measures mood, vegetative, and psychotic symptoms commonly seen in major depression

Hamilton Anxiety Rating Scale
Measures emotional and somatic symptoms of anxiety

Yale-Brown Obsessive-Compulsive Scale (Y-BOCS)
Measures both obsessive and compulsive symptoms

Should I Use Rating Scales for My Patients?

Rating scales are not routinely used in clinical practice for patients who are not part of research protocols. However, for the sake of your personal experience and education, you might want to administer a rating scale to one or more of your patients to provide documentation of the patient's change in clinical status. Three of the most commonly used rating scales, the Scale for the Assessment of Negative Symptoms (SANS), the Scale for the Assessment of Positive Symptoms (SAPS), and the Hamilton Rating Scale for Depression, are included in Appendices B through D.

KEY POINTS

◆ Psychological testing cannot provide a psychiatric diagnosis for your patient.

◆ Psychological testing is not routine. Referral should include a specific question to be answered.

Symptoms, Signs, and Abnormal Laboratory Values

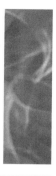

11

Hallucinations

MYRL R. S. MANLEY

What Are Hallucinations?

Hallucinations are sensory perceptions that occur without external stimuli; they are generated wholly within the central nervous system (CNS). They can occur in any sensory modality: sight, sound, touch, smell, or taste. Hallucinations are distinguished from *illusions,* in which a real external stimulus initiates a perception that is distorted or misinterpreted.

What Causes Hallucinations?

The neuropathology is not fully understood, and there are probably several different biologic mechanisms that result in hallucinations. They occur in a large number of psychiatric and medical conditions and drug-related states. Hallucinations are common in schizophrenia and occur in episodes of major depression and mania. They are often seen in patients with delirium, patients with CNS tumors, and patients with migraine headache. People with seizure disorders may experience hallucinations in the aura preceding a seizure. Among the common drug causes of hallucinations are hallucinogens such as lysergic acid diethylamide (LSD) or phencyclidine, intoxication with CNS stimulants, withdrawal from CNS sedatives such as alcohol, and sometimes marijuana intoxication. These causes are summarized in Table 11-1.

Are Hallucinations Ever Normal?

It is a common experience for people who are grieving to hallucinate the voice or the image of the departed loved one. This is not usually experienced as troublesome or symptomatic by the individual (some people find such hallucinations comforting) and is not regarded as pathologic. In addition, many people experience hallucination-like perceptions as they are falling asleep (*hypnagogics*) or as they are waking up (*hypnopompics*). Hypnagogics and hypnopompics are symptoms of narcolepsy, but they are

Table 11-1

Some Common Causes of Hallucinations

Psychiatric Disorders
Schizophrenia
Schizoaffective disorder
Major depression
Bipolar disorder

Medical Conditions
Seizure disorders
Delirium
Central nervous system tumors
Migraine headaches

Drug-Related States
Alcohol
   Major withdrawal
   Hallucinosis (hallucinations in a clear sensorium)
Central nervous system stimulant intoxication (cocaine, amphetamines)
Anticholinergic intoxication
Hallucinogenic drug intoxication (LSD)
Marijuana intoxication

Normal, Nonpathologic
Grief
Hypnagogics (while falling asleep), hypnopompics (while waking up)

also reported by people with no diagnosable sleep disturbance or other psychiatric disorder.

EVALUATION

How Do I Know if My Patient Has Hallucinations?

Although some patients report the presence of hallucinations, you should ask about them as part of the complete psychiatric and medical assessment of all patients. Patients with hallucinations experience them as full sensory perceptions, indistinguishable from true perceptions. Patients with auditory hallucinations truly *hear* what they are reporting; they are not making it up or speaking metaphorically. Some useful opening questions are "Have you ever heard things or seen things that other people could not?" and "Have you heard voices talking when there was no one else around? Have you had visions? Have you smelled things when you couldn't figure out where the odor was coming from?" It is usually not helpful to start by asking, "Have you ever had hallucinations?" Patients may be uncertain of the medical meaning of the term, and if it is perceived to have derogatory connotations, the patient may not acknowledge the presence of hallucinations.

What Should I Ask Patients Who Tell Me They Have Hallucinations?

Try to get the fullest possible description of the hallucination. Find out the modality (e.g., sight, sound), the content, and the circumstances in which it occurred. Was the person fully awake? Did some event immediately precede the perception? How long did it last? Did it occur only in the context of medical illness or drug use? What was the individual's reaction? Was there an emotional or behavioral response? It is also helpful to find out the patient's understanding by asking, "What did you make of it?" or "What did you think was going on?"

How Can I Tell if My Patient's Hallucinations Are Caused by a Psychiatric Disorder or an Underlying Medical or Drug-Related Condition?

Sometimes patients provide clear histories of preexisting medical or psychiatric disorders or of drug use. Although the information is helpful, it will not give you the diagnosis. As is always true in establishing a differential diagnosis, you need to draw on all elements of the history, mental status examination, and physical examination. Find out if there are other psychotic symptoms. Ninety percent of patients with hallucinations caused by a psychiatric disorder also have delusions. Look for a significant mood disturbance or the presence of vegetative symptoms suggesting a psychotic mood episode. On the other hand, an altered level of consciousness and disorientation are more suggestive of medical and drug causes than of primary psychiatric disorders. Any abnormalities noted during the physical examination increase the likelihood of an underlying medical or substance-related condition. Look for elevated blood pressure, heart rate, and temperature; dilated pupils; increased deep tendon reflexes; heavy sweating or dry skin; skin flushing or jaundice; abnormalities of gait or movement; and any focal neurologic signs (Table 11-2).

Table 11-2

Distinguishing Psychiatric from Medical Hallucinations

Factors Associated with Hallucinations Caused by Psychiatric Disorders	Factors Associated with Hallucinations Caused by Medical Conditions or Drug Use
Chronic, long-standing symptoms	Acute onset in a middle-aged or old person with no previous psychiatric history
No abnormal physical findings	Presence of physical signs
No laboratory test abnormalities	Laboratory test abnormalities
Mood and vegetative symptoms	Disorientation, memory impairment, altered level of consciousness
	Absence of other psychotic symptoms, such as delusions

Is the Presence of Hallucinations Ever an Emergency?

Hallucinations often occur with delirium, and depending on the underlying cause, delirium can be a medical emergency with significant morbidity and mortality if not treated promptly. The delirium of major withdrawal from alcohol (*delirium tremens*, or DTs) includes heavy sweating, tremulousness, an altered level of consciousness, and increased heart rate, blood pressure, and temperature. *Anticholinergic delirium* is marked by warm dry skin, dilated pupils, absent bowel sounds, tachycardia and other arrhythmias, and mental changes. Both types of delirium can lead to cardiovascular collapse and death.

Are There Laboratory Tests That Will Help with the Diagnosis?

There are no laboratory tests for the diagnosis of primary psychiatric disorders. Laboratory investigations are used to rule out nonpsychiatric causes of hallucinations and should be guided by the information in the history, mental status examination, and physical examination. A basic electrolyte and metabolic panel helps to establish the overall state of physical health and may help determine the presence or absence of encephalopathy caused by failure of a major organ system such as the kidneys or liver. Brain imaging studies may be useful and are necessary if there are localizing neurologic findings. An electroencephalogram may help if you suspect a seizure disorder. However, keep in mind that a seizure disorder is a *clinical* diagnosis and is not ruled out by a normal electroencephalogram.

Does a Urine or Blood Toxicology Screen Help?

Toxicology screens are of some help, but you must be cautious in interpreting the results. A positive drug screen means that the person has the drug in his or her system, not necessarily that the drug has caused the hallucinations. A negative toxicology screen does not rule out a drug-related cause of hallucinations because some substances, such as cocaine or amphetamines, can cause hallucinations that persist after the drug has been cleared. Moreover, a negative toxicology screen is common in patients whose hallucinations are caused by drug withdrawal because, by definition, they result from the *absence* of the drug. You must interpret the results of a toxicology screen in the context of all of the information you have obtained in the course of evaluating your patient. For example, if the patient's urine is positive for cocaine, check for physical findings such as dilated pupils, increased heart rate, and elevated blood pressure that are consistent with cocaine intoxication. Does the appearance of the hallucinations coincide with the drug use? Has there been a history of hallucinations in the past, when the patient was not using drugs?

Does the Modality of Hallucination Help Make the Diagnosis?

No. One of the most tenacious pieces of folk wisdom in clinical psychiatry is that auditory hallucinations suggest a primary psychiatric disorder such as schizophrenia and that visual hallucinations suggest medical and drug conditions. All modalities are seen in both psychiatric and medical or drug states, and by itself the modality has no diagnostic significance.

Twenty-five percent of patients with schizophrenia report visual hallucinations, as do sizable numbers of people with psychotic depression or mania. Of the psychiatric patients who have hallucinations, 20% experience them in more than one sensory modality, most often auditory and visual. Olfactory hallucinations are seen in tumors of the cribriform plate and lesions of the uncus, but they also are found in psychotic depression. One exception to the generalization that modality has no diagnostic significance is the tactile hallucination called *formication*, in which the patient feels bugs crawling over his or her skin. Formication is common in alcohol withdrawal and CNS stimulant intoxication and rare in other conditions.

Does the Content of the Hallucination Help with the Diagnosis?

There are no pathognomonic symptoms in psychiatry. However, there are characteristic patterns that, although they do not make the diagnosis, may suggest that one diagnosis is more likely than another. For example, certain types of auditory hallucinations are strongly suggestive (but not by themselves diagnostic) of schizophrenia: hearing one's thoughts being spoken aloud, hearing a voice making a running commentary on one's actions, and hearing two or more voices arguing with each other about oneself. Hallucinations in schizophrenia tend to be mood neutral, whereas hallucinations in psychotic mood disorders characteristically fit the mood. Depressed patients may hear derogatory, belittling voices, whereas manic patients might hear voices of extravagant praise.

What Are Command Hallucinations?

As the term suggests, *command hallucinations*—usually auditory—tell the patient to do something. Sometimes the instructions are benign, such as writing a letter or calling a friend. More alarmingly, voices may tell patients to hurt themselves or to hurt someone else. Patients describe varying degrees of ability to resist the commands. At least some patients find the hallucinations extremely difficult to ignore and feel that they must act on the command even though their conscious wish is to resist. Although one study has reported no increased risk for suicide or violence in the presence of command auditory hallucinations, they must be taken very seriously, and the degree of risk must be assessed for the individual patient.

Are Hallucinations and Flashbacks the Same Thing?

A *flashback* is the vivid reliving of previous emotionally intense experiences. Although flashbacks are conceptually different from hallucinations because they originate from earlier experience rather than arising de novo, the subjective and sensory experiences reported by the patient with flashbacks may be indistinguishable from those of the patient with hallucinations. Unlike true hallucinations, flashbacks are not well controlled with antipsychotic medication. Flashbacks are common in post-traumatic stress disorder and are associated with some drug states.

TREATMENT

How Are Hallucinations Treated?

The main thrust of treatment must be of the underlying condition, whether psychiatric, medical, or drug related, but antipsychotic medications are effective in controlling hallucinations arising in most diagnoses. An antipsychotic agent is often used along with other treatment modalities.

Are There Contraindications to the Use of Antipsychotics for Hallucinations?

The contraindications are not absolute, but two conditions with hallucinations for which an antipsychotic would not be first-line treatment are DTs and anticholinergic delirium. There is a risk of seizure with DTs, and many antipsychotic drugs lower the seizure threshold. In addition, drugs that are cross-tolerant with alcohol, such as the benzodiazepines, control not only the hallucinations but also the other signs and symptoms of DTs and at the same time decrease the likelihood of seizures. Similarly, many antipsychotic agents have anticholinergic properties that exacerbate an anticholinergic delirium. Physostigmine, a cholinesterase inhibitor, counters the effects of anticholinergic toxicity.

KEY POINTS

◆ The modality of hallucinations does not have diagnostic significance.

◆ A negative toxicology screen does not rule out a drug-related cause of hallucinations.

◆ Suspect an underlying medical or drug-related cause for hallucinations in patients with physical signs or those who are disoriented and have an impaired level of alertness.

Case 11-1

A frightened 24-year-old man is brought to the emergency department by his friend because the patient has had threatening visual hallucinations during the past 24 hours.

    A. How should he be evaluated?
    B. How should he be treated?

Case 11-2

A 26-year-old woman is brought to the physician's office by her parents because of her strange behavior during the past 6 weeks. She had grown increasingly isolative, stopped going to her job, and during the past 2 days has complained of hearing voices. The mental status examination reveals auditory hallucinations of different voices that speak her thoughts out loud and comment on her.

A. What is the diagnosis?
B. What additional information do you need?
C. How should she be managed?

Case Answers

11-1 A. *Learning objective:* **Be familiar with the differential diagnosis of hallucinations.** The possible causes of hallucinations are multiple and varied. Much more additional information is needed. An important point in diagnostic thinking is to determine whether the hallucinations are due to a primary psychiatric disorder or to an underlying medical or drug-related condition. A full history, physical examination, and mental status examination are needed. These, in turn, may indicate specific laboratory investigations. The presence of physical signs, an altered level of consciousness, and disorientation suggest a medical or drug-related cause.

11-1 B. *Learning objective:* **Understand how the cause of hallucinations guides treatment decisions.** Although antipsychotics treat most hallucinations regardless of cause, it is better to hold off on treatment until you have a better understanding of the etiology. If the man is very frightened and agitated, a benzodiazepine may give symptomatic relief while you conduct your evaluation. If you diagnose a delirium, urgent treatment will focus on the cause, not the symptoms. On the other hand, steroid intoxication (e.g., from excessive use of anabolic steroids) poses little acute medical risk, and the frightening symptoms can be well controlled with antipsychotic medication.

11-2 A. *Learning objective:* **Understand how the content in hallucinations is used in making a diagnosis.** You cannot know the diagnosis from the information given. Although the content of her hallucinations suggests schizophrenia, it does not establish it.

11-2 B. *Learning objective:* **Understand how pertinent positives and negatives guide a diagnostic evaluation of hallucinations.** Although you have little information, you do have some. You are given a time course of about 6 weeks, the presence of hallucinations that suggest schizophrenia, and no altered level of consciousness. At this point your evaluation will do two things: look for other evidence of schizophrenia and rule out other possible causes. The time course of 6 weeks is less likely for a drug or medical cause than for a primary psychiatric disorder. A medical history, review of medical symptoms, and physical examination will support or contradict this impression. A past psychiatric history, family history, and mental status examination (delusions, formal thought disorder) will help rule in or out a diagnosis of schizophrenia.

11-2 C.   *Learning objective:* **Be familiar with the treatment of hallucinations.** Her management will depend on your further evaluation. If there is no evidence of an underlying medical or drug-related cause, an antipsychotic can be prescribed. The medication will reduce psychotic symptoms, including hallucinations, and may make it easier to obtain additional history.

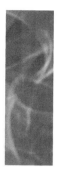

12

Delusions

MYRL R. S. MANLEY

What Are Delusions?

Delusions are false beliefs. However, unlike most of the mistaken ideas people have from time to time, delusions are held with a tenacity that resists change, no matter how much contradictory evidence the person receives. Delusions can be about realistic, everyday matters, such as the belief that one's spouse is having an affair, in which case they are called nonbizarre. Or they can be wildly fantastic such as the belief that one has been impregnated by space aliens, in which case they are called bizarre. In all cases, the belief is held with fixed rigidity: patients cannot be reasoned out of delusions. Religious beliefs and shared cultural beliefs are usually not regarded as delusional.

What Causes Delusions?

Delusions are seen in a large number of unrelated psychiatric and medical conditions. Although the precise neurobiologic mechanisms by which delusions are produced are poorly understood, it is clear that they can arise not only from purely biologic causes such as cocaine intoxication or cerebral malaria but also from environmental events. Some of the circumstances associated with delusion formation are social isolation, sensory deprivation, and geographic immigration, especially when language fluency is lacking.

In What Psychiatric Disorders Are Delusions Seen?

Delusions are nonspecific psychotic symptoms. They can be seen in any disorder with psychotic symptoms. In delusional disorder, they are the only symptom. In other psychotic disorders, they coexist with symptoms such as hallucinations, formal thought disorders, and bizarre behavior (Table 12-1).

Table 12-1

Some Psychiatric Disorders That Can Include Delusions

Schizophrenia
Schizoaffective disorder
Bipolar disorder (I and II)
Major depression
Delusional disorder

What Medical and Drug-Related Conditions Cause Delusions?

Virtually any illness or medication that alters perception or distorts reason has the potential to result in delusions. Delusions are seen as one feature of the syndromes of global impairment: delirium and dementia. They may also be the only psychiatric manifestation of a medical illness or drug-related state (Table 12-2).

Table 12-2

Some Common Medical and Drug-Related Causes of Delusions

Neurologic
Brain tumors
Huntington's disease
Alzheimer's disease

Infections
Cerebral malaria
Viral encephalitis
Tertiary syphilis

Metabolic and Endocrine Disorders
Acute intermittent porphyria
Cushing's disease
Encephalopathy caused by major organ system failure
   (e.g., liver, kidney, pancreas)
Hyponatremia
Thyroid disorders

Drugs
Intoxication with central nervous system stimulants (e.g., cocaine, amphetamines)
Withdrawal from central nervous system sedatives (e.g., alcohol, benzodiazepines)
Marijuana intoxication
Steroids (androgenic and corticosteroids)
Anticholinergic drugs
Dopamine agonists (L-dopa)

EVALUATION

How Do I Ask My Patient about Delusions?

Because the patient with a delusion firmly believes it to be true, you cannot ask, "Do you have any delusions?" Moreover, because the patient's subjective experience is that the belief is a reality, he or she rarely presents a delusion as a symptomatic complaint. Instead, there are two complementary approaches for eliciting delusions. The first is simply to give your patient the time and safety to talk openly and spontaneously, while you listen for evidence of delusional thinking and follow up on the patient's leads. For example, if a young man mentions in passing, "They don't want me to succeed," you would quite naturally ask, "Who are 'they'?" The second approach is to ask gently probing questions in clinical circumstances where delusions may exist, taking care to ask in a manner that does not challenge the validity of the belief. Examples of such screening questions are shown in Box 12-1.

Does the Content of a Delusion Help with the Diagnosis?

A little bit. The content of delusions is nonspecific. Virtually any belief can be found with any diagnosis. However, certain delusions are seen much more frequently in some diagnoses than in others and, although not establishing the diagnosis, strongly suggest it. For example, delusions of control (e.g., that a machine is controlling one's thoughts or movements from a distance) are more commonly seen in patients with schizophrenia than in patients with other psychotic disorders. When delusions occur in the major mood disorders, they are often mood congruent: grandiose delusions occur with manic episodes, and delusions of guilt or body decay occur with depressive episodes. Delusions commonly seen in certain psychiatric disorders are summarized in Table 12-3.

Some disorders include beliefs that are difficult to distinguish from delusions, sometimes called "near delusions." Examples include obsessive-compulsive disorder, in which the individual lacks insight into the purposelessness of symptoms, and hypochondriasis, in which the fear of illness is deeply entrenched.

Delusions

BOX 12-1

SOME SCREENING QUESTIONS FOR DELUSIONAL BELIEFS

1. Are there people who want to hurt you or cause you trouble?
2. Have you had unusual experiences? Things you couldn't discuss with other people?
3. Do you have special powers?
4. Have you ever received special messages from television or newspapers?

Delusions

Table 12-3

Delusions Common to Some Diagnosis

Patient's Delusion	Diagnosis
Mind or body control	Schizophrenia
Grandiose special powers	Manic episode
Guilt or body decay	Major depression
Persecution	Manic episode, schizophrenia, or delusional disorder

How Can I Tell if My Patient's Delusion Is Caused by a Psychiatric or a Medical Condition?

Every thorough assessment must include a good history and an attentive physical examination. Primary psychiatric disorders do not include physical signs. The presence of dilated pupils, high blood pressure, localizing neurologic signs, or an abdominal mass cannot be explained by a psychiatric diagnosis only and must be investigated further. Similarly, laboratory test abnormalities raise the suspicion of a medical process. The history also helps; the abrupt onset of symptoms in a previously healthy and emotionally stable adult suggests a medical or drug-related cause. Abnormalities of the sensorium such as disorientation, impaired alertness, and memory problems may signal an underlying medical condition.

What Laboratory Studies Should Be Ordered for a Delusional Patient?

It is not possible to describe a single standard battery of tests that is appropriate for all patients. The studies you choose will be based on your patient's history, review of systems, and examinations. Reasonable screening tests for many patients include a complete blood cell count, electrolytes, glucose, calcium, and renal and liver function tests. Routine use of neuroimaging studies such as computed tomography or positron emission tomography has an extremely low yield and should be reserved for patients for whom the tests are indicated by history (e.g., seizures or head trauma) or by physical findings (e.g., localizing neurologic signs) or when the diagnosis remains unclear and the patient is not responding to conventional therapies.

How Can I Tell if My Patient's Weird Belief Is Delusional or True?

It is not always easy. You need to convince yourself of the two essential elements of all delusions: falseness and fixity. The unreality of bizarre delusions is often readily apparent. Assessing nonbizarre delusions is more difficult and sometimes requires corroboration from outside sources.

For example, an impoverished, disheveled homeless man was admitted to the medical service of a city hospital for treatment of tuberculosis. The man claimed he was in a major Academy Award–winning movie. An enterprising resident rented the videotape of the movie and discovered that her patient did indeed have a small but important part, as he had claimed.

Does Calling a Patient "Paranoid" Mean That the Person Has Delusions?

Not necessarily. Paranoid is a general term for exaggerated suspiciousness that is used in several diagnoses. Patients diagnosed with paranoid schizophrenia or paranoid delusional disorder (delusional disorder of the persecutory type) do have delusions. People with paranoid personality disorder do not. The term paranoia is not itself a standard psychiatric diagnosis.

If Two or More People Believe the Same Thing, Can It Still Be a Delusion?

Yes. By definition, delusions do not include religious or cultural beliefs. It is possible, however, for more than one person to have the same delusion, in which case it is called a shared psychotic disorder (or, more popularly, folie-a-deux if shared by two people, folie-a-trois if shared by three people, and so on). Very commonly in shared psychotic disorder, the delusion originates with one strong-willed, charismatic individual and is then adopted by more subordinate, impressionable people.

How Can I Determine Which Psychiatric Disorder My Delusional Patient Has?

As with all psychiatric disorders, the diagnosis is based only on symptoms and course. You need to pay particular attention to the presence or absence of other psychotic symptoms such as hallucinations and disorganized thinking and to the prominence of mood symptoms. Delusional disorder includes no other psychotic symptoms and usually runs a chronic, unvarying course. Schizophrenia is a chronic, relapsing illness with episodes of (often multiple) psychotic symptoms followed by residual periods of negative symptoms. Bipolar disorder and major depression are episodic and usually include normal mood and functioning between episodes.

Does Distinguishing between "Bizarre" and "Nonbizarre" Delusions Help in Making the Diagnosis?

Yes, to a degree, if you are using DSM-IV-TR. The delusions of delusional disorder cannot be bizarre. On the other hand, a diagnosis of schizophrenia requires the presence of fewer symptoms if delusions are bizarre rather than nonbizarre. Not everyone, however, agrees on what is bizarre and what is not. Some beliefs have high levels of reliability—for example, most psychiatrists rate "A machine has been implanted in my brain that is

Delusions

controlling my thoughts" as bizarre and "My husband is having an affair" as nonbizarre. Even seasoned experts are split, however, on other beliefs, such as "Queen Elizabeth is personally involved in an international drug ring."

Are Delusional Patients Dangerous?

They can be. People who feel threatened may lash out and attack others; people who feel nihilistic or delusionally guilty may hurt themselves. An important part of your assessment will be your patient's response to delusions. Does the patient feel compelled to respond? What response is likely? How much restraint is the person capable of?

TREATMENT

How Are Delusions Treated?

Most delusions, like other psychotic symptoms, respond well to antipsychotic medication regardless of the cause. Anecdotal reports have suggested that the older, typical antipsychotic pimozide is more effective than other medications in controlling delusions, but there are no controlled studies. If the delusion results from a medical or drug-related state, the treatment will be directed to the underlying condition, but judicious use of an antipsychotic may be a useful adjunct. The delusions of delusional disorder are less likely to get better with medication than are those seen in other psychiatric conditions. This has led some observers to speculate that delusional disorder is more likely a learned condition without the substantial genetic and biochemical components seen in schizophrenia and the major mood disorders.

What Should I Do if My Patient's Delusions Don't Go Away with Medication?

Some patients who show no improvement on antipsychotic medication, especially those with delusional disorder, benefit from cognitive-behavioral therapy. They learn techniques for minimizing the disruptiveness of the delusion and may eventually be able to encapsulate it. The delusion does not disappear, but the patients are better able to control with whom they do and do not discuss it, control the urge to act on the belief, and learn how to redirect their thinking to other issues.

KEY POINTS

- ◆ Delusions are fixed false beliefs. Patients cannot be talked out of them.
- ◆ The distinction between bizarre and nonbizarre delusions has diagnostic significance but lacks reliability.
- ◆ You cannot assess for delusions by asking your patient if he or she has any.

Case 12-1

A 32-year-old woman is brought to the emergency department by a friend because of bizarre behavior. For the past 12 hours, the woman has refused to leave her house, has insisted that all curtains and blinds be closed although it is daytime, and has insisted that all appliances be unplugged. She insists that her life is threatened by a religious cult and that cult members are monitoring her 24 hours a day. The woman has no prior medical or psychiatric history. Her blood pressure is 150/110 mm Hg, and her heart rate is 100 beats per minute. Her pupils are dilated, and deep tendon reflexes are increased.

    A. Does the woman have a psychiatric diagnosis?
    B. What additional assessment is needed?
    C. How can she be managed?

Case Answers

12-1 A. *Learning objective:* **Be familiar with the findings that suggest a medical or drug-related cause for symptoms.** The woman has a delusion of persecution. Her age, the sudden onset, absence of a previous psychiatric history, and the physical findings all suggest that the delusion is caused by an underlying medical condition or drug use.

12-1 B. *Learning objective:* **Be familiar with the medical evaluation of psychiatric patients.** A good history and physical are the necessary starting points. Specific laboratory tests will be suggested by the findings. Her signs and symptoms are consistent with central nervous system stimulant intoxication, and a good substance use history is needed. A urine toxicology screen may help confirm the presence of central nervous system stimulants, but a negative screen will not rule out a drug-related cause. Additional tests that may be indicated, depending on the history, are electrocardiography, thyroid studies, and complete blood cell count.

12-1 C. *Learning objective:* **Know how delusions are treated.** Antipsychotics are usually effective in treating delusions, even if they result from medical conditions or drug use. Treating the delusion (e.g., with risperidone or haloperidol) may resolve the delusion and help obtain a more accurate history, although the benefit from antipsychotics is usually not immediate.

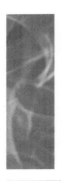

13

Disorganized Thinking and Speech

MYRL R. S. MANLEY

What Causes Disorganized Speech?

Disorganized speech is sometimes caused by brain damage, as in the aphasias. Or, because speech reflects thoughts, it may be caused by disorganized thinking. A formal thought disorder is a common psychiatric cause of disorganized speech.

What Is a Formal Thought Disorder?

A disorder of thought form—the way ideas are connected as opposed to the ideas themselves—is referred to as a formal thought disorder. It represents a breakdown in the goal directedness or internal logicality of thinking. The term is commonly abbreviated in day-to-day medical conversations as "thought disorder." Thought disorders that are sufficiently serious to impair communication are usually considered psychotic symptoms. Figure 13-1 is a copy of a letter requesting discharge that was submitted by a hospitalized patient with schizophrenia. The letter's incoherence and disorganization reflect underlying disorganized thinking.

What Causes Formal Thought Disorders?

Because the brain mechanisms by which ideas are associated in normal thinking are poorly understood, the mechanisms for formal thought disorders are equally obscure. They occur in many psychiatric disorders ranging from the benign (adjustment disorder with anxiety) to the most serious (disorganized schizophrenia) as well as in medical conditions such as delirium.

Are Formal Thought Disorders Always Pathologic?

Hardly. Verbatim transcripts of normal conversations reveal speech—and presumably thinking—that is often illogical, repetitive, digressive, and emotionally driven. What may seem shockingly incoherent on the printed page, however, can be easily understood by the participants, who rely on a multiplicity of signals such as facial expression, vocal tone, body posture,

```
 t  to  the  public    all   you   known   me   talks   in  all   you
you  minds  ovrer      over   new  york                seemly  out   to  hel
   me  in  i love    that  i want  to  be  are  the  person  you  people

want  mmee  toto  be  music  artist    that  im   for    newyork   i
                                          that
love  you  people  the  glitter     i get   from  aii  you   help   me

---so--mue--      —   somush  im  new   place  i  always   draem ed  orf

  the   builting   all  that   happen   i beeb  right  here   in  themi

middile   so  all this  harmony  that  move     me   i  like  it   to

  keepgoing       the  love  yt  to  keep  going   thej   joy   smlies

 subpost    that  i  have   throught   you   we  all   as  a  term   need

   to  work  to gather  to  subpost  us  aii   your   jial      yourb
villle

to   sing  asong    to  save  aworld   to  live  a   life   without
   fear  is  to  homeerbly   and  kno wn  thatlovve  has  came   in
     gone--k--i  still  be  loving  you  tomorrowin  aii  allall  you
 sir   mainer  time  so  i  want  give  youall  me   all  allme

 judge   lawyer     in  all    im  thebest  ican  be  loving  all

 in  stay  on  my  medicine   thanks  to  all  'you
```

FIGURE 13-1 A letter requesting release from the psychiatry inpatient service submitted by a 43-year-old man with schizophrenia. The incoherence of the letter reflects the underlying disorganization of the man's thinking.

and gestures to understand one another. Not infrequently, two or more independent lines of reasoning are discussed simultaneously. In addition, normal people in abnormal circumstances of intense anxiety or fear may lose their usual fluency and become disorganized in thinking and speech. To qualify as a thought disorder, the disturbance must impair communication and understanding and not be limited to specific situations. A list of common thought disorders is presented in Table 13-1.

EVALUATION

What Questions Should I Ask to Evaluate a Formal Thought Disorder in My Patient?

Thought disorders reveal themselves when patients are given the chance to speak spontaneously. There are no specific questions or tests for thought disorders: you need to listen to your patient. Open-ended questions that ask a patient to talk freely about a general topic ("How were things for you in high school?") are much more likely to reveal thought disorders than

Disorganized Thinking

Disorganized Thinking

Table 13-1

Some Common Formal Thought Disorders

Name of Disorder	Description	Characteristic of
Derailment	A breakdown of the overall logicality and goal directedness of thinking	Schizophrenia
Thought blocking	A sudden disruption of the flow of thoughts	Schizophrenia
Tangentiality	Answering a question with a response that is appropriate to the general topic without giving a substantive answer (e.g., "What time did you go to bed?" "I slept on the sofa last night.")	Schizophrenia, mood disorders, anxiety disorders, personality disorders, dementia
Clang associations	Words are linked by their sounds rather than their ideas such as by rhyming or assonance	Mania
Flight of ideas	Multiple simultaneous associations	Mania
Perseveration	Repetition of words, phrases, or ideas	Delirium, dementia
Word salad	Complete incoherence, a seemingly random jumble of words without meaning	Expressive aphasia, delirium, dementia
Circumstantiality	Overinclusion of unnecessary detail that delays getting to the main point	Mild dementia, anxiety disorders, personality disorders

are closed-ended questions that ask for specific factual information ("Which high school did you attend?"). Some patients, but not all, are aware of their difficulty with thinking and may be able to respond to direct inquiries, such as "Are you having trouble thinking clearly?" or "Are your thoughts racing?" Most people, healthy or psychotic, have a finely developed social reflex to fill in meaning in conversations in which meaning is unclear. Try not to do this as you are listening to your patient. You are more interested in your patient's ability to organize thoughts clearly than in your ability to interpret what the patient probably means. When something is unclear or inconsistent, ask about it. For example, "I didn't understand what you meant when you used the phrase 'all of it is none of it'."

How Can I Distinguish Disorganized Speech Caused by Aphasias from That Caused by Thought Disorders?

Aphasias are language problems caused by brain dysfunction. The symptoms of the aphasia change when different areas of the brain are affected.

Patients with Wernicke's aphasia, for example, typically can speak fluently but have difficulty understanding someone else's speech. On the other hand, patients with lesions in Broca's area understand others without difficulty but cannot speak fluently themselves. The ability to name objects and to read and write is much less likely to be impaired in patients with a psychiatric thought disorder than in patients with a neurologic aphasia. Although the ability to use language effectively is impaired in aphasic patients, the ability to think and reason usually is not.

Is the Kind of Thought Disorder Diagnostic?

Only as a very rough guide. Some thought disorders are more commonly seen in certain disorders than in others, but there are numerous exceptions. In general, perseveration and incoherence are more common in medical conditions than in psychiatric conditions. Derailment and thought blocking are characteristic of schizophrenia; flight of ideas and clang associations are often seen in manic states. These generalizations alert you to possibilities. No psychiatric diagnosis can be made on the basis of the thought disorder alone.

Are the Physical Examination and Laboratory Test Results Important in Evaluating Patients with Disorganized Thinking?

They are extremely important in ruling out medical conditions. This is especially true for delirium, a medical emergency with high morbidity and mortality in which disorganized speech and thinking may be the most prominent mental status finding. Psychiatric disorders do not arise with physical signs and do not cause laboratory abnormalities.

TREATMENT

How Are Thought Disorders Treated?

The treatment is that of the underlying condition, whether medical or psychiatric. In addition, antipsychotic medication may be useful.

KEY POINTS

- ◆ Open-ended questions help reveal formal thought disorders.
- ◆ In formal thought disorders both speech and reasoning are affected; in aphasias only speech is affected.
- ◆ Disorganized thinking is not always pathologic.

Case 13-1

A 76-year-old woman is brought to the physician's office by her daughter, who is concerned about the woman's erratic behavior. She has left on the gas burner and was found wandering outside her home at night wearing only a robe. The physician asks the woman what she had for breakfast that morning. She replies, "Eggs and toast." When he asks her what she had for dinner the night before, she says, "Eggs and toast." The physician then asks her to add 2 plus 2. She answers, "4." He asks her to add 4 plus 1, and she replies, "4." The woman has no significant medical or psychiatric history.

   A. Is the woman's condition more likely to be medical or psychiatric?
   B. What is the most likely diagnosis?

Case Answers

13-1 A.   *Learning objective:* **Be familiar with the diagnostic implications of different formal thought disorders.** The woman demonstrates *perseveration*—the inappropriate repetition of words or ideas. Perseveration is much more likely to be due to medical or neurologic conditions than to primary psychiatric disorders. The suspicion of a medical condition is also increased by her age and absence of any psychiatric history.

13-1 B.   *Learning objective:* **Recognize the diagnostic limitations in identifying specific thought disorders.** Although her condition is more likely medical than psychiatric, a more specific diagnosis cannot be made without additional information. Her age, forgetfulness, and current perseveration are all consistent with dementia, but more complete cognitive testing is needed.

Disorganized Thinking

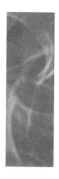

14

Mood Symptoms

MICHAEL DULCHIN

What Causes Mood Changes?

Mood changes are among the most commonly reported psychiatric symptoms, but there are many things besides psychiatric disorders that can result in mood changes, including drug and medication use, medical illnesses, and normal life events. Seasonal changes in sunlight and menstrual changes are associated with mood swings in some individuals, even when no other psychiatric or medical condition is present. Although the neurobiologic mechanisms of mood change are poorly understood, environmental, medical, and psychiatric events can all serve as triggers; these are summarized in Table 14-1.

What Is the Difference between "Mood" and "Affect"?

Mood is best thought of in its colloquial sense: the predominant feeling or emotion that a person is having. It is the answer usually given by the patient when asked, "How do you feel?" The term affect is used to distinguish the inner, subjective experience of mood from the ways in which emotions are externally conveyed through facial expression, body posture, and tone of voice. Affect is described in three ways: range, congruence with mood, and the emotion being displayed. For instance, a depressed patient reporting a sad mood might have an affect described as constricted, mood congruent, and sad. A manic patient could also be described as having a constricted and mood-congruent affect, but in this case the affect might be constricted to happy, elated, or angry. Mood and affect are terms that lack precision, and there are no universally agreed-on meanings. No research has demonstrated that even experienced clinicians can reliably rate affect.

What Psychiatric Disorders Commonly Present with Mood Symptoms?

The list includes but is not limited to the mood disorders: major depression, bipolar disorder, and dysthymia. Patients with schizophrenia sometimes

107

Table 14-1
Some Common Causes of Mood Disturbance

Psychiatric Disorders
Mood disorders
   Bipolar disorder
   Major depression
   Dysthymia
Psychotic disorders
   Schizophrenia
   Schizoaffective disorder
Personality disorders
   Borderline
   Dependent
   Histrionic
   Narcissistic
Adjustment disorders with mood disturbances

Medical Conditions
Endocrine disorders
Thyroid abnormalities
Adrenal abnormalities
Parathyroid abnormalities
Neurologic conditions
Stroke
Parkinson's disease
Multiple sclerosis
Frontal lobe damage

Drug and Medication Induced
Central nervous system (CNS) stimulant withdrawal
CNS sedatives
Opioid intoxication
Corticosteroids
Anabolic steroids
Interferon
Antihypertensives

Mood Symptoms

experience depression in the period after resolution of a psychotic episode (the period during which the risk for suicide is highest in patients with schizophrenia) or as a prodromal symptom. Patients with schizoaffective disorder have prominent mood symptoms in addition to psychotic symptoms. Patients with adjustment disorders can have significant mood symptoms in response to difficult life circumstances, and individuals with personality disorders may experience seriously depressed moods or anger in response to interpersonal difficulties. For example, a person with narcissistic personality disorder may become enraged and depressed after a perceived slight, even if relatively trivial, such as failing to get a desired seat assignment on a heavily booked flight. A person with borderline personality disorder is vulnerable to feeling despair at perceived abandonment. Patients with substance abuse problems also frequently have mood symptoms.

Does Culture Shape Mood?

Culture probably does not affect the emotions that people feel so much as the ways in which emotions are expressed. Facial expressions for basic emotions (happiness, fear, sadness) are the same in all countries, but there is wide variation in the amount of emotional display that is considered culturally appropriate. Consequently, the intensity of expression is not always an accurate guide to the degree of subjective distress. This is especially important in evaluating patients from cultures that encourage stoicism, where the absence of visible distress may tempt you to minimize the significance of mood symptoms.

Is Anxiety a Mood State?

For many patients, anxiety can be a symptom of a mood disorder. Patients in the midst of depressive episodes and bipolar episodes can have anxiety as a prominent part of the presenting picture. Patients can also have anxiety symptoms that are independent of mood symptoms and thus receive diagnoses such as generalized anxiety disorder and panic disorder.

Are Menstrual Mood Changes Normal or Abnormal?

Both. There are certain times in the reproductive cycle during which a woman is more vulnerable to mood swings than during other times. The vulnerability is normal; the mood swings themselves may or may not be, depending on their severity. If the depressive symptoms are severe, they may meet criteria for premenstrual dysphoric disorder. Women with a preexisting mood disorder, or the predisposition to one, are at increased risk. Times of vulnerability are just before and after menses, the postpartum period, and at menopause. Pregnancy does not appear to increase risk, although current research suggests that pregnancy does not protect against mood swings, as was once thought. Interestingly, women who have had episodes of major depression tend to experience the most pronounced premenstrual mood symptoms, whereas women with bipolar disorder are most symptomatic in the immediate postmenstrual period. Both are at risk for serious postpartum mood disorders.

How Do I Distinguish between Normal Emotional Reactions and Pathologic Mood States?

Grief, joy, sorrow, and contentment are inextricably part of the human condition. At times, however, even normal events can provoke abnormal reactions. Grief can become so overwhelming, prolonged, and disabling that a person can no longer cope with life and manifests the symptoms of major depression. Postpartum blues can become so intense that a mother is unable to care for her baby or tries to harm the baby—she then has postpartum depression or psychosis. In general, the distinction between

Mood Symptoms

normal and abnormal mood is based on the degree of distress and disability. Although the distinction is admittedly somewhat arbitrary, it is not trivial because it helps identify conditions that are unlikely to resolve spontaneously and are more likely to require medical intervention.

EVALUATION

How Do I Assess My Patient's Mood?

By asking and observing. Information about mood is obtained from the present and past psychiatric histories and from the mental status examination. If your patient has significant mood symptoms at the time of your interview, these symptoms can be used as a reference for exploring the past: "Have you ever felt this way before? When did it start? How long did it last?" If your patient has a normal mood (euthymia), you need to explain what you mean when asking about prior mood symptoms. If you ask "Have you ever been depressed?" the answer will almost always be yes. You can follow up with more discriminating questions such as "Have you ever felt bad all day, day after day, for weeks at a time? Was it so bad that you couldn't enjoy anything? Couldn't work? Did you feel life was not worth living?" In your mental status examination, you need to assess both how your patient feels and how he or she looks. Good initial questions are "How are you feeling?" and "What's your mood like these days?" to be followed with more detailed questions depending on the patient's response. Aspects of emotional expression that you need to assess are the range (how many emotions), the lability (how quickly the patient moves from one emotion to another), the intensity, and the appropriateness, both to the topic being discussed and to the setting. It is important in patients who are currently depressed to ask about past symptoms that may be part of a bipolar disorder including mania, euphoria, irritability, unusual productiveness, and racing thoughts.

How Can I Tell If My Patient's Mood Symptoms Are Caused by Drugs or a Medical Condition?

As is always true in psychiatric assessments, the history and physical examination are important in detecting a potential underlying medical illness. Hair loss may arouse suspicion of hypothyroidism in a depressed patient. Hyperreflexia and Chvostek's sign suggest hypocalcemia in a patient with anxiety. In addition, extreme emotional lability—rapid movement from one emotional state to another with little or no provocation—suggests a medical condition and is especially associated with frontal lobe dysfunction caused by infarcts, tumors, neurodegenerative diseases, or drugs that affect the frontal lobes. Patients with frontal lobe damage may be laughing heartily and then, within seconds, crying inconsolably. Some bipolar patients, especially with mixed states, may also demonstrate lability.

Are Laboratory Tests Helpful in Evaluating Mood Disturbances?

Laboratory tests may be necessary to establish a medical diagnosis. For example, hyperthyroidism cannot be diagnosed just on the basis of history and physical findings; the measurement of thyroid function is

Mood Symptoms

required. There are, however, no laboratory tests to confirm the diagnosis of a primary psychiatric disorder. You can make the diagnosis of a mood disorder such as major depression only after you have convinced yourself that the disturbance is not caused by drugs or a medical illness.

My Patient Seems to Have No Emotions. Is That Pathologic?

It may be; it is as important to evaluate the absence of normal emotions as it is to evaluate the presence of abnormal or exaggerated ones. Keep in mind, though, that the external manifestation of mood may not accurately reflect what the person is actually feeling. Blunted emotional expression is not uncommon in patients with schizophrenia or Parkinson's disease, and it may be seen in patients who are unusually stoic. An absence of subjectively experienced emotions is associated with some personality disorders (especially obsessive-compulsive and antisocial personality disorders) and chronic intoxication with certain drugs such as benzodiazepines. Alexithymia is a word used to describe the inability to name one's own emotions. If you ask an alexithymic individual what he is feeling, the usual (and honest) answer is, "I don't know." Alexithymia is not diagnostically specific.

TREATMENT

Can My Patient's Mood Symptoms Be Treated if It Is Unclear if the Diagnosis Is Primarily Psychiatric or Medical?

Antidepressants and mood-stabilizing drugs are usually ineffective until taken for several days or weeks. Consequently, the focus of treatment in medical diseases with mood symptoms is usually the underlying illness. The appropriate treatment for depression caused by hypothyroidism is thyroid hormone replacement, not antidepressant medication. For patients in severe emotional distress, the physician often temporizes with a much more quickly acting drug such as an antipsychotic or a benzodiazepine anxiolytic agent while the medical work-up proceeds.

Does That Mean That Antidepressants and Mood-Stabilizing Drugs Are Not Used for Medically Caused Mood Symptoms?

Not necessarily. There are some medically related disorders such as a postpartum depression that can be effectively treated with antidepressant medication. In addition, people can develop emotional reactions to the knowledge of having a serious illness. In those cases, medication may be useful.

Is It Important to Clarify the Psychiatric Diagnosis before Treating Depression?

Yes, because treating a bipolar patient with an antidepressant can induce mania or irritability. Bipolar depression is ideally treated with mood stabilizers, but sometimes an antidepressant becomes necessary despite the risk of mania or inducing mood cycling. In this case, there should always be a mood stabilizer in addition to the antidepressant.

Mood Symptoms

KEY POINTS

◆ Mood lability suggests a medical or drug-related condition affecting the frontal lobes.

◆ An assessment of mood should include both how the patient feels and how she looks.

◆ A clear diagnosis that rules out medical causes of mood disorders is indicated before treatment.

Case 14-1

A 63-year-old man is brought to the emergency department by police after he was found wandering in a confused state in a park. The man is tearful and sighs heavily. At times he wrings his hands and moans. Twice during the interview, he suddenly burst into laughter for no clear reason. He denies any suicidal thoughts or plans. He walks with a broad-based and slightly unsteady gait.

A. What is the cause of the man's mood symptoms?
B. What further assessment do you want?
C. How would you treat his mood symptoms?

Case Answers

14-1 A. *Learning objective:* **Recognize when mood symptoms suggest an organic etiology.** Although we know very little about this man, there is enough information to suggest an underlying medical or neurologic problem. He was confused at the time he was brought in and he has a gait abnormality. In addition, his mood is labile, strongly suggesting frontal lobe dysfunction.

14-1 B. *Learning objective:* **Know how to evaluate mood disturbances.** Because a neurologic abnormality is implicated, neurologic investigations must receive a top priority. If they have not been completed, a careful neurologic physical examination and mental status examination are needed to clarify the type and extent of problems. Locating friends or family for additional history is vitally important. A computed tomography scan of his head will identify trauma, space-occupying lesions, or neurodegeneration. Laboratory studies will help in looking for infections and evidence of drug or alcohol use.

14-1 C. *Learning objective:* **Understand the principles of treating mood symptoms caused by medical conditions.** The focus of treatment will be on his underlying medical or neurologic condition. There is no reason to give an antidepressant because the benefit—if any—would not be seen for 2 weeks or longer. If he is very agitated, impulsive, or in distress, an antipsychotic such as haloperidol may help. Benzodiazepines should be used cautiously because they can cause disinhibition and increased agitation in patients with frontal lobe damage.

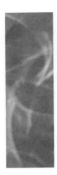

15

Anxiety Symptoms

MOLLY E. POAG

ETIOLOGY

How Common Is Anxiety?

Anxiety is a common emotion that is experienced at times by everyone and is often related to an identifiable stress. Patients with anxiety are ubiquitous in a general medical practice. The task for the physician is to understand the nature of the anxiety and whether it is normal or pathologic. Appropriate ("normal") anxiety is often adaptive and can lead to learning or self-protection. Anxiety is somewhat different from fear, which is an innate sense of dread and excitation in response to a specific external threat.

When Is Anxiety Considered Normal versus Pathologic?

Anxiety is a normal part of human development. Common growth experiences that often generate anxiety include starting school, forming relationships, and changing careers. Some anxiety, like moderate level stress, can actually promote learning. It is when anxiety is excessive that it interferes with learning, concentration, and memory. Anxiety is considered pathologic when it seems to have no identifiable trigger, when it is excessive in magnitude or duration, or when it impairs a person's ability to cope or function. A patient who can no longer concentrate at work or sleep well weeks after receiving the diagnosis of diabetes, for example, is experiencing pathologic anxiety. Anxiety disorders are syndromes with specific patterns of pathologic anxiety, and as a group they constitute the most common of all psychiatric disorders.

What Do We Know about the Neurobiology of Anxiety?

The amygdala is one of the major brain structures involved in fear processing and is sometimes referred to as the heart and soul of fear. The amygdala receives sensory input and coordinates autonomic and behavioral responses through projections to other key regions (Fig. 15-1).

114

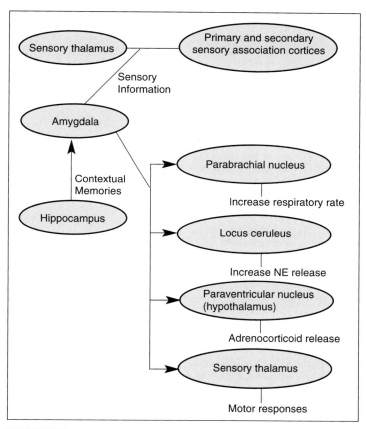

FIGURE 15-1 Brain areas and circuits in fear and anxiety. (From Stein DJ. "The neurobiology of panic disorder." CNS Spectr 2005;10[Suppl 12]:15.)

Major neurotransmitter systems involved in fear and anxiety appear to be norepinephrine (NE), serotonin (5-HT), and gamma-aminobutyric acid (GABA). Abnormalities in this neuroanatomy and neurochemistry probably contribute in pathologic anxiety states.

What Causes Anxiety Symptoms?

Anxiety falls into two categories: cognitive anxiety such as worry or nervousness and physical anxiety such as palpitations, dizziness, tremor, nausea, or sighing. A patient's neurobiology and psychological events often converge, resulting in signs and symptoms of anxiety. Conflicted feelings often cause anxiety. For example, a patient may have conflicting emotions about marriage and present to your office with fatigue, weakness, insomnia, and nervousness after recently becoming engaged. Losses, such as the loss

Anxiety Symptoms

of a relationship, a job, or physical vitality, are common triggers. Drug intoxication or withdrawal states are among the most common causes of anxiety symptoms and should be considered in virtually every patient (Table 15-1). Anxious patients often "self-medicate" with alcohol and other drugs, which over time results in a worsening of the anxiety or a frank anxiety disorder. People with a variety of medical conditions can also present with anxiety symptoms.

What Medical Conditions Cause Anxiety Symptoms?

The relationship between anxiety symptoms and medical conditions is complex because numerous physiologic derailments produce physical or even cognitive anxiety symptoms. In addition, physical anxiety symptoms may mimic medical illness. A patient's psychological reaction to a medical illness and the associated treatments and side effects must also be examined. The meaning of a particular medical condition may cause anxiety symptoms for a particular patient. For example, a patient with hepatitis C infection may have anxiety symptoms caused by metabolic abnormalities, side effects from α-interferon, self-blame, and fears of transmitting the illness. The physician must recognize and address each of these factors to treat this patient's anxiety symptoms successfully. Common medical conditions that can cause or are associated with anxiety symptoms are listed in Table 15-2.

How Can I Tell if My Patient's Anxiety Symptoms Are Due to a Medical Problem or to a Primary Anxiety Disorder?

A thorough medical and psychosocial history has the highest yield in making this determination. A complete physical and neurologic examination may reveal a medical illness that is associated with anxiety symptoms. Urine toxicology and other laboratory tests may also be helpful and in some cases (e.g., hypocalcemia) will give you the answer. Factors associated with medical causes of anxiety are given in Box 15-1.

Table 15-1
Some Drug-Related Causes of Anxiety Symptoms
Intoxication Caffeine Cocaine Phencyclidine Club drugs (e.g., ecstasy [MDMA]) ***Withdrawal*** Alcohol Sedative-hypnotics Club drugs (gamma-hydroxybutyrate [GHB], ketamine)

Table 15-2

Some Medical Causes of Anxiety Symptoms

Cardiovascular	Hypoxia, arrhythmias, angina, congestive heart failure
Neurologic	Temporal lobe epilepsy, demyelinating diseases, traumatic brain injury, stroke, vitamin B_{12} deficiency, Parkinson's disease, early degenerative dementias
Endocrine	Hyperthyroidism, hypoparathyroidism, pheochromocytoma, hyperinsulinemia, perimenopause
Metabolic	Acidosis, hypoglycemia, hypocalcemia, hyperthermia
Other	Anemia
	Human immunodeficiency virus infection
	Hepatic disease
	Chronic obstructive pulmonary disease
	Collagen vascular disease
	Fibromyalgia
	Gastroesophageal reflux disease
	Irritable bowel syndrome

BOX 15-1

SUSPECT A MEDICAL CAUSE OF ANXIETY WITH

Late onset of symptoms (past age 35)
No family history of anxiety or childhood anxiety symptoms
Physical anxiety symptoms without accompanying psychic anxiety
No avoidant behaviors
Poor response to anxiolytic medications

Can Medications Cause Anxiety?

Many prescribed medications, over-the-counter drugs, and herbal remedies can trigger physical (and, less often, psychic) anxiety symptoms and even mimic a primary anxiety disorder. When evaluating a patient with anxiety, especially one with somatic symptoms, it is critical to inquire about all medications and supplements. Often the offending agents are linked temporally with the onset of the anxiety symptoms. If a medication is suspected, the risk-benefit ratio of discontinuing the drug must be weighed carefully. It is ideal to withdraw or change the drug. If this is not medically possible, such as with a necessary course of steroids, the anxiety may be treated symptomatically with psychotropic medication such as a benzodiazepine. Table 15-3 provides a partial list of frequently offending agents. Remember that because countless medications can have neuropsychiatric side effects, it is best to review all medications that a patient is taking.

Anxiety Symptoms

Table 15-3	
Some Medications That Can Cause Anxiety Symptoms	
Prescribed Medications	**Herbal Supplements**
Sympathomimetics	Yohimbe bark
Steroids	Creatine
Estrogen and progestins	SAMe (S-adenosyl-L-methionine)
Theophylline	Goldenseal
Thyroid hormone	
Selective serotonin reuptake inhibitors	
Bronchodilators	
Caffeine	
Levodopa and bromocriptine	
Stimulants	
Digitalis	
Nonsteroidal anti-inflammatory drugs	
Sumatriptan	
Captopril	

Can Other Primary Psychiatric Disorders Present with Anxiety?

Yes. Patients with major depression frequently have anxiety or agitation as the most prominent symptom of their illness, especially those with the melancholic type. Asking about sadness, hopelessness, and lack of enjoyment can point to depression as the primary problem. Other psychiatric disorders that have anxiety as a feature or have high rates of comorbid anxiety include bipolar disorder, substance abuse disorders, and schizophrenia (especially in the prodromal phase). A positive family psychiatric history may raise the likelihood of a primary mood or psychotic disorder as the primary diagnosis in your patient, with anxiety as the chief complaint.

EVALUATION

Where Do Patients with Anxiety Symptoms Seek Help?

Most patients who are experiencing anxiety symptoms do not seek help from a psychiatrist. Because many of the symptoms are experienced as physical, the initial presentation is usually to a primary care physician, emergency department, or medical subspecialist such as a cardiologist, neurologist, or gastroenterologist.

How Do I Ask a Patient about Anxiety without Causing Offense?

It is helpful to ask patients the questions necessary to rule in or out a medical diagnosis when they present with physical anxiety symptoms, even if they appear objectively worried or nervous. This will assure them that you are taking their symptoms and distress seriously and are not prematurely suggesting an emotional illness. You can ask about common physical measures of anxiety such as muscle tension, headaches, insomnia, fatigue, palpitations, and gastrointestinal symptoms, explaining to the patient that you are also interested in possible "stress-related symptoms." It is helpful to explain that there is a physiologic connection between the brain and the body. This will pave the way for asking the patient about worries, recent stress or losses, and common cognitive anxiety symptoms such as fear of dying or dread.

What Physical Signs and Symptoms Can Be Caused by Anxiety?

Anxiety can produce physical symptoms associated with virtually every organ system. Very common are tachycardia, shortness of breath, dizziness, fatigue, weakness, nausea, muscle tension, and paresthesias. On the physical examination, the physician may note a rapid pulse or respiratory rate, cold clammy hands, tremulousness, or a moderately elevated systolic blood pressure. Abnormal laboratory findings can include a respiratory alkalosis with associated hypocalcemia and a sinus tachycardia on the electrocardiogram. Table 15-4 outlines common physical symptoms caused by anxiety.

Should I Check Specific Laboratory Tests in Patients with Anxiety Symptoms?

There are no specific laboratory tests that can be used to diagnose anxiety. If a patient describes a clear stress, loss, or psychological conflict that seems to be temporally related to the onset of anxiety symptoms, a physician may defer laboratory studies and address the anxiety symptoms in psychological or behavioral ways. Typically, however, at least general medical screening laboratory tests are important so as not to miss a medical or substance abuse cause for the anxiety. These tests include urine toxicology, blood chemistries, thyroid and liver function tests, complete blood cell count, vitamin B_{12} level, and an electrocardiogram. Additional tests are indicated only if the clinical assessment suggests a medical illness.

TREATMENT

Why Is It Important to Treat Anxiety?

There is enormous morbidity associated with untreated anxiety, including impaired functioning on the job, interpersonal difficulties, increased use of medical services, and serious substance abuse problems. Anxiety often causes noncompliance with medical treatments because of exaggerated fears of tests or medication while at the same time leading to excessive health care utilization. Anxious patients are often exquisitely sensitive to medication side effects, abandoning one trial after another and frustrating both the physician and the patient.

Can Anxiety Be Treated by a Primary Care Physician?

Often yes, and it should be. Most patients with anxiety are seen in primary care settings, and primary care physicians provide psychiatric treatment in general to more patients than do any other group of clinicians, including psychiatrists. If there is acute stress in the patient's life, crisis

---

Table 15-4

Physical Symptoms of Anxiety

Cardiovascular
Palpitations
Tachycardia
Feeling of impending heart attack
Flushing

Neurologic
Dizziness or lightheadedness
Fatigue and/or weakness
Paresthesias
Headaches
Muscle pain or stiffness
Tremor
Impaired memory and concentration
Insomnia
Feeling that one is going to fall down

Pulmonary
Shortness of breath
Tightening of throat or chest
Sighing

Gastrointestinal
Nausea or "butterflies in stomach"
Diarrhea
Anorexia or binge eating
Abdominal pain or fullness
Feeling one is going to choke or cannot swallow

Genitourinary
Urinary frequency
Decreased libido
Impotence or anorgasmia

---

intervention may alleviate the anxiety. Scheduling more frequent and regular office visits may help decrease anxiety and related emergency visits. Teaching the patient relaxation techniques such as slow abdominal breathing and meditation exercises can be helpful. Even if the cause of the anxiety is a medical condition, benzodiazepines can be used to provide symptomatic relief.

Does the Treatment of Anxiety Differ if Substance Abuse Is Present?

Because patients with anxiety frequently abuse alcohol and other substances, often in an effort to dampen the anxiety, both problems require treatment interventions. It is always a mistake to treat the patient's anxiety pharmacologically and ignore the substance abuse problem. The treatment will be unsuccessful, and the substance abuse can cause severe morbidity and mortality. In fact, the substance abuse disorder should usually be treated first. The treatment of drug- and alcohol-related disorders is discussed more fully in Chapter 26.

What Types of Psychotherapy Are Most Useful for Anxiety?

Cognitive-behavioral psychotherapy is the best studied and has efficacy rates roughly equal to those for medication. Time-limited (often about 12 sessions) anxiety management group therapy teaches techniques to reduce anxiety, and patients benefit from working with others who share symptom patterns. Insight-oriented therapy is often appropriate for patients with chronic anxiety related to their personality. Meditation and exercise programs, although not forms of psychotherapy, are also helpful anxiety reduction modalities. Psychoeducation—naming the symptoms and explaining the etiology and treatment—is also important.

KEY POINTS

◆ Substance abuse and undiagnosed medical conditions are often the cause of anxiety symptoms.

◆ Prescribed and over-the-counter medications can cause anxiety symptoms.

◆ Anxiety disorders often run in families.

◆ Untreated anxiety can interfere with medical treatments and result in excessive health care utilization.

◆ Treating anxiety often improves school, work, and social functioning.

Case 15-1

A 43-year-old female lawyer with no prior medical problems or psychiatric history presents on an emergency basis to her internist fearing she is about to have a heart attack. Earlier that day she experienced rapid heart palpitations, which abated after about 10 minutes. She has had two similar, but shorter, episodes in the past month. She has always had a stressful career but in general reports feeling more "on edge" during the past 2 months, with intermittent insomnia, which is new for her. She has also lost a few pounds but denies changing her diet. Her physical examination is essentially normal other than a heart rate of 96 beats per minute, a mildly elevated temperature of 99.8 °F, and some tremulousness.

    A. What further questions do you wish to ask?
    B. What laboratory tests are indicated, if any?
    C. How should you treat this patient's symptoms?

Case 15-2

A 22-year-old male college senior comes to the university health service with his girlfriend early in the morning. He is acutely anxious and mildly tremulous and says he "thinks he's going crazy." His heart rate is 120 beats per minute and regular; blood pressure, 140/80 mm Hg; respirations, 28; and he is afebrile. He lives in a fraternity house off campus and volunteers that he was "partying more than usual last night" for a friend's birthday. His girlfriend adds that daily drinking is nothing new but that for months he has been increasingly anxious and jumpy. Recently, he has not been leaving the house. He has not attended his morning classes since the time he had "an attack" in a class earlier in the semester.

A. What is the most likely contributing factor to this man's anxiety?
B. What laboratory tests are important?
C. What short- and long-term treatments are indicated?

Case Answers

14-1 A. *Learning objective:* **Recognize patterns of symptoms suggesting a medical cause of anxiety symptoms.** The patient is older than 35 and has never had anxiety or panic symptoms before. Although tachycardia and tremor can be seen with anxiety disorders, hyperthermia is not usual. This patient also has little in the way of cognitive anxiety symptoms. She thought she might be having a heart attack when she was having cardiac symptoms but has otherwise been without worries or fears. She has not been avoiding work or any other situations, even though she had two prior episodes.

14-1 B. *Learning objective:* **Understand the usefulness of laboratory tests in evaluating anxiety.** This patient has several medical issues that should be addressed. Her recent history of "being on edge," weight loss, insomnia, and mild hyperthermia may be due to hyperthyroidism; therefore, a thyroid-stimulating hormone (TSH) level should be obtained. Because her palpitations could be due to an arrhythmia, an electrocardiogram with rhythm strip and possibly a Holter study should be done, as well as basic chemistries to rule out metabolic causes for the palpitations. Given the mild fever, a complete blood cell count with differential is also indicated.

14-1 C. *Learning objective:* **Understand that symptoms can be treated symptomatically while the underlying medical cause is being addressed.** If this patient is hyperthyroid, treatment and adjustment of thyroid levels may take time, and neuropsychiatric symptoms can persist despite euthyroid laboratory values. Short-term treatment with a benzodiazepine would be a good choice, and there is no contraindication such as substance abuse or other medical compromise.

14-2 A. *Learning objective:* **Recognize that substance abuse, dependence, and withdrawal are common causes of anxiety symptoms.** This patient has a history of regular heavy alcohol use. His anxiety symptoms have been most severe in the mornings, after his blood alcohol level has fallen—consistent with minor withdrawal. His current vital signs do not indicate major withdrawal or delirium tremens, but he is at risk for this over the next week, despite his young age.

14-2 B. *Learning objective:* **Understand the appropriate use of urine toxicology and blood alcohol levels in evaluating anxiety.** Toxicology screens should be done as soon as possible or positive results may be missed. This young man would probably have a low blood alcohol level because the withdrawal may be causing the anxiety. Other drugs including cocaine and stimulant intoxication can cause a similar picture. Liver function tests are also important.

14-2 C. *Learning objective:* **Be familiar with the basic treatment approaches of anxiety.** The patient has some symptoms of minor withdrawal, including elevated heart rate and systolic blood pressure, mild tremor, and agitation. A clonazepam taper will decrease his acute anxiety and minimize the risk of lethal withdrawal. Benzodiazepines should be avoided in the long term, however, as this patient would be at high risk for addiction. He primarily needs intensive treatment for his alcohol abuse. If his anxiety persists after substance abuse treatment and a period of sobriety, selective serotonin reuptake inhibitor (SSRI) treatment may be a good choice.

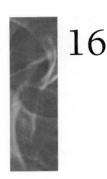

16

Memory Loss

MICHELLE IZMERLY

What Is Memory?

Human memory is a complex process of cognition, and it manifests in multiple pathways. Memory can be divided into many different categories: by the amount of time that elapses between presentation and recall (e.g., immediate versus remote recall), by the means by which the information was remembered (e.g., free recall versus recognition), or by the type of information that was stored (e.g., declarative versus procedural.) Some memories are brief in duration and need constant rehearsal to be recalled (e.g., remembering a phone number), whereas others last long after the experience leaves our awareness (e.g., remembering a past experience or your own telephone number). Table 16-1 lists the ways in which memory is classified. Memories are formed and stored in different areas of the brain; injuries to different areas cause different kinds of memory problems.

Where in the Brain Are the Memories Stored?

Areas of importance include the medial temporal lobe (the hippocampus, the surrounding cortex, and the amygdala), the midline diencephalon (which includes the thalamus, hypothalamus, and the mammillary bodies), and the cerebral cortex. Injuries to these regions can lead to clinical syndromes. For example, when the medial temporal lobe is removed (for control of treatment-resistant epilepsy), patients have trouble transferring newly learned information into long-term memory. These patients have immediate recall and can remember remote events prior to surgery but have trouble remembering what happened yesterday. When the right side of the medial temporal lobe is affected, there are often problems with non-verbal memory, whereas the left temporal lobe is associated with verbal memory.

Table 16-1

Classifications of Memory

I. By type of information that is stored
  A. Explicit (or "declarative"): Consciously recalled events and facts
  B. Implicit (or "procedural"): Unconscious retention of motor skills, habits, and emotional responses to stimuli (e.g., riding a bicycle)
II. By how the information was stored
  A. Free recall: Recalling information without prompts, making clues to remember this information, for example, using a mnemonic
  B. Recognition: Recalled information with prompts
III. By the amount of time that information is stored
  A. Immediate: Information stored for seconds to minutes
  B. Recent (or short term): Information stored for minutes
  C. Remote (or long term): Information stored for years

What's the Difference between Verbal and Nonverbal Memory?

Verbal memory refers to events and facts that can be stated in words. Nonverbal memories are those that cannot be encoded in words such as recognizing a person's face or remembering a piece of music.

How Are Memory Impairments Classified?

They are broadly divided into two syndromes—amnestic disorders and dementias. Amnestic disorders involve the inability to recall past experiences despite otherwise normal sensory and intellectual functioning. Retrograde amnesia refers to the loss of memories that were formed before an injury, and anterograde amnesia refers to the loss of the ability to retain new information. In dementias, memory loss is accompanied by impairment in other areas of cognition such as language, motor skills, planning, and comprehension of sensory stimuli. The dementias are covered more extensively in Chapter 27.

What Causes an Amnestic Disorder?

Brain injury from neoplasms, head trauma, and ischemia (from either strokes or myocardial infarctions) may cause amnesia. Basilar artery ischemia can produce a phenomenon called transient global amnesia, which lasts 3 to 24 hours. Other possible causes include metabolic abnormalities, seizures, and infectious and postinfectious conditions. Iatrogenic causes include anesthesia, electroconvulsive therapy, and medications. Alcohol can induce amnesia for the period of intoxication ("blackouts"). Alcohol-related thiamine deficiency leads to long-term memory impairment resulting from damage to the mammillary bodies; this is Korsakoff's syndrome. Table 16-2 lists some common memory syndromes associated with alcohol use. Amnesia may also be due to a purely psychiatric cause, in which case it is referred to as a dissociative amnesia.

Table 16-2

Alcohol-Related Memory Syndromes

Blackouts	Amnesia for the period of intoxication; person was awake but now has no recollection of the events
Korsakoff's syndrome	Memory loss and other cognitive impairments caused by damage to the mammillary bodies from thiamine deficiency; key feature is confabulation, or filling in memory gaps with inaccurate information; syndrome preceded by Wernicke's encephalopathy: delirium, oculomotor abnormalities, ataxia
Alcoholic persisting dementia	More global cognitive impairment caused by cumulative effects of repeated head injuries and long-term exposure of the central nervous system to alcohol

What Is Dissociative Amnesia?

Dissociative amnesia—formerly called a functional amnesia—involves the inability to recall personal life events, usually of a traumatic or an upsetting nature. Dissociative amnesia is rarely diagnosed because patients who present with functional amnesia typically have other psychiatric disorders, and those disorders are often judged to be the cause of the amnesia. Moreover, the amnesia does not always impair social or occupational functioning—a threshold required for the diagnosis of any psychiatric disorder. Dissociative amnesias are more common among women and are thought to occur more in adolescents and young adults than elderly persons. Most cases show rapid recovery of memory. DSM-IV-TR lists four dissociative disorders (in addition to a residual category of dissociative disorder not otherwise specified). These are discussed more fully in Chapter 33.

Can There Be Memory Problems That Are Neither Amnestic Disorders Nor Dementias?

Yes, it is possible to see a full spectrum of memory problems from the disabling to the very mild, in which case the symptoms may not reach the level of amnesia or dementia. In addition, memory problems may be symptoms of an underlying medical or psychiatric disorder. Many drugs produce memory loss with other cognitive symptoms. Also consider metabolic and endocrine abnormalities, such as thyroid disease, estrogen loss, hyperparathyroidism, Addison's disease, Cushing's syndrome, hypernatremia, and renal failure. It has been repeatedly demonstrated that patients experiencing depression or mania have a reduced capacity to learn new information and often have deficits in retaining the new information they learn. Major depression may manifest with cognitive and memory symptoms that can be severe enough to resemble dementia. People with generalized anxiety disorder may have memory problems caused by impaired concentration. Schizophrenia is often associated with disturbance in attention, motor skills, abstraction, learning, and memory. Table 16-3 provides some common causes of memory problems, and Table 16-4 lists some causes of transient memory loss.

Is It Normal for People to Lose Memory as They Grow Old?

Memory problems with normal aging tend to reflect a decrease in the efficiency with which information is encoded and retrieved. Encoding refers to the process in which information is acquired, processed, and

Table 16-3

Common Causes of Memory Problems

I. Drugs
  A. Antiadrenergics (e.g., clonidine, reserpine)
  B. Anticholinergics (e.g., benztropine)
  C. Antihistamines (e.g., diphenhydramine)
  D. Anticonvulsants (e.g., phenytoin, phenobarbital, valproic acid, carbamazepine [Tegretol])
  E. Benzodiazepines (e.g., temazepam, lorazepam)
  F. β-Blockers (e.g., centrally acting such as propranolol)
  G. Corticosteroids (e.g., prednisone)
  H. Interferons
  I. Lithium
II. Medical conditions
  A. Hypothyroidism
  B. Estrogen loss
  C. Hyperparathyroidism
  D. Addison's disease
  E. Hypernatremia
  F. Renal failure
  G. Traumatic brain injury
III. Psychiatric conditions
  A. Major depressive disorder
  B. Generalized anxiety disorder
  C. Schizophrenia

Table 16-4

Some Causes of Transient Memory Loss

Alcoholic blackouts
Transient ischemic attack
Epilepsy
Head trauma
Electroconvulsive therapy
Dissociative amnesias

transformed into stored data. Retention refers to the process in which encoded information is retained over time in the absence of rehearsal, and retrieval is bringing this retained information back into consciousness when needed. Short-term memory is usually well preserved in healthy old people and can be tested with repeating a set of six numbers. However, when asked to manipulate the information being held in short-term memory, such as repeating the six numbers backward, older people tend to do worse than their younger counterparts. There is also some deficit in the retrieval process of long-term memory. Older individuals have more difficulty in recalling stories or word lists when tested but are able to do so when cues are used. Many old people (and not a few middle-aged people) have trouble recalling a name, only to have it pop into mind an hour later when they are thinking of something else. These memory problems are not considered pathologic. More serious and persistent memory deficits—especially those affecting functioning—should never be dismissed as merely the consequence of growing old. Regardless of a person's age, memory complaints deserve a thorough assessment.

EVALUATION

How Should I Assess Memory in the Mental Status Examination?

You should always include tests for immediate, recent, and remote memory. Immediate verbal recall can be evaluated by having the patient repeat sequences of digits forward and backward. A normal adult can repeat about six digits forward and four digits backward. Recent memory can be tested by having the patient repeat three words and then remember them 5 minutes later. Assess visual recall by having the patient copy drawings from memory. Examples of remote memory include remembering the name of the city where the patient was married, the name of a fifth-grade teacher, or family vacations from childhood.

What Questions Should I Ask My Patient with Memory Loss?

Ask about the onset, circumstances, severity, and duration. (It is often necessary to obtain information from a family member if the patient is severely impaired.) Is there a discrete loss of memory for a period of time, or is the disturbance persisting? Was the onset abrupt or gradual? Are some types of information spared while others are lost? Does the patient have difficulty in other areas of cognition? Are emotional or other psychiatric symptoms present? Was there a physical or psychiatric trauma preceding the memory loss? Review the patient's medical conditions, menopausal status, current medications, substance use, and psychiatric history.

What Should I Look for on the Physical Examination of My Patient with Memory Complaints?

A physical examination should include an inspection for evidence of falls, head trauma, and drug intoxication, use, or withdrawal. A detailed neurologic examination can reveal focal deficits suggestive of strokes, mass lesions, and brain injury. Movement abnormalities visible on examination may be associated with certain dementias such as Huntington's or Parkinson's disease. Cardiac, pulmonary, abdominal, and extremity evaluation may point to systemic illness that contributes to memory impairment. Vital signs may reveal risk factors for stroke, such as hypertension or an irregular heartbeat. Carotid bruits can suggest an increased risk factor for an ischemic event. Psychogenic causes of memory loss are diagnosed only after physical examinations, laboratory tests, and neuroimaging studies are negative.

Are There Tests That Help Determine the Cause of Memory Impairment?

Yes. A basic laboratory work-up (Box 16-1) should be ordered. This can be followed up with additional tests when there are clinical indications. An electrocardiogram should be obtained to assess for heart disease. Certain diseases of the heart (arrhythmias, vascular disease, emboli) can affect the blood flow to the brain, leading to ischemic events. Carotid bruits on physical examination should be followed up with carotid artery studies, such as Doppler studies or magnetic resonance angiography (MRA). Neuroimaging studies such as computed tomography and magnetic resonance imaging reveal evidence of structural brain damage. Electroencephalography can help determine whether seizures are the cause of memory loss. For a more detailed evaluation of specific areas of memory impairment, consider requesting formal neuropsychological tests (see Chapter 10). One example is the Wechsler Memory Scale–

BOX 16-1

LABORATORY WORK-UP OF MEMORY LOSS

Routine

- Complete blood count
- Basic metabolic panel
- Liver function tests
- Thyroid function tests
- Rapid plasma reagin
- Vitamin B_{12} and folic acid levels
- Urine toxicology
- Human immunodeficiency virus

When Clinically Indicated

- Serologies of other infectious disease
- Cerebral spinal fluid tap evaluation for herpes virus
- Hormone levels (thyroid, cortisol, parathyroid, and estrogen)
- Infections disease such as Lyme titers

Revised, which includes subtests for general, verbal, and visuospatial memories. Some disorders such as Alzheimer's disease, multiple sclerosis, and Korsakoff's syndrome show classic patterns on neuropsychological testing. (However, the diagnoses are always based on clinical signs and symptoms and clinical course, not neuropsychological test results.)

TREATMENT

Is Memory Loss Treatable?

Whether memory loss is treatable depends on the cause. Reversible causes of dementia and amnesia should, of course, be treated by correcting the underlying condition. The treatment of dementia is covered in Chapter 27. Psychotherapy can be useful for people with dissociative amnesia. Some women report improvement in perimenopausal memory symptoms with conjugated estrogens, although there are limited data published on this matter. Providing patients who have significant memory problems with a stable, structured, and stimulating environment is an important intervention. One useful strategy is to furnish the home with reorienting cues such as clocks, calendars, and fresh newspapers. Enlisting the help of available family members while providing support and education is a critical component of treatment.

KEY POINTS

◆ Memory is not a unitary phenomenon. Memory formation involves many brain structures, but the medial temporal lobes and midline diencephalon are particularly important.

◆ Both dementias and amnestic disorders are characterized by memory loss, but a diagnosis of dementia requires impairment in other areas of cognition such as speech, language, motor tasks, and executive function.

◆ To diagnose a psychogenic cause of memory loss, medical conditions and substance-induced conditions must be ruled out.

Case 16-1

A 64-year-old woman is taken to the emergency department by a neighbor who finds her wandering in the street, unable to recall her name or where she lives. The neighbor tells you she is not aware of any medical or psychiatric history, but the patient's Medic-Alert bracelet states that she takes Coumadin (warfarin). On the mental status examination, the patient performs normally on almost all tests, including short-term and long-term memory for world events. However, she is disoriented to person and can recall only a few vague memories from childhood. A brief neurologic examination is unremarkable. She appears somewhat anxious and tachypneic.

    A. How would you obtain further history about this patient?

    B. What additional work-up would you do?

    C. How might you distinguish between a dementing condition and a psychological amnesia?

Case Answers

16-1 A.   *Learning objective:* **Recognize that collateral sources of information are usually necessary when evaluating patients with memory loss.** The neighbor may know family members who can provide a more complete history. Identification cards or other papers in the patient's possession may also provide useful clues.

16-1 B.   *Learning objective:* **Know that memory loss is a symptom and is not diagnostic of any one condition.** The absence of neurologic signs or other cognitive impairment is suggestive of a psychiatric disorder, but you must first assess the patient for medical and substance-induced conditions. A physical examination with careful inspection for evidence of a fall, an electrocardiogram, an electroencephalogram, laboratory studies, and a urine drug screen should be performed. A neuroimaging study of the brain is indicated, especially for a patient taking an anticoagulant.

16-1 C.   *Learning objective:* **Know the difference between amnestic disorders and dementia.** Amnestic disorders are characterized by a relative absence of other cognitive impairments and usually have a more abrupt onset. In this patient, the loss of personal identity suggests a dissociative amnesia, which may have resulted from an emotional trauma.

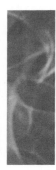

17

Suicide

VAN YU AND HEATHER LEWERENZ

How Common Is Suicide?

Suicide is the eighth cause of death among adults in the United States and the third cause for people between the ages of 15 and 25. In the United States there are about 30,000 suicides per year, a rate of 12.5 per 100,000. The yearly rate has been stable for as long as suicide statistics have been kept in this country (about 100 years). The suicide rate varies considerably from country to country, with a range of about 5 to 50 per 100,000 population per year.

What Causes People to Commit Suicide?

There is no cause of suicide per se. Rather there are traits that make some people more susceptible to suicide than others. This is evidenced by the fact that completed suicides are not assorted randomly in the population but can be grouped into a subpopulation of people who share certain risk factors. These risk factors include the presence of a psychiatric illness and demographic traits such as age, sex, and ethnicity.

What's the Relationship between Suicide and Psychiatric Disorders?

Ninety percent of people who complete suicide meet criteria for an Axis I condition including alcohol and drug use. The reason for this is that significant suicide attempts almost always occur in the context of impaired impulse control and judgment or with the distortions of psychotic thinking, which in turn are most commonly the result of psychiatric disorders. Conditions with particularly high risk for suicide are major depression, bipolar disorder, schizophrenia, mania, intoxication, and delirium. Of these, recent alcohol use is the factor most associated with completed suicides. For patients with a psychiatric disorder, the risk changes with symptom severity and course. Depressed patients with psychotic symptoms are

132

at especially high risk. In schizophrenia, however, the risk is highest during nonpsychotic prodrome or residual periods.

What Other Factors Are Associated with Higher Rates of Suicide?

A number of demographic factors have been identified, but it is important to understand that they are not necessarily an index of misery. For example, more men than women take their lives (by a factor of 3 to 1), but this does not mean men are unhappier than women. Men are more likely to choose guns or jumping from high places—methods with a high likelihood of a fatal outcome. Women more often use pill overdoses or gas inhalation. In fact, although men complete suicide more than women, women make more attempts (4:1). Over 50% of completed suicides are by gunshot. Similarly, old people take their lives more often than young people, but elderly people actually make fewer attempts than other age groups. (The higher completion rates may be attributable to elderly persons more often living alone or the physical health of old people already being compromised.) Factors associated with increased suicide rates are listed in Table 17-1.

Have Any Biologic Markers for Suicide Been Identified?

There are no markers, but there does appear to be a genetic predisposition for suicide. Among families with genetic loading for psychiatric disorders, suicide distributes to only some of the families instead of being evenly distributed to all. Moreover, within families with psychiatric loading, the risk for suicide and the risk for the phenotypic expression of the disorder vary separately. A first-degree relative of a patient with schizophrenia who commits suicide is at increased risk for suicide, even if the relative does not have schizophrenia. At this time it is not at all clear what the genetic predisposition might be, although studies of cerebrospinal fluid transmitter metabolites in people who have made serious suicide attempts suggest that impaired serotonin transmission may be a factor.

EVALUATION

How Do I Assess the Potential for Suicide in My Patient?

You must be able to talk about suicide in an open, direct, nonjudgmental, and noneuphemistic manner. Some good screening questions are "Have you ever felt that life wasn't worth living?" and "Have you ever thought about hurting yourself? About taking your life?"

Aspects of suicidal thinking to assess in your patients are intent, plans, means, preparations, and consequences. These are discussed in Table 17-2.

Should I Ask about Suicidal Thoughts in a Patient Who Doesn't Seem Depressed?

Absolutely. Suicide assessment must be included in every complete psychiatric evaluation. Suicidality is not a marker for depression. It occurs in many diagnoses.

Suicide

Suicide

Table 17-1

Factors Associated with Increased Risk of Suicide

Factors	Comments
Age: Age:Risk increases with advancing age and during adolescence.	Elderly people make fewer attempts than younger people but complete the attempt more often.
Sex: Males are at greater risk than females (3:1).	Women make more attempts than men (4:1).
Race: Whites are at greater risk than blacks.	Suicide rate is increasing among nonwhites in the United States. Rates for black and white adolescent males are equal. Higher rates are seen among recent immigrants compared with the general population.
Marital Status: Risk is highest for divorced, separated, or widowed; next highest for single; and lowest for married people.	Suicide rates have not been well established for alternative families and partnerships. Some observers believe that any committed, emotionally reciprocal relationship protects.
Work: Work protects. Rates are lower among the employed. Rates are higher among certain occupations: doctors, lawyers, dentists, police, insurance agents.	Occupational risk is probably a result of access to means of suicide (drugs, guns) or the ability to manipulate the consequences of suicide (lawyers, insurance agents) rather than of job stress.
Prior suicide attempt	The risk is increased even if the previous attempt appeared superficial.
Presence of a psychiatric disorder	Especially: major depressive disorder, bipolar disorder, schizophrenia, drug and alcohol abuse, delirium

My Patient Cut Herself on the Thigh and Insists This Was Not a Suicide Attempt. Could She Be Telling Me the Truth?

Quite possibly. For some psychiatric patients—notably, but not exclusively, people with a diagnosis of borderline personality disorder—compulsive acts of self-mutilation appear to relieve anxiety and are not intended to be fatal.

Will Asking about Suicidality Make It More Likely That a Patient Will Attempt Suicide?

Although students often worry that in asking about suicide they will raise the possibility for a patient who was not previously suicidal, this is virtually never the case. On the contrary, most patients are relieved to be able to talk about such deeply troubling thoughts.

Table 17-2

Suicide Assessment

Intent

Does the patient truly want to die? To relieve suffering any way possible? To punish family and friends? Does the patient feel compelled to commit suicide because of hallucinations or delusions? What degree of ambivalence exists? It's helpful to ask, "What has kept you from acting on these feelings so far?"

Plan

Does the patient have a clearly thought out plan for suicide (e.g., pills, jumping, gunshot, cutting)? Patients who have no specific plan but who say, "I just wish I were dead" or "I wish I'd get hit by a truck," are said to have passive suicidal ideation.

Means

Does the patient have the means to carry out the plan? Access to guns? Living on a high floor with a balcony? Availability of potentially lethal drugs?

Preparations

Has the patient been taking steps to carry out the plan? Has he or she stockpiled drugs? Made arrangements to obtain a gun? Are preparations being made for an anticipated death? A will being drawn up? Property being disposed of? A business being closed or child care arranged?

Consequences

What does the patient see happening as a result of his or her death? The end of suffering? Reunion with a deceased loved one? Unbearable suffering for the family left behind?

Does a Past Suicide Attempt Increase the Risk for Future Attempts?

Yes. People who have attempted suicide have a higher risk for completing suicide in the future than those who have not. (On the other hand, about 60% of people who complete suicide do so on the first attempt.) If you discover that your patient has attempted suicide in the past, you should take a careful history of those attempts. Two features of previous attempts to assess are intent and seriousness (both medical and psychiatric). Your questions should include what a person actually did in an attempt to kill himself, what he was thinking during the attempt, where it was made, what his expectations of discovery were, and what were the medical sequelae. For example, if the patient took a pill overdose, you can ask, "How many pills did you take? Over what period of time? How sick did you get? How sick did you think you would get? Where were you when you took the pills? Was anyone around? Did you think anyone would try to find you?" For the patient who cut herself ask, "Where did you cut yourself? How deep and long was the cut? Did it require sutures? Was there any nerve or vascular damage?"

Suicide

How Can I Use Demographic Risk Factors in Assessing a Patient?

The increased risk for suicide among particular groups based on age, sex, ethnicity, or marital status applies to populations, not individuals. Use demographic factors to rule in risk, not to rule it out. If your depressed patient fits the profile of a high-risk individual (for example, an elderly, recently divorced, alcoholic man with chronic medical problems), you need to keep a high index of suspicion, even if your patient dismisses your questions about suicide. On the other hand, the patient who clearly states strong intent and available means cannot be considered low risk no matter what the demographic factors.

Can Suicide Be Predicted?

Although a great deal is known about who completes suicide, it is nearly impossible to predict. Our ability to prevent is currently greater than our ability to predict. Prevention is more likely with a trusting doctor-patient relationship and an awareness of the risk.

Should I Trust a Patient Who Is Telling Me He Is Not Suicidal?

Psychiatrists often ask a patient, "If you feel suicidal, will you tell someone or go to the emergency room?" This is referred to as a "contract for safety." Studies have shown this to be a very unreliable method of assessing a patient's suicidal thoughts and predicting behavior. A patient who "contracts for safety" may not be able to keep his contract when he feels suicidal. The only real usefulness of this is if the patient tells you she is unable to contract. This gives you an indication that the patient is feeling too vulnerable even to trust herself. You must consider the whole picture—recent actions, history, personal circumstances—and err on the side of keeping the patient safe.

TREATMENT

How Is Suicidality Managed?

A person who is at significant risk for suicide should be observed in a safe environment. Often this means admission to a psychiatric emergency department or inpatient unit. Suicidal patients may be admitted involuntarily in all 50 states. If a patient has reliable, strong primary social support, consideration may be given to allowing the person to be observed in the community with the help of family and friends. Even the close supervision of the inpatient unit may be inadequate to protect a patient, and the patient may warrant around-the-clock "one to one" supervision by nursing staff. After attending to the person's immediate safety, you must treat the underlying psychiatric disorder that is causing suicidal thoughts. To date, the only medication that has been shown in clinical trials to be specifically effective against suicide (not just mood disorders) is lithium—obviously not an appropriate choice for all psychiatric disorders that increase risk. Psychosocial interventions may also be helpful. Especially among socially isolated suicidal patients, efforts to reintegrate them into a community and to establish social ties will be protective.

Can I Send a Patient Home after a Suicide Attempt If I Don't Believe There Is a Risk of Another Attempt?

Yes, there are times when discharge from the emergency room is more appropriate than admission to an inpatient service. However, the decision must be made with great caution because our ability to predict future suicide attempts is so uncertain. The decision will be guided by the medical sequelae of the attempt and the current psychiatric status. A general rule is to require that something in the person's life or environment must be different from when the person made the attempt. For example, an individual who was living alone may now be planning to live temporarily with family whose concern was aroused by the attempted suicide. The student must never make the decision for discharge alone without consultation and approval by the attending in charge. If in doubt, err on the side of safety.

KEY POINTS

◆ An assessment of suicidal thoughts and plans must be included in every psychiatric evaluation.

◆ Suicide is not diagnostically specific; it should not be interpreted as a measure of depression or misery.

Case 17-1

A 35-year-old married, employed, Catholic woman with two children who has no previous psychiatric history is brought to an emergency room after she is found unresponsive on a bed in a hotel by a maid. On the bed the maid found empty bottles of diazepam, diphenhydramine, aspirin, and vodka. The patient's husband reports that she left home this morning as usual and he assumed she was at work until he was phoned from the emergency room. Hotel staff report that the woman paid for the room in cash and used a false name. When interviewed hours later, the woman denies dysphoric mood or any other signs or symptoms of depression or any other psychiatric disturbance. The woman is released to her husband. A week later she successfully commits suicide by shooting herself.

    A. With few identifiable risk factors, how could the seriousness of the suicide attempt be assessed?
    B. How could the case have been managed differently?

Suicide

Case Answers

17-1 A. *Learning objective:* **Be familiar with the appropriate use of risk factors in assessing suicide.** Risk factors are used to rule in risk for suicide, not to rule it out. Although this woman had no known history of psychiatric illness and no demographic risk factors usually associated with suicide, the seriousness of the attempt should outweigh all else in your assessment. Two aspects of the first attempt that resulted in her coming to the emergency room were the medical seriousness and the likelihood of her not being found. Not only did she take a great deal of drugs and alcohol, but she mixed different agents. This is usually more dangerous than an overdose with a single drug, especially when central nervous system depressants such as alcohol and benzodiazepines are combined. The woman appeared to have no expectation of being discovered in time to be rescued. She rented a hotel room without identifying herself or telling anyone where she was going.

17-2 B. *Learning objective:* **Understand the need for hospitalization as a first-line treatment for suicidality.** Because the woman died, it is obvious that the case should have been managed differently. The circumstances of the first attempt were very serious, and it is likely that there were other factors that were not immediately evident but that needed to be considered in her evaluation. She may, for example, have had more psychiatric symptoms than she was willing to acknowledge. Alternatively, there may have been something in her life—for example, domestic abuse or recent diagnosis of a serious illness—that she was responding to. There was not enough information to send her home with confidence. The only way to "treat" suicidality acutely is to prevent the person physically from acting on suicidal impulses. This often requires hospitalization.

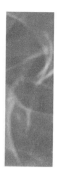

18

Violence

VAN YU AND HEATHER LEWERENZ

What Causes a Patient to Be Violent?

It is probably not useful to talk about a cause of violence in the same way we talk about atherosclerotic plaque as the cause of coronary artery disease. Violence is not a symptom like chest pain or a diagnosis like hypertension but is a behavior that people are more or less prone to under different circumstances. It is better to ask about the conditions in which a person is more or less likely to be violent. For a psychiatric patient, the risk of violence is influenced not only by the diagnosis but also by the intensity of symptoms and specific mental status findings such as whether or not hallucinations are present. A person is more likely to be violent if he feels threatened, has poor judgment, and has impaired impulse control. Among the psychiatric disorders commonly associated with an increased risk for violence are paranoid states, drug-related conditions, manic episodes, delirium, and certain personality disorders (Table 18-1).

Have Any Biologic Factors Been Associated with Violence?

Yes. People who have committed impulsive violent or self-destructive acts have been found to have significantly lower levels of serotonin metabolites in their spinal fluid than control subjects. This finding is sometimes interpreted as indicating that lowered serotonin transmission may increase the risk for violence. It has no diagnostic significance.

EVALUATION

How Can I Ask My Patient about Violent Tendencies?

An assessment of violent behavior or the likelihood of violence is a necessary part of all psychiatric evaluations. You will want to know about both the past history and the current mental status. In both cases, it is best to start with general screening questions, followed by more specific and detailed questions that follow your patient's leads. For the past

139

Violence

Table 18-1
Some Conditions with an Increased Risk for Violence

Delirium
Drug intoxication
   Cocaine
   Alcohol
   Phencyclidine
   Steroids
Paranoid states
   Paranoid schizophrenia
   Paranoid delusional disorder
   Paranoid personality disorder
Mania
Personality disorders
   Antisocial
   Borderline
   Paranoid

history, a good introductory question is, "Do you ever have trouble with your temper?" or "Does your temper ever get the best of you?" These questions sound nonjudgmental and are therefore more likely to get an honest response. Follow-up questions can include, "Have you ever gotten so mad that you broke something? Have you ever hurt somebody? What happened?" Similarly, for the current mental status, a good screening question could be, "Are you feeling irritable?" or "Are you having trouble keeping your temper under control? Do you think you might get so mad that you could hurt somebody? Do you want to hurt somebody? Do you have any plans? What are they?" If your patient makes a credible threat against a specific third party, you have a legal obligation to notify that person and the threat should be discussed as quickly as possible with your supervisor or attending. Because the attending also has a legal liability for what happens on her service, you must not act unilaterally. Of course, there are some patients whose behavior is so obviously hostile and threatening that careful questioning about the possibility for violence is unnecessary.

How Can I Tell if My Patient Will Become Violent?

You can't always. You need to recognize the potential with any psychiatric patient, maintain a high level of suspicion, and trust your instincts. Some belligerent patients make overt threats or talk openly about violent or homicidal ideas. Other warning signals include irritability, suspiciousness, agitation, inability to cooperate with the interview, disorientation, and intoxication. Random violent outbursts are commonly preceded by a period of increasing psychomotor agitation: pacing, talking more and more loudly, glaring, uttering expletives, and pounding one's fist into one's hand or against a wall or door. Patients with psychotic symptoms may feel danger where none exists. Intoxicated and delirious patients have impaired judgment and poor impulse control.

TREATMENT

How Do I Manage a Violent Patient?

There are some general guidelines for use with all patients that help decrease the likelihood of violence erupting. These are outlined in Table 18-2. Do not attempt to manage violence alone. Depending on your location and situation, you should push the panic button to alert security or involve staff. On the inpatient service or in the emergency room, with plenty of staff and security at hand, violent patients are usually restrained with injections of medication or with physical restraints, or both. Physicians (and students) are sometimes uncomfortable with the physical coercion of restraint, seeing it as violent and punitive. Regrettably, it is sometimes necessary. Patients cannot be cared for under threat of violence. If you are afraid, you will not be able to think and reason clearly. Other patients and staff must know they are protected. The violent patient may need restraints in order to be adequately assessed. Some violent patients are suffering from a delirium and in need of urgent medical attention. A full, accurate, and potentially lifesaving assessment may be possible only if the patient is restrained.

In the outpatient clinic or private office, there is usually no way chemically or physically to restrain a patient. Most clinics have security staff who can physically remove a violent patient, and you should know how to get their help quickly. This may include the use of panic buttons

Violence

Table 18-2

Guidelines for Interviewing Potentially Violent Patients

Trust your instincts. If a situation feels unsafe, it should be treated as such.

Interview in a calm, quiet place. Decreased environmental stimulation decreases the risk of violence.

Keep a respectful distance from the patient and do not touch the patient. If touching is necessary, for example, to take a blood pressure, explain calmly in advance what is being done and be certain the patient is cooperative before proceeding.

Do not block the exit. Patients who feel trapped and threatened are at greater risk for violence. (In the psychiatric emergency room, security guards may block the exit, especially if a patient has been brought in by police, but this is not your job.)

Ask if the patient is carrying a weapon. If he is, ask to have the weapon left with a third party or in an inaccessible place such as a car out on the street. Do not attempt to take weapons from your patient. If the patient has a weapon and will not relinquish it, end the interview.

Do not reason, argue, or bargain. If the decision to use restraints is made, it must be massive, quick, and irrevocable. Reconsider the decision after restraints are in place, not during the process of restraint.

strategically placed in clinic offices. Where security is not available (e.g., a private office) or where the security staff cannot act quickly enough to remove a patient, you should remove yourself. To give yourself the best chance, sit near the office door and make sure your exit is not blocked. Know the escape routes out of the clinic or building. Be aware of who besides clinic or office staff may be available to help you. And try always to be near a phone in case you need to call for emergency medical services or police.

How Should I Physically Restrain a Patient?

You shouldn't! Restraint is a job for the experts—people with the experience and training to be able to do it with minimal risk of harm. The best thing a student can do is to get out of the way. Make yourself available to the team—they may ask you to alert your attending to the situation, call the hospital security, or ask nurses for medications. Procedures vary from hospital to hospital. At our institution, patients are physically restrained on a stretcher. It requires team coordination, usually with a team captain who assigns other team members to be responsible for one of the patient's limbs. When the team leader gives the signal, team members approach the patient, secure their assigned arm or leg, and carry the patient to the stretcher. When the decision to restrain a patient has been made, it must be done with a large enough number of people to guarantee safety and speed. Very often, agitated patients become more subdued when confronted with overwhelming force. A variety of devices are used to attach a person to a stretcher, and you should familiarize yourself with what is in use at your institution and learn how to tie appropriate knots or use fasteners. A spitting patient may require a mask. If a patient who is physically restrained on a stretcher continues to struggle and threatens to overturn the stretcher, a second stretcher can be tied to the first and the two placed securely against a wall. Figure 18-1 illustrates the use of physical restraints.

How Are Violent Patients Medicated?

Choice of medication for agitated or violent patients is a topic of some debate, and even within a given institution, clinicians disagree. Antipsychotics (chlorpromazine, thioridazine, droperidol, and haloperidol), benzodiazepines (diazepam and lorazepam), and other nonbenzodiazepine sedative-hypnotics including diphenhydramine are used alone or in combinations. Literature comparing efficacy and safety of these agents, alone and combination, is not conclusive. At our institution, we predominantly use the combination of haloperidol 5 mg and lorazepam 2 mg intramuscularly because we believe this is effective and safe for the vast majority of patients. Even though either of these agents alone or in smaller doses would be effective for some patients, we believe the risk of having to give intramuscular injections on two occasions outweighs the risk of overmedication. Intramuscular medication requires 5 to 30 minutes to take effect. Therefore, we try to not give a second injection for at least 15 minutes, even if the

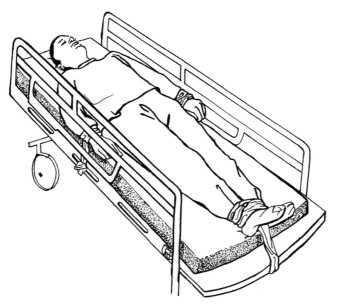

FIGURE 18-1 A violent patient is physically restrained with four-point restraints.

patient remains agitated. Intravenous lines are not allowed in most psychiatric units, eliminating the choice of intravenous chemical restraint such as diazepam. You should become familiar with the preferred chemical restraint and mode of administration at your institution.

KEY POINTS

◆ The risk for violence is not diagnostically specific; it can occur in multiple psychiatric and drug-related conditions.

◆ Trust your instincts. You cannot adequately assess a patient if you are afraid.

◆ Physical restraint is sometimes necessary but is never the responsibility of the medical student.

Case 18-1

A 56-year-old man is brought to an emergency room by police after he threatened to attack several people in a train station. He appears confused and sleepy. His speech is slurred and he is disoriented to time and place. He walks with an unsteady, broad-based gait. In the course of his evaluation, he becomes aroused and agitated. He begins pacing back and forth, pounding the wall with his fist, and shouting obscenities at staff and other patients. When a nurse approaches him in an effort to redirect him, he yells at her, threatens to hit her, and throws a chair against the wall.

A. What is your diagnosis?
B. What do you do next?

Case Answers

18-1 A.   *Learning objective:* **Recognize the need for urgent medical evaluation in some violent patients.** Although you do not know much about this man, there is enough information to conclude that he is probably suffering from a delirium: his altered and fluctuating level of consciousness, disorientation, and the neurologic signs (unsteady gait and slurred speech). Delirium is one of the conditions associated with an increased risk for violence. It may also be a medical emergency, depending on the underlying cause.

18-1 B.   *Learning objective:* **Be familiar with the ways of safely assessing violent patients.** Because of the likelihood of delirium, this man urgently needs a quick medical assessment. It cannot wait until he calms down, and there is no reason to think that he will become more cooperative with time. His potential for violence has already tipped over into manifest behavior. He must be physically restrained and possibly pharmacologically sedated in order to proceed with the necessary and potentially lifesaving investigations.

Violence

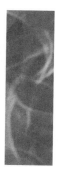

19

Sleep Disturbances

MYRL R. S. MANLEY

What Causes Problems with Sleep?

Almost anything. Sleep is one of the biologic functions most easily perturbed by emotional or environmental events. When sleep problems are caused by an underlying psychiatric or medical condition, the disorder is secondary. When there is no apparent medical or psychiatric condition, the sleep disturbance is primary. Almost any medical condition that causes physical discomfort (e.g., fever, pain, diarrhea, nausea) will interfere with sleep. In addition, there are some medical conditions in which abnormalities of sleep are symptoms of the syndrome itself. Delirium typically causes a breakdown in the normal sleep/wake cycle: the patient falls fitfully in and out of sleep throughout the day. Milder forms of delirium may result in sleep reversal, with the patient sleeping during the day and being awake all night. Some infectious diseases, such as influenza, cause hypersomnia (Table 19-1).

What Psychiatric Disorders Cause Sleep Problems?

Episodes of major depression often include early morning awakening. The depressed patient falls asleep with no difficulty but wakes after only a few hours and cannot get back to sleep. Less often with adults and more typically with children and adolescents, depression can cause hypersomnia. Manic or hypomanic episodes usually result in a decreased need for sleep. Anxiety states make falling asleep difficult.

What about Drugs?

Drugs are a common cause of sleep complaints. People who use caffeine or other stimulants late at night have trouble falling asleep. People who drink alcohol before going to bed are likely to experience rebound insomnia in the middle of the night. Lithium and diuretics may interfere with sleep by causing frequent night-time urination.

Table 19-1

Some Causes of Secondary Insomnia

Psychiatric Disorders
Major depression: Cannot stay asleep, hypersomnia in some
Bipolar manic: Decreased need for sleep
Generalized anxiety disorder: Trouble falling asleep and staying asleep
Situational anxiety: Trouble falling asleep

Medical Conditions (for All, Trouble Falling Asleep and Staying Asleep)
Any condition causing discomfort, such as pain, nausea, diarrhea, or fever
Hyperthyroidism
Nocturnal angina
Orthopnea
Delirium
Prostatism (frequent nighttime urination)

Drugs
Withdrawal from central nervous system sedatives such as alcohol: Middle of the night rebound insomnia
Central nervous system stimulants (e.g., methylphenidate, caffeine): Trouble falling asleep and staying asleep
Bronchodilators: Trouble falling asleep and staying asleep
Selective serotonin reuptake inhibitors: Trouble falling asleep and staying asleep
Lithium and diuretics: Night-time urination

What Are the Most Common Causes of Sleep Problems?

For healthy young adults, situational anxiety (e.g., pretest anxiety) is the most common cause of insomnia. For middle-aged individuals, especially if overweight, obstructive sleep apnea—usually experienced as heavy daytime sedation—is the most common cause. Other frequent causes are drugs, mood disorders, and anxiety disorders.

EVALUATION

What Questions Should I Ask?

Sleep is a barometer of physical and emotional health. You should ask about sleep in every medical and psychiatric assessment you perform. In the review of systems, start with a general screening question such as, "Have you noticed any change in your sleep?" or "How are you sleeping these days?" If your patient has had trouble sleeping, you first need to clarify the main symptomatic complaint: insomnia, hypersomnia, or nonrestful sleep. Then follow up by asking for more descriptive details. If the trouble is insomnia, ask whether the patient has trouble falling asleep or staying asleep. If staying asleep is the problem, ask when the patient wakes up. Can she get back to sleep? After how long? For how many times a night? A good history of the sleep complaint includes when it started, how it has changed, whether anything makes it better or worse, and what the patient thinks is causing it. Keep in mind that to distinguish between a primary and secondary sleep problem, you will need to perform a general medical, psychiatric, and substance use assessment.

How Much Sleep Is Too Much or Too Little?

The range of normal variations in sleep patterns is considerable. Although 7 to 8 hours per night is an average, some people are happy and fully functional after 5 hours, whereas others need 10 hours to feel fully rested. The absolute length of sleep is less important than is any change in the length of sleep and whether sleep is restorative. The person who normally sleeps 11 hours at night and is now sleeping 7 hours and feels exhausted throughout the day has insomnia. In addition, sleep patterns change with age. Children and adolescents sleep more than adults. Old people sometimes have biphasic sleep: two consolidated periods of sleep in 24 hours instead of one.

What Laboratory Studies Help in Evaluating Sleep Problems?

Laboratory studies can be extremely important in establishing the cause of a secondary sleep disturbance, such as insomnia caused by hyperthyroidism. Determination of the tests that should be ordered will be guided by the history, review of systems, and physical and mental status examinations. Sleep laboratory studies provide the most thorough investigations. For these studies, the patient spends an entire night—sometimes two or more nights—at a sleep laboratory center. While the patient sleeps, multiple functions are monitored: blood pressure, heart rate, temperature, muscle tone, breathing, and sometimes others. In addition, electroencephalography is performed. Understandably, the studies are time consuming and expensive, but the results provide a detailed, minute-by-minute picture over an entire night of the physiology of an individual's sleep.

When Are Sleep Laboratory Studies Indicated?

They should be considered for severe persistent sleep disorders when the underlying cause cannot be established and when conventional therapies are not working. Sleep laboratory studies are used to confirm the diagnosis of narcolepsy and sleep apnea.

TREATMENT

Do All Sleep Problems Need Treatment?

Not at all. Transient situational insomnia is a near-universal experience. Most people are able to function adequately (although uncomfortably) after a night or two of poor sleep and to make up the deficit in the following nights. However, for some people, a sleepless night initiates a vicious cycle in which anxiety about not being able to sleep interferes with falling asleep. The judicious use of medication can help prevent this cycle.

What Sleeping Pills Should I Prescribe?

The term sleeping pill is nonspecific. A number of different drugs and drug classes are sedating and may help patients sleep. Benzodiazepines are anxiolytic agents that are sometimes also used for sleep, depending on the time of onset of the pharmacologic effect and half-life of the drug. Zolpidem and zaleplon are used only as hypnotics. Barbiturates and chloral hydrate are effective sleep agents, but because of the danger of tolerance, addiction, and adverse effects, they should be reserved for severe cases that do not respond to other treatments. The sedating properties of some antidepressants and histamines can be exploited to help with sleep and pose a lesser problem of dependence. Over-the-counter sleep aids are usually effective only for mild insomnia. Melatonin has received much press as a "natural" sleep regulator, but so far there has been little research confirmation. Medications that are used to treat insomnia are summarized in Table 19-2.

How Do I Choose Which Medication to Prescribe?

The choice of medication will be guided by your patient's symptoms and the results of your evaluation. When the sleep disturbance is secondary, you will want to treat the underlying medical or psychiatric cause.

Table 19-2

Drugs Used to Treat Insomnia

Drug	Possible Problems
Sedative-Hypnotics	
Benzodiazepines	Dependence, respiratory depression when combined with alcohol
Zolpidem (Ambien)	Waking up too soon, drug hangover, impaired memory
Zaleplon (Sonata)	Waking up too soon, drug hangover, impaired memory
Eszopiclone (Lunesta)	Daytime sleepiness, memory problems
Ramelteon (Rozarem)	Daytime sleepiness, increased prolactin and decreased testosterone levels
Chloral hydrate	Dependence, tolerance, gastrointestinal symptoms
Barbiturates	Dependence, tolerance, respiratory depression
Sedating Antidepressants	
Trazodone	Daytime sleepiness
Mirtazapine (Remeron)	Daytime sleepiness, weight gain
Tricyclic antidepressants	Cardiotoxicity; anticholinergic and other side effects
Antihistamines	
Diphenhydramine	Ineffective for serious insomnia
Over-the-Counter	
Melatonin	Uneven effectiveness
Night-time sleep aids	Usually contain antihistamines; only moderately sedating

The short-term use of zolpidem or zaleplon for both primary and secondary insomnia is an effective first choice. When there is associated anxiety, choose a benzodiazepine. Sedating antidepressants are not addictive and can be considered for longer term use, regardless of whether the patient is depressed. Antihistamines are less effective in promoting sleep but are relatively benign and worth a try.

Can't I Just Give Sleeping Pills to Everyone Who Has Insomnia?

Insomnia is a symptom, not a diagnosis. There are serious potential difficulties with the indiscriminate use of sedative-hypnotics. Tolerance and dependence can develop. Even with nonaddictive drugs, patients can become habituated to their use and find it hard to sleep without them. Once they are started, it may be very difficult to wean patients off the drugs. In addition, although the sedative-hypnotics are usually effective for people with anxiety, they can be harmful to patients with other causes of sleep problems, such as sleep apnea. Finally, there are some people—especially elderly people or other people with cognitive impairment such as delirium—who become confused and agitated with sedative-hypnotics and whose sleep is made worse by their use. These individuals often do better with a low-dose antipsychotic agent such as haloperidol.

Are Any Sleeping Pills Safe for Long-Term Use?

Yes, two newer agents have been approved for chronic use. Eszopiclone (Lunesta) is a gamma-aminobutyric acid (GABA) agonist. Clinical trials of eszopiclone have shown no evidence of tolerance or withdrawal. Nevertheless, like the benzodiazepines, zolpidem and zaleplon, it is classified as a controlled substance. Unlike zolpidem and zaleplon, which are effective in initiating sleep but not sustaining it through the night, eszopiclone does both. Ramelteon (Rozarem) is the first prescription hypnotic that is not a controlled substance. It targets receptors in the suprachiasmatic nucleus, an area of the brain that regulates circadian rhythms. Although both eszopiclone and ramelteon are available for long-term use, they should still be prescribed with care. The need for continued medication should be periodically reevaluated and the presence of an underlying medical condition or psychiatric disorder thoroughly investigated.

Are There Other Treatments for Poor Sleep Besides Drugs?

There are several measures that can be taken to promote better sleep, commonly referred to as "sleep hygiene." These measures are summarized in Box 19-1. In addition, some patients benefit from the use of meditation, relaxation exercises, or yoga. When you are treating someone whose sleep difficulties are clearly not secondary, be sure to try all nonmedication approaches first.

Should I Tell My Patients Not to Nap?

There are no hard and fast rules. You need to consider the circumstances and the effects of napping for your individual patient. People who nap in the afternoon and are troubled by difficulty falling asleep

---

BOX 19-1

SLEEP HYGIENE

Go to bed and wake up at regular times.
Do not use stimulants such as coffee or tea at night.
Avoid eating large meals and exercising just before going to bed.
When possible, use the bedroom only for sleep and sex.
Do not drink alcohol at bedtime.

---

at night should try doing without a nap. Other people, however, find an afternoon nap refreshing, rejuvenating, and untroubling to night-time sleep. If their schedules permit it, there is no reason to interfere. In fact, there is evidence that many people in the United States are chronically sleep deprived. Some sleep specialists have advocated the addition of a daytime nap for more people. Scheduled daytime naps sometimes help people with narcolepsy avoid sudden unwanted sleep attacks.

KEY POINTS

Diagnose the cause of insomnia before treating it.

If your patient has:	*Think:*
Trouble falling asleep	Anxiety
	Stimulant drug use
Trouble staying asleep	Prebedtime alcohol use
	Depression
Daytime sedation	Sleep apnea
	Central nervous system depressant drug use

Request sleep laboratory studies
For severe, intractable insomnia
To establish a diagnosis of sleep apnea or narcolepsy

Case 19-1

A 26-year-old woman complains to her physician about difficulty falling asleep. For the past year, it has taken her 1 to 2 hours to fall asleep after going to bed. In the past month, the insomnia has worsened; sometimes she takes as long as 4 hours to fall asleep. She is extremely tired throughout the day and has had increasing difficulty at work.

    A. What evaluations do you recommend?
    B. What treatment strategies do you propose?

Case Answers

19-1 A. *Learning objective:* **Be familiar with the differential diagnosis of insomnia.** There are many medical and psychiatric causes of insomnia, and the evaluation must include a thorough history, physical examination, and mental status examination and a careful review of drug use, both prescription and recreational. Laboratory testing will be guided by the history and physical examination and should be used to screen for common causes of insomnia such as hyperthyroidism. Sleep laboratory studies should be reserved for individuals with severe, persistent insomnia not responsive to treatment.

19-1 B. *Learning objective:* **Know the range of treatments available for sleep complaints.** If her sleep disorder is found to be secondary to a medical, drug, or psychiatric condition, treatment must be directed to the primary disturbance. However, short-term use of zolpidem may give initial relief and may help break the cycle in which fear of insomnia becomes self-fulfilling. The principles of sleep hygiene should be reviewed and implemented before starting chronic therapy for a primary sleep disturbance.

Sleep Disturbances

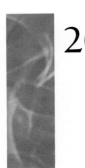

20

Sexual Symptoms

MICHELLE ROTTENSTEIN

How Do Sexual Symptoms Develop?

Sexual symptoms may last a lifetime. More commonly, they develop as a result of medical illness, as the direct effect of drugs or medication, or for psychological reasons. These reasons include psychiatric syndromes such as anxiety and depression, which can interfere with an individual's interest in and focus on sexual activity, as well as thoughts, feelings, or actions that distract the person from the sexual moment and interfere with her ability to involve herself in and derive pleasure from sexual activity.

How Do Sexual Symptoms Appear?

Sexual symptoms may be either primary (lifelong), which means that they have always existed without a period of normal functioning, or secondary (acquired), which means that they appeared after a period of normal functioning. They may be global, occurring in all sexual situations, or situational, occurring only with a particular partner, but not with others, or only when the patient is with a partner and not when he or she is masturbating. Sexual symptoms are not always apparent unless specifically elicited because patients are often embarrassed to bring up sexual matters. Consideration should be given to obtaining a sexual history for every patient, and it is important that the physician or medical student feel comfortable in discussing such matters with patients of various ages and sexual orientations to put the patient at ease and to communicate that sexual problems are something that can be addressed in the physician-patient interaction. Sexual history taking is discussed more fully in Chapter 31.

EVALUATION

What Are Sexual Symptoms?

Sexual symptoms consist of anything that interferes with sexual pleasure and functioning. They may be purely psychological (decreased libido), purely physiologic (retrograde ejaculation), or, more often, a combination.

152

It is convenient to think of symptoms as they occur in a particular stage of the sexual response cycle, outlined in Table 20-1. Sexual symptoms can arise from any area of sexual functioning. In men, common presenting symptoms are impaired libido, erectile dysfunction, premature ejaculation, and retarded ejaculation. In women, common presenting symptoms are impaired libido, lack of lubrication, pain on intercourse, and anorgasmia.

What Organic Factors Need to Be Considered?

Organic factors should always be considered in patients with sexual symptoms. As many as 20% of patients presenting with sexual symptoms have dysfunction related to an organic cause. However, in some cases, an organic cause can be ruled out on the basis of history alone, such as in the case of a clearly situational disturbance or in the case of premature ejaculation, which is rarely, if ever, due to any cause other than psychological. Physical illnesses that can affect sexual functioning include diabetes, cardiovascular disorders, genital pathology, neurologic disease, and hormonal problems. Drugs of abuse that may impair sexual functioning include opioids, alcohol, sedative-hypnotics, and stimulants, such as cocaine. Medications may also have a profound effect on sexual functioning. Selective serotonin reuptake inhibitors (SSRIs) cause sexual dysfunction in as many as 40% of women who take them, as well as a smaller proportion of men. Other drugs that may cause sexual dysfunction include other antidepressants (monoamine oxidase inhibitors, tricyclic antidepressants) and antipsychotic, antihypertensive, and anticholinergic agents. Of the antidepressants, bupropion is considered the least likely to cause sexual side effects. Some common organic causes of sexual symptoms are listed in Table 20-2.

What Causes Sexual Symptoms When They Are Not Organic?

Sexual responses are very sensitive to emotional stress. Chronic stress and depression result in decreased levels of circulating testosterone, which are associated with decreased libido (sexual interest) in both

---

Table 20-1

Stages of the Sexual Response

There are four stages of the sexual response.

Excitement occurs with the onset of erotic feelings. In men, this is characterized by an erection. In women, this is characterized by lubrication.

Plateau is the stage of greater arousal that precedes orgasm. It involves an increase in vasocongestion. In men, the erection becomes firmer. In women, there is increased swelling and lubrication.

Orgasm consists of rhythmic contractions of the vas and seminal vesicles, prostate, and urethra in men, resulting in ejaculation, and of the lower third of the vagina and the uterus in women. In men, there is a refractory period after orgasm during which they are unable to have another erection. The length of the refractory period increases with age.

Resolution is the reversal of the changes of these previous stages and results in the return of the body to its resting state.

Table 20-2

Some Common Causes of Sexual Symptoms

Causes	Symptoms
Medical Conditions	
Diabetes mellitus	Decreased libido
	Decreased arousal
	Erectile dysfunction
	Anorgasmia
Cardiac disease	Decreased libido
	Decreased arousal
	Erectile dysfunction
Menopause	Decreased libido
	Decreased lubrication/arousal
	Dyspareunia
	Anorgasmia
Psychiatric Disorders	
Major depression	Decreased libido
Anxiety disorders	Decreased libido
	Decreased arousal
	Erectile dysfunction
	Anorgasmia
Drugs	
Alcohol	Erectile dysfunction
Cocaine	Retarded ejaculation
	Anorgasmia
Heroin	Decreased libido
Antidepressants	Erectile dysfunction
(especially SSRIs and MAOIs)	Anorgasmia
	Retarded ejaculation
Antipsychotics	Decreased libido
	Erectile dysfunction
	Retarded ejaculation
Oral contraceptives	Decreased libido
	Decreased arousal
Antihypertensives	Decreased libido
	Erectile dysfunction
	Decreased arousal
	Impaired ejaculation

MAOI, monoamine oxidase inhibitor; SSRI, selective serotonin reuptake inhibitor.

men and women. Anxiety can interfere with both interest and arousal. Sexual reactions are also responsive to behavioral conditioning; there may be learned inhibition if arousal is associated with negative feelings such as guilt or fear.

Anxiety and learned inhibitions are usually the immediate causes of sexual dysfunction. That is, they occur at the moment the patient is engaging in sexual activity, distracting him and resulting in interference with the sexual response. These may occur at (and disrupt) any stage of the sexual response. Deeper intrapsychic conflicts, the remote causes of sexual problems, are often involved, although often not immediately apparent. There may, for example, be unresolved hostility toward one's parents. If the dysfunction is clearly situational, a nonorganic pathology is likely; for example, the patient who experiences normal morning erections but has erectile dysfunction when attempting sexual intercourse is likely to have a functional (nonorganic) sexual disorder.

TREATMENT

How Are Sexual Symptoms Treated?

The treatment of organic sexual symptoms consists of identification and treatment of the underlying condition or a change in medication. The treatment of other sexual disorders usually involves the treatment of both the immediate-behavioral and the remote-psychodynamic causes. Treatment of sexual dysfunction is discussed more fully in Chapter 31.

KEY POINTS

◆ There are four stages to the sexual response, and specific sexual symptoms relate to the various stages.

◆ The patient may not volunteer information about sexual symptoms unless specifically asked. A sexual history should be elicited as part of the general medical or psychiatric history.

◆ Consider organic causes unless the sexual symptom is clearly situational.

Case 20-1

A 35-year-old single woman with a history of major depression presents with the complaint that she is unable to reach orgasm. She also reports a decrease in desire, although lubrication is normal. The symptoms occur during masturbation, oral sex, and vaginal intercourse. She states that the symptoms first occurred 9 months ago, when she became increasingly depressed after the loss of her job as a Web designer, with worsening of her depression after her fiancé ended their relationship. At that time, she noticed difficulties with sleep and appetite, impaired concentration, and lack of interest in sexual activity. She denies any previous difficulties with sexual functioning. After seeking treatment with a psychiatrist, she was prescribed fluoxetine 20 mg daily, with resolution of all of her symptoms after 4 weeks except for the sexual ones.

A. Are the woman's sexual symptoms likely to have a physiologic or psychological cause?
B. Are the sexual symptoms primary or secondary?
C. What is likely to be causing the current symptoms?
D. What treatment do you recommend?

Case 20-2

A 42-year-old married woman presents complaining of difficulty reaching orgasm. She states that the symptom first occurred 2 years ago and denies any difficulty with sexual functioning before that time. On further inquiry, the woman admits that her anorgasmia began after she discovered that her husband was having an extramarital affair while she was pregnant with their second child. She thought about ending the marriage at that time but decided against divorce because she wanted to keep the family intact and because her husband promised to end the extramarital relationship. When asked about her current relationship with her husband, she tearfully states that she is still very angry with her husband and that she thinks about his infidelity whenever they have sexual relations.

A. What is the immediate cause of the woman's sexual symptom?
B. What treatment do you recommend?

Case Answers

20-1 A. *Learning objective:* **Recognize that sexual symptoms may have both physiologic and psychological components.** The onset of the woman's initial sexual symptoms occurred at the same time that she began to experience an episode of major depression, with a variety of neurovegetative symptoms including decreased libido. With treatment, her depression resolved; however, she has ongoing problems with desire and with orgasm, now most likely related to side effects of her antidepressant. Of note, patients may not complain of sexual side effects related to antidepressants until after their depression has resolved, when there is some return of their interest in sexuality.

20-1 B. *Learning objective:* **Know the difference between primary, or lifelong, and secondary, or acquired, sexual symptoms.** In this case, the woman's complaints follow a history of normal functioning. Therefore, her symptoms are secondary. Secondary sexual disorders often have a better prognosis than sexual disorders that have been of lifelong duration.

20-1 C. *Learning objective:* **Know that antidepressants commonly cause sexual symptoms.** This is especially common in women, particularly with the SSRIs, such as fluoxetine. Unlike this particular case, patients do not generally volunteer information about medication-induced sexual side effects, and this should be routinely inquired about when indicated by the side effect profile of the particular drug.

20-1 D. *Learning objective:* **Know that antidepressant-induced side effects can and should be treated.** Options include switching to an antidepressant without potential sexual side effects, such as bupropion or nefazodone.

20-2 A. *Learning objective:* **Know the difference between immediate and remote causes of sexual symptoms.** In this case, it is apparent that the woman's anger with her husband and her thoughts about his affair while they are having intercourse are distracting her from sexual fantasies and sexual feelings during sexual activity. The remote psychodynamic causes are not immediately apparent in this case.

20-2 B. *Learning objective:* **Know that treatment of sexual disorders involves treatment of the couple.** In this case, sex therapy addressing the immediate and remote causes of the woman's complaints and involving her husband as a partner in the therapy is indicated. In addition, couple's therapy would be useful to address the relationship difficulties apart from the sexual problems.

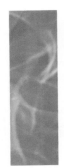

21

Changes in Appetite and Eating Disturbances

NATALIE GLUCK

What Can Cause a Change in Appetite?

Changes in appetite can occur with many medical and psychiatric disorders. However, in a majority of cases, the cause is not related to a pathologic condition. For example, change in appetite may be attributable to increased exercise or a change in routine. However, when a patient's appetite is either increased or decreased from baseline for several days to weeks or when changes result in a loss or gain of more than 5% of body weight, consider the possibility that there may be an underlying medical or psychiatric condition.

What Psychiatric Disorders Cause Changes in Appetite and Weight?

Different forms of depression can lead to changes in appetite and weight. For example, melancholic depression is often associated with a loss of appetite, whereas atypical depression is often associated with increased appetite, often accompanied by hypersomnia. Although not a mental illness, bereavement shares many characteristics with depression and can lead to increases or decreases in appetite and weight. Mania, and occasionally hypomania, may also be associated with loss of appetite. Table 21-1 summarizes the psychiatric disorders commonly associated with appetite and weight changes.

Does Weight Loss Always Suggest Decreased Appetite?

No. *Anorexia nervosa*, which in Greek translates to "a nervous loss of appetite," is actually a misnomer. Patients with anorexia nervosa often suffer extreme hunger but refuse to eat because of a distorted body image and an intense fear of being fat. Patients who have gastrointestinal diseases with malabsorption syndromes also lose weight without necessarily losing their appetite.

Table 21-1

Psychiatric Disorders Commonly Associated with Appetite and Weight Changes

Mood disorders
  Major depressive disorder
  Dysthymic disorder
  Adjustment disorder with depressed mood
  Bipolar I disorder
  Bipolar II disorder
  Schizoaffective disorder
Bereavement
Anorexia nervosa*

*Weight loss is not due to a decrease in appetite.

Does Weight Gain Always Result from an Increase in Appetite?

Not always. Sometimes a change in appetite results from changes in body size and activity. For example, an athlete's body may change dramatically while he trains, and his appetite may naturally increase as he builds muscle.

What Medical Conditions Can Cause Weight Loss?

Many medical conditions can cause weight loss, including cancer, chronic obstructive pulmonary disease, peptic ulcer disease, acquired immunodeficiency syndrome, and liver disease. Table 21-2 summarizes the major medical causes of weight loss.

Table 21-2

Medical Causes of Weight Loss

Cancer
Infections
  HIV and AIDS
  Intestinal parasites
Endocrine disorders
  New-onset diabetes mellitus
  Hyperthyroidism
  Addison's disease
Gastrointestinal disorders
  Malabsorption syndromes
  Liver disease
  Peptic ulcer
Chronic obstructive pulmonary disease

AIDS, acquired immunodeficiency syndrome; HIV, human immunodeficiency virus.

Are There Medical Conditions That Cause Weight Gain?

Yes, but not many. Weight gain is often the result of a sedentary lifestyle. However, some endocrinologic disorders, such as hypothyroidism and Cushing's syndrome, can cause weight gain and should be ruled out.

Can Medications Induce Changes in Weight?

Yes. Most antipsychotic and antidepressant agents can cause weight gain. Notable exceptions of agents that do not increase weight are the typical antipsychotic agent molindone, the atypical antipsychotic agents ziprasidone and aripiprazole, and the antidepressant bupropion. Mood stabilizers, including lithium and the anticonvulsants valproate and carbamazepine, are also associated with weight gain. Other medications that commonly cause an increase in appetite and weight are oral contraceptives and glucocorticoids. See Table 21-3 for a list of common medications associated with weight gain.

What Drugs of Abuse Affect Appetite and Weight?

Stimulants such as cocaine, methamphetamine ("speed"), 3,4-methylene-dioxymethamphetamine (Ecstasy [MDMA]), methylphenidate, and "diet pills" are appetite suppressants. Caffeine and nicotine are also mild stimulants and suppress appetite. When people abruptly stop using stimulants, their appetite increases and they often gain weight. Some smokers are reluctant to give up cigarettes because of the weight they put on when they try to quit. Cannabis, on the other hand, increases appetite during intoxication, and people who use marijuana usually report a strong carbohydrate craving when they smoke.

Table 21-3
Common Medications (and Examples) Associated with Weight Gain

Psychiatric
    Atypical antipsychotics (clozapine, olanzapine)
    Typical antipsychotics (chlorpromazine)
    Lithium
    Anticonvulsants (valproic acid, carbamazepine)
    TCAs (amitriptyline, clomipramine)
    MAOIs (phenelzine)
    SSRIs (paroxetine)
    Atypical antidepressants (mirtazapine)
Medical
    Oral contraceptives
    Glucocorticoids (prednisone)

MAOI, monoamine oxidase inhibitor; SSRI, selective serotonin reuptake inhibitor; TCA, tricyclic antidepressant.

What Is Binge Eating?

Binge eating is not simply overeating. It is a disordered type of eating characterized by repeated episodes of excessive consumption of food in a brief period of time (usually 1 to 2 hours) during which the individual experiences a loss of self-control. Binge eating can occur in anorexia nervosa (binge eating/purging type) and bulimia nervosa. When the binge eating is not followed by any compensatory behaviors, as in anorexia and bulimia, it is classified under the DSM-IV category of eating disorder not otherwise specified. Binge eating can also be seen in patients with borderline personality disorder who have poor impulse control. Women with premenstrual dysphoria sometimes binge eat and often experience intense carbohydrate cravings.

Does Self-Induced Vomiting Always Indicate an Eating Disorder?

Almost. Although it is true that self-induced vomiting is characteristic of anorexia nervosa (binge eating/purging type) and of bulimia nervosa (purging type), there are still some conditions to be ruled out. Some patients with a pathologic need to assume the sick role intentionally induce vomiting to convince their physicians that they are sick (factitious disorder), and some other people make themselves vomit to avoid school, work, court, or other obligations (malingering).

What Is Pica?

Pica is the eating of non-nutritive substances, typically paint, plaster, animal feces, sand, or soil. It usually occurs in children with mental retardation or developmental disorders, but it occasionally affects adults. Eating disturbances are summarized in Table 21-4.

Table 21-4

Common Causes of Eating Disturbances

Binge eating
  Anorexia nervosa, binge eating/purging type
  Bulimia nervosa, purging and nonpurging types
  Borderline personality disorder
  Premenstrual dysphoric disorder (possibly)
  Marijuana intoxication
Self-induced vomiting
  Anorexia nervosa, binge eating/purging type
  Bulimia nervosa, purging type
  Factitious disorder
  Malingering
Pica
  Mental retardation
  Pervasive developmental disorder
  Pregnancy
  Iron deficiency anemia
  Idiopathic

EVALUATION

What Do I Ask My Patient Who Has Lost or Gained Weight?

When confronted with a patient whose weight has changed significantly, you should start by assessing how much weight was lost or gained and the time course over which the changes in weight occurred. You should then assess the circumstances under which these changes occurred. For example, you should screen for psychiatric conditions that may lead to changes in appetite, such as depression. In addition to interviewing the patient, you may need to talk to members of the patient's family because some patients with severe depression or anorexia nervosa may not be able to provide an accurate, complete history. On the other hand, patients who are good historians, are appropriately concerned about the weight change, and appear to be perplexed should raise your level of suspicion for medical causes.

Are There Any Physical Findings That Are Helpful in the Diagnosis?

The presence of dental erosions, calluses on the back of the hand, and salivary gland hypertrophy highly suggests repeated self-induced vomiting and the presence of an eating disorder. In addition, patients with anorexia, restrictive type, can have various findings on physical examination, including orthostatic hypotension, bradycardia, and evidence of hair loss.

How Can I Distinguish between Changes in Weight Caused by a Psychiatric Illness and Those Caused by a Medical Disease?

Most medical conditions (with the exception of many types of cancer) arise with a constellation of physical signs and symptoms. In contrast, physical signs are uncommon in patients whose weight changes are related to psychiatric disorders. In general, you should rule out a medical disease with appropriate history, physical examination, and laboratory and radiographic studies before diagnosing a psychiatric illness in a patient with changes in weight.

What Laboratory Studies Should Be Ordered for a Patient with Changes in Appetite and Weight?

Routine tests include complete blood cell count, electrolytes, calcium, magnesium, glucose, renal panel, liver and thyroid function tests, and erythrocyte sedimentation rate. A urine toxicology examination and human immunodeficiency virus antibody test can be helpful to complete the evaluation. Patients with severe weight loss should also have an electrocardiogram to evaluate for cardiac arrhythmias.

TREATMENT

How Are Changes in Appetite and Weight Treated?

If the weight change is due to a medical condition, treatment of the underlying disorder often restores appetite and weight. Depression with neurovegetative symptoms is treated with antidepressant medications and psychotherapy. Severe depression may require the addition of antipsychotic medications or electroconvulsive therapy. For anorexia nervosa, the primary goal is weight restoration followed by psychotherapy. Antidepressants such as selective serotonin reuptake inhibitors are not generally helpful in restoring weight during the acute stages of anorexia but may be useful for anxiety or depression that persists after weight stabilization.

Are There Treatments for Other Eating Disturbances?

Yes. Binge eating, self-induced vomiting, and pica often respond to cognitive-behavioral psychotherapy. The aim is to teach healthier behaviors and routines (behavioral modifications) while making the patient aware of his or her distorted perceptions and thoughts (cognitive restructuring). Antidepressant medications such as selective serotonin reuptake inhibitors, nutritional counseling, and self-help groups can also assist as adjunctive treatments. Eating disorders and their treatments are discussed more fully in Chapter 29.

KEY POINTS

◆ Many medical conditions, such as cancer or thyroid abnormalities, cause a disturbance of appetite and should be ruled out before making the diagnosis of an eating disorder.

◆ Psychiatric illnesses, such as depression, may cause increases or decreases in appetite and weight.

Case 21-1

A 39-year-old general physician presents to the emergency department after an overdose of sleeping pills. Although the patient denies all symptoms and insists that it was "just an accident," his partner tells you that the patient has lost more than 40 lb in the past 2 months and now weighs 165 lb. The partner also tells you that the patient hardly sleeps at night, that he has stopped playing soccer on Saturdays as he always did, and that during the past 2 weeks he has started to believe that his internal organs are rotting. The partner reports that 10 years ago, the patient had a similar episode but they did not come to the hospital. The patient's vital signs are stable.

A. What else do you want to ask the partner?
B. What is the next step?
C. How will you treat the patient?

Case Answers

21-1 A. *Learning objective:* **Be familiar with the medical and psychiatric differential for weight loss.** Although the history given by the partner is very consistent with the diagnosis of major depressive disorder, recurrent and severe with mood-congruent psychotic features, you also need to ask the partner about the patient's medical history and any use of illicit or prescription drugs. You should also consider medical causes as well as drug-related causes of severe weight loss, remembering that physicians have easier access to scheduled drugs and are thus at increased risk. You would also like to know about any history of mania, psychosis in the absence of depression, and eating disturbances because the patient may suffer from bipolar disorder, schizoaffective disorder, or a primary eating disorder.

21-1 B. *Learning objective:* **Recognize the importance of a mental status examination in assessing weight changes.** Talk to the patient and obtain a mental status examination to check the patient's orientation and basic cognitive functioning. If the patient has an altered level of consciousness or is disoriented, you must consider delirium in addition to more chronic processes as a cause of the 40-lb weight loss. Follow up with a thorough physical examination and laboratory studies. The patient is likely to be admitted to a psychiatric unit and will also require an electrocardiogram and a chest radiograph.

21-1 C. *Learning objective:* **Be familiar with treatments for severe depression and serious weight loss.** If you conclude that the patient has depression with psychotic features, he will need antidepressant medications with adjunctive antipsychotic medications. Remember, however, that antidepressants take several weeks to take full effect. If your patient is at very high risk for suicide or starvation, you may consider electroconvulsive therapy to bring the patient out of his severe depression more quickly. You will then follow up with medications and psychotherapy.

Patients with a Known Condition

22

Schizophrenia and Other Psychotic Disorders

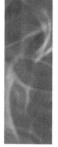

MYRL R. S. MANLEY

How Common Is Schizophrenia?

In the United States and throughout most of the world, about 0.5% to 1% of the population have the diagnosis of schizophrenia some time during their lifetime. Schizophrenia has been found in every country and every culture that has been studied. Higher rates are found in large cities. Men are affected as often as women.

What Causes Schizophrenia?

Nobody knows. There is strong evidence for a genetic factor, although specific genes or chromosomes have not been identified. What is inherited is probably a vulnerability to the disorder, not the disorder itself. Among monozygotic twin pairs, if one twin has schizophrenia, the other twin has the disorder only 40% to 50% of the time. Because monozygotic twins are genetically identical, this is strong evidence that the etiology involves more than abnormal genes. This has variably been referred to as the "stress-diathesis" model or the "two-hit" theory: a genetic vulnerability activated by an environmental trigger.

Do We Know What the Trigger Is?

No, but the risk for developing schizophrenia appears to be increased in a variety of circumstances, raising the possibility of multiple triggers. Among those circumstances are obstetric and perinatal complications, perhaps resulting in hypoxia to the infant's brain, and a maternal viral infection during pregnancy. Increased risk is also correlated with birth during the late winter and early spring months, presumably because of the increased risk of colds and influenza at that time of year. One study found a correlation between increased risk for schizophrenia and paternal age, possibly because of random mutations in spermatic genes.

Can Any Abnormalities Be Seen in the Brains of People with Schizophrenia?

Yes, although not consistently enough to serve as diagnostic markers. Overall brain volume is reduced by about 5% compared with control subjects without schizophrenia. In some brain regions, such as the prefrontal cortex and the mesial temporal cortex, the loss of volume is greater—as much as 15%. Correspondingly, the lateral ventricles are often slightly enlarged. In addition, functional imaging studies show a tendency toward decreased metabolic activity in the frontal lobes, a finding referred to as "hypofrontality."

Doesn't This Mean That Schizophrenia Is a Degenerative Disorder like Alzheimer's Disease?

Not necessarily. The observed structural brain changes could result from degeneration of a previously normal brain but could also be the result of a brain that develops abnormally. Most available evidence supports abnormal development as opposed to degeneration. For example, degeneration is accompanied by gliosis, a neural scarring involving glial cells. Gliosis is not found in the brain of individuals with schizophrenia. Moreover, prospective studies of children at high risk (because of family members with schizophrenia) have demonstrated abnormalities in social interactions and minor neurologic abnormalities among children who are subsequently diagnosed with schizophrenia but years before the disorder becomes clinically apparent.

A model of schizophrenia with wide acceptance suggests abnormal brain development in genetically vulnerable individuals. The abnormality is postulated to be in the interconnections of various brain regions—neural networks. Schizophrenia may prove to be a syndrome with multiple etiologies. It is not caused by bad parenting.

How Does Schizophrenia First Appear?

Although the first psychotic episode often occurs in early adulthood, in the late teens into the mid-20s, it can occur any time throughout life. Stress such as separation from family, financial hardships, fights, and arguments may help to precipitate a psychotic episode. Sometimes the first episode is preceded by a long insidious prodrome of withdrawal from friends and family and deterioration in school or work performance, in which case the prognosis is worse than if the episode occurred acutely. For the individual with an established diagnosis of schizophrenia, recurrent psychotic episodes are most commonly related to cessation of antipsychotic medication.

Are There Medical Conditions or Drug-Related States That Mimic Schizophrenia?

Yes, at least in the short term. Many conditions cause psychotic symptoms; fewer cause the combination of psychotic symptoms and a long-term waxing and waning course. However, in the evaluation of a patient, the long-term course may not be apparent. One relatively uncommon medical condition that mimics both the symptoms and course in schizophrenia is acute intermittent porphyria; the "madness" of King George III of England who presided over the loss of the American colonies is now believed to have been porphyria.

What Is Schizoaffective Disorder?

This diagnosis applies to people who have both prominent mood symptoms and prominent psychotic symptoms. DSM-IV-TR distinguishes a mood disorder with psychotic features from schizoaffective disorder by requiring the latter to include a period of at least 2 weeks in which there are psychotic symptoms with no mood disturbance.

Is Schizoaffective Disorder Related to Schizophrenia?

Probably, although the exact relationship is still not clear. Several large-scale studies have demonstrated an increased prevalence of schizophrenia in first-degree relatives of patients with schizoaffective disorder. An increased prevalence of psychotic mood disorders has also been found.

Does That Mean That People with Schizoaffective Disorder Have a Mood Disorder Superimposed on Schizophrenia?

That certainly is one possibility, although not the most likely. An alternative explanation is that mood and psychotic symptoms coexist on a spectrum with variable clinical expression. At one extreme are mood disorders and at the other extreme is schizophrenia. In between are psychotic mood disorders, schizoaffective disorder, and schizophrenia with prominent mood symptoms. The more emotional features a person has, the better the prognosis. Schizoaffective disorder has a prognosis between that for mood disorders and that for schizophrenia.

Is Delusional Disorder a Variant of Schizophrenia?

It doesn't appear to be. Delusional disorder is monosymptomatic: the only feature is a delusion. There are no prominent hallucinations, disorganization, or negative or cognitive symptoms. Unlike schizophrenia, the disorder does not have clinical phases. The delusion is always there. By definition, it must be "nonbizarre', that is, something that could actually happen in real life. Examples include the (false) belief that one's spouse is having an affair or that one has become the target of a plot by an organized crime syndicate. The belief that a microchip has been implanted in one's brain to control thoughts and actions is "bizarre" and is inconsistent with a diagnosis of delusional disorder. (See Chapter 12 for further discussion.) Some studies have found an increased family prevalence of schizophrenia in patients with delusional disorder; others have not.

EVALUATION

Are There Blood Tests or Imaging Studies That Help Make a Diagnosis of Schizophrenia?

Not yet, although the search for laboratory markers is intense. The structural brain abnormalities mentioned earlier (decreased cortical volume,

Schizophrenia

enlarged ventricles, abnormal cerebral blood flow) are neither sensitive nor specific enough to make a diagnosis. In the absence of external markers, schizophrenia is a diagnosis that can be made only on the basis of *clinical* criteria: characteristic symptoms and characteristic course.

What Points in the History and Mental Status Examination Help in Making a Diagnosis of Schizophrenia?

Schizophrenia is a disorder of recurrent psychotic episodes followed by residual phases of diminished function. The first episode often occurs in late adolescence or early adulthood and may be preceded by a prodrome. During the psychotic episode, *positive* (or psychotic) symptoms predominate: hallucinations, delusions, disorganized thinking, or disorganized bizarre behavior. During the prodrome and residual phases, *negative* symptoms predominate: social withdrawal, emotional blunting, decreased motivation, and anhedonia (the inability to achieve pleasure).

Many patients also have *cognitive* symptoms: impaired attention, trouble learning new information, and difficulty recognizing social cues such as the emotional meaning of facial expression. The cognitive symptoms are present during both the acute and residual phases of the disorder.

The *absence* of certain symptoms also helps with the diagnosis. There are usually no prominent mood symptoms. Significant changes in sleep and appetite are not typical. Abnormalities in the sensorium—alertness, orientation, and memory—do not usually occur. Because schizophrenia is a chronic disorder with waxing and waning symptoms, evidence of the disturbance must be present for at least 6 months. People who appear to have schizophrenia but have had symptoms for less than 6 months are given a diagnosis of *schizophreniform disorder*. This diagnosis is changed to schizophrenia if the disorder continues beyond 6 months.

Are There Any Pathognomonic Symptoms?

Sadly, no. However, it has been recognized that certain symptoms, while not establishing the diagnosis, may suggest it. Especially characteristic are delusions of control (e.g., believing that a machine is controlling one's thoughts or actions) or of thoughts being inserted into or withdrawn from the patient's mind. Hearing voices is common, especially voices talking about the patient and commenting on his or her actions. Derailment or loosening of associations and thought blocking are often present.

How Do I Rule Out Medical and Drug-Related Conditions?

A good physical examination is essential. Schizophrenia does not arise with neurologic or other physical signs. (There may, however, be physical signs caused by antipsychotic drugs, such as tremor, rigidity, or muscle spasms.) Similarly, abnormalities in laboratory testing cannot be explained on the basis of schizophrenia alone. If abnormalities are present, the possibility of a medical or drug-related condition must be investigated. A history of physical illness and treatment in the presence of physical symptoms suggests an underlying medical condition. Urine toxicology screens are of some, but limited, use. A positive test result indicates only that the drug is present, not that it caused the patient's symptoms. Moreover, a negative test does not rule out a drug-related syndrome. Some drugs, such as cocaine, can cause psychotic symptoms that persist even after the drug has been cleared. Psychotic symptoms caused by drug withdrawal result from the *absence* of the drug after prolonged use, in which case the toxicology screen is most likely to be negative.

A sudden onset of symptoms in an older person with no previous psychiatric history raises the suspicion of a medical or drug-related cause, as do the presence of disorientation, significant memory problems, and an altered level of consciousness. In addition to an attentive physical examination, a careful history of previous medical illnesses and of prescription and recreational drug use and a review of physical symptoms are necessary.

Are There Sex Differences in Schizophrenia?

There are, but they are most clearly seen when looking at large populations and are less useful in evaluating a particular patient because of considerable individual variability. The first psychotic episode generally occurs at an earlier age for boys (late teens to early 20s) than for girls (early to mid-20s). In addition, men typically have a more difficult course, with more frequent and more severe episodes, and they have a greater likelihood of increasingly impaired ability to function independently as time passes.

How Is Schizophrenia Distinguished from Other Psychotic Disorders?

Schizophrenia is distinguished on the basis of symptoms and course (Table 22-1).

TREATMENT

What Drugs Are Used to Treat Schizophrenia?

Antipsychotic agents form the mainstay of pharmacotherapy for most people with schizophrenia. They are used to treat psychotic symptoms

Table 22-1	
The Psychotic Disorders	
Schizophrenic	Recurrent episodes of psychotic symptoms, with negative symptoms and cognitive symptoms between acute episodes
Schizophreniform	Symptoms like those of schizophrenia but lasts less than 6 months
Schizoaffective	Psychotic symptoms and mood symptoms occur together, and at another time during the same episode, psychotic symptoms occur without mood symptoms
Delusional	Delusions only (no hallucinations)
	Delusions must be of something that could really happen in everyday life

Schizophrenia

and do so, for the most part, regardless of the cause. The older antipsychotic agents are called "typicals," and the newer agents are called "atypicals" (Table 22-2). The typical agents can be subdivided on the basis of potency. High-potency and low-potency antipsychotic agents are equally effective but must be administered in different strengths. Because of the greater potency of the high-potency drugs, effective doses are often in multiples of 10 mg or less. Low-potency antipsychotic agents are administered in

Table 22-2

Antipsychotic Medications

Drug Class (Examples)	Typical Doses[*]	Common Side Effects	Potential Problems
Typical: Low Potency			
Chlorpromazine (Thorazine)	500–1000 mg/day	Sedation Anticholinergic effects (dry mouth, constipation, urinary retention, blurred vision) Sexual dysfunction Orthostatic hypotension Extrapyramidal symptoms (less than high-potency agents)	Tardive dyskinesia with long-term use Seizures
Typical: High Potency			
Haloperidol (Haldol)	5–20 mg/day	Extrapyramidal symptoms (dystonias, Parkinson's disease-like symptoms, akathisia)	Tardive dyskinesia with long-term use
Fluphenazine (Prolixin)	5–20 mg/day	Anticholinergic symptoms (less than low-potency agents)	Neuroleptic malignant syndrome
	Both Haloperidol and Fluphenazine are available in long-acting intramuscular decanoate forms	Sedation (less than low potency agents) Orthostatic hypotension (less than low-potency agents) Sexual dysfunction	
Atypical			
Aripiprazole (Abilify)	10–30 mg/day	Dizziness Constipation Akathisia	Neuroleptic malignant syndrome

(Continued)

Table 22-2			
Antipsychotic Medications (Continued)			
Drug Class (Examples)	**Typical Doses***	**Common Side Effects**	**Potential Problems**
Clozapine (Clozaril)	150–300 mg/day	Sedation Orthostatic hypotension Anticholinergic side effects Weight gain	Agranulocytosis Seizures
Olanzapine (Zyprexa)	5–20 mg/day	Sedation Weight gain Dizziness	Metabolic syndrome
Quetiapine (Seroquel)	200–400 mg/day	Sedation Postural hypotension Dizziness	Possible cataract formation
Risperidone (Risperdal)	4–6 mg/day	Extrapyramidal symptoms Sedation Dizziness	Neuroleptic malignant syndrome
Ziprasidone (Geodon)	20–80 mg/day	Sedation Dizziness Nausea	QT prolongation

*Doses for individual patients may vary considerably.

Schizophrenia

doses of multiples of 100 mg. Low-potency typical antipsychotic agents tend to be more sedating and to have more anticholinergic side effects than high-potency antipsychotic agents. On the other hand, the high-potency drugs are more likely to cause acute movement abnormalities, such as dystonias, akathisia, and Parkinson's disease-like symptoms. Both high- and low-potency antipsychotic agents have a risk of tardive dyskinesia. (See Chapter 36 for further discussion of medication-induced movement disorders.)

The atypical agents are the newer generation of antipsychotic drugs. They tend to cause fewer movement abnormalities and to have a significantly decreased risk for tardive dyskinesia. They are often effective for a patient who has not responded to multiple trials of typical drugs, and there is growing evidence that at least some atypical agents, such as clozapine and olanzapine, are effective in treating negative symptoms as well as positive symptoms in schizophrenia.

Other medications are used on an adjuvant basis. A benzodiazepine anxiolytic helps to decrease anxiety and agitation and may be especially helpful during acute psychotic flare-ups. An antidepressant medication helps people with schizophrenia who also experience periods of depression. Additional medications are often used to counteract side effects of the antipsychotic agents. Anticholinergic, anti-Parkinson's drugs such as benztropine or trihexyphenidyl decrease movement abnormalities.

Schizophrenia

Do Typical and Atypical Antipsychotic Medications Act in Different Ways?

Yes, the pharmacodynamics are different but overlapping. The typical drugs block dopamine D2 receptors and their potency is directly related to their effectiveness in doing so. Atypicals are weaker D2 antagonists and stronger serotonin 5HT-2A receptor antagonists.

Do Atypicals Have Fewer Side Effects than Typicals?

They have different side effects. The commonest side effects of the older, typical medications (especially high-potency drugs) are extrapyramidal symptoms (EPSs). The atypicals cause far fewer EPSs but carry a greater risk for metabolic problems: type 2 diabetes mellitus, hypercholesterolemia, and hyperlipidemia, sometimes referred to as a "metabolic syndrome." In addition, olanzapine has a greater likelihood than typical agents of causing significant weight gain. The EPSs of typical medications are commonly present from the start of treatment. Metabolic problems from the atypicals may not be apparent for many months.

How Do I Know Which Antipsychotic Drug Is Right for My Patient?

The antipsychotic agents are broadly effective, but there is no way to predict which individual patient will improve best with which drug. Prior experience is helpful. If the patient has been treated with a certain drug in the past, did well, and tolerated the side effects, that is a good medication with which to start. Similarly, a family history of effective drug treatment may help. If there is no individual or family medication history on which to draw, the side effect profile is a useful guide. Because the atypical agents tend to have fewer and less severe initial adverse effects, they are sometimes thought of as first-line agents. However, a large-scale study comparing perphenazine—a mid-potency typical—with the atypicals olanzapine, ziprasidone, quetiapine, and risperidone showed similar rates of discontinuation and little difference in therapeutic efficacy between the older and newer generations of antipsychotics. (Olanzapine appears to have slightly greater efficacy but also greater risk of severe and potentially fatal metabolic problems.) In addition, the atypical antipsychotics are usually vastly more expensive than generic versions of the older drugs. Table 22-3 lists some differences between typical and atypical antipsychotics.

The available routes of administration and the ease of dosing schedule may also help you choose an antipsychotic drug. Once-a-day dosing is easier than multiple doses throughout the day and enhances compliance. Haloperidol and fluphenazine (both high-potency typical antipsychotic agents) and the atypical risperidone are available in an injectable decanoate form in addition to the regular oral form. Some patients who have been unable or unwilling to maintain a daily regimen of medications do well with a once-a-month injection of one of these drugs. (You must remember, however, that once the injection is administered, it cannot be removed; the patient is left with whatever adverse effects occur for several weeks.)

Table 22-3

Differences between Typical and Atypical Antipsychotics

	Typical Antipsychotics	Atypical Antipsychotics
Examples	Chlorpromazine (Thorazine) Haloperidol (Haldol) Fluphenazine (Prolixin) Perphenazine (Trilafon) Thiothixene (Navane)	Aripiprazole (Abilify) Clozapine (Clozaril) Olanzapine (Zyprexa) Quetiapine (Seroquel) Risperidone (Risperdal) Ziprasidone (Geodon)
Mechanism of Action	Dopamine D2 receptor antagonist	Weaker D2 antagonism, stronger 5HT-2A antagonism
Efficacy	Good control for positive symptoms Less benefit for negative symptoms	Good control of positive symptoms Some benefit for negative and cognitive symptoms, especially olanzapine and clozapine
Common Reasons for discontinuation	Extrapyramidal symptoms Tardive dyskinesia Other side effects (especially sexual side effects, weight gain, gynecomastia, sedation)	Metabolic syndrome Other side effects (especially weight gain and sedation)

Schizophrenia

How Long Will My Patient Have to Take Medication?

A puzzling minority of patients with schizophrenia—perhaps as many as 10%—recover from their symptoms and remain unimpaired for the rest of their lives. For most patients, however, schizophrenia is a chronic, relapsing condition that requires long-term medication. Stopping the drug for short or long periods is not helpful and increases the risk of relapse. Long-term, quite possibly lifelong, medication treatment at the lowest possible dose consistent with symptom control is necessary for most people.

Does Psychotherapy Help?

The right kind of psychotherapy can help considerably in treating people with schizophrenia; the wrong kind can make things worse. Psychodynamic psychotherapies are usually contraindicated. The lack of structure is disorganizing, the therapist's neutrality can heighten paranoia, and meaningful self-reflection may be impossible. More helpful therapies are discussed in Box 22-1.

Do I Need to Distinguish Subtypes of Schizophrenia?

You may. It is still unclear whether they are true subtypes of a common disorder or different conditions that look alike only superficially. Some studies have shown that subtypes for individuals can change over time. The subtypes are diagnosed on the basis of which symptoms are most prominent; they are summarized in Table 22-4.

Schizophrenia

BOX 22-1

SOME PSYCHOTHERAPIES THAT ARE HELPFUL IN TREATING SCHIZOPHRENIA

Psychoeducation

This teaches patients and families about the disorder. They learn to identify and recognize symptoms, the circumstances that trigger them, and the effect of prescribed medications. They come to better understand and control the kinds of life stresses that can trigger relapses, and they recognize the hoped-for benefit in complying with treatment recommendations.

Social Skills Training

This helps patients with schizophrenia to dress appropriately, to interact with others, and to behave in public in ways that make independent living and work more possible.

Supportive Psychotherapy

This seeks to strengthen existing adaptive capacities and coping skills and to minimize maladaptive ones. The patient and therapist look at what worked or what did not work in the past to come up with strategies for dealing with current problems. In addition, supportive therapy can be extremely helpful in offering an island of safety, predictability, and emotional stability to a person whose psychic world is chaotic and frightening.

Family Therapy

This helps family members understand the patient's condition, the need for medication, and the significance of symptoms. Family therapy can help reduce stresses at home that worsen symptoms. (Family therapy exploring family dynamics is not helpful.)

The purpose of a diagnosis is to make predictions about treatment response and outcome, and there are some differences among the subtypes. People with paranoid schizophrenia tend to have the best prognosis with the least overall impairment; people with disorganized schizophrenia usually have the most impairment and the worst long-term outcome. Individuals with catatonic schizophrenia often respond to electroconvulsive therapy; people with other subtypes usually do not. Most cases of schizophrenia diagnosed in the United States are the undifferentiated subtype and are treated with a combination of long-term antipsychotic medication and therapeutic intervention such as psychoeducation or psychosocial rehabilitation.

Are the Other Psychotic Disorders Treated the Same Way as Schizophrenia?

Because antipsychotic medications are effective for most psychotic symptoms regardless of the diagnosis, they are the foundation of treatment for the entire group. However, antipsychotic agents often are not effective

Table 22-4

Schizophrenia Subtypes

Subtype	Features
Paranoid	Prominent delusions or hallucinations (do not have to be persecutory)
	No disorganized speech or behavior
	No blunted emotions
Disorganized	Prominent disorganization of speech and behavior
Catatonic	Prominent abnormalities of behavior
	Immobility
	Mutism
	Echolalia and echopraxia (purposeless mimicking of what someone else says or does)
	Excessive purposeless movement
Undifferentiated	No single predominant symptom or a mixture of features found in other subtypes
Residual	Prominent negative symptoms, no current psychotic symptoms

Schizophrenia

for the delusions in delusional disorder, and behavioral interventions are required. Patients may learn how to minimize the impact of a delusion by not discussing it with others. Patients with shared delusional disorder may be helped only by separation from one another. Schizoaffective disorder is often treated with the combination of an antipsychotic and a mood stabilizer, sometimes with the addition of antidepressant medication.

What's the Prognosis for My Patient with Schizophrenia?

When a diagnosis of schizophrenia is established, the prognosis is always guarded but, contrary to popular misconception, not invariably poor. Only about a third of people with a diagnosis of schizophrenia show chronic, progressive deterioration with increasing difficulty living independently, managing their own affairs, and maintaining social and family contacts. Others stabilize with greater or lesser degrees of residual symptoms. For most patients, the disorder lasts a lifetime with a chronic risk for recurrent psychotic episodes. Some factors suggest a better outcome (Table 22-5). Risk of suicide in patients with schizophrenia is 15 times that seen in the general population.

What Kind of Follow-up Should I Arrange for My Patient with Schizophrenia Who Is Ready for Discharge?

In an ideal world, every patient with schizophrenia would have a safe, comfortable place to live, the chance to interact with others and to work constructively, access to medical care, medications as needed, and regular psychiatric follow-up with a trusted individual with whom the patient can develop a relationship over time.

In the real world, the availability of these ideals may be compromised by cost, politics, and public policy. Nonetheless, some solutions are

Table 22-5

Prognosis in Schizophrenia

Better	Worse
Acute onset	Insidious onset
Onset in old age	Onset in childhood
Emotions intact	Emotional blunting
No disorganization of speech or behavior	Disorganization present
Female	Male

better than others: family involvement is better than estrangement, social opportunities are better than isolation, a sheltered workshop or vocational training is better than idleness, and for patients with schizophrenia who are homeless, assisted living and halfway houses are better than the streets or public shelters.

At the minimum, at the time of discharge, a patient needs a safe place to live, a supply of medications and a way to continue to receive them, and an opportunity for follow-up in the near future.

KEY POINTS

◆ Symptoms that increase the suspicion of schizophrenia:

Delusions of control (body or mind)
Delusions of thoughts being put into or taken out of the patient's mind
Auditory hallucinations that comment on the patient's actions
Derailment and thought blocking

◆ Consider an underlying medical or drug-related condition if

There are physical signs
You find abnormal laboratory results
The onset was abrupt in an older person with no psychiatric history
The patient has impaired alertness, memory, and orientation

◆ Neuroimaging studies such as computed tomography and positron emission tomography do not rule in schizophrenia; they rule out other potential causes of symptoms, such as tumors.

◆ Choose an antipsychotic agent based on

Patient's previous medication experience
Family medication experience
Side effects
Dosing schedule
Cost
Routes of administration

◆ Schizophrenia is differentiated from other psychotic disorders on the basis of symptoms and clinical course

Case 22-1

A 19-year-old man is accompanied by his parents to your office because of his bizarre behavior. He has been increasingly isolative during the preceding 4 months, and he stopped attending community college classes 3 weeks ago. He acknowledges hearing voices talking about him, and he believes that a microchip was implanted in his brain while he was sleeping and that it is now controlling his thoughts. He appears apprehensive. His heart rate is 110 beats per minute, and his blood pressure is 150/100 mm Hg; his pupils are dilated.

    A. What additional work-up do you want to do?
    B. What treatment, if any, do you recommend?
    C. What do you tell the man and his parents?

Case 22-2

A 32-year-old woman is admitted to your service after a suicide attempt. She has had two previous admissions to control psychotic episodes and has a diagnosis of chronic undifferentiated schizophrenia. She has responded well to haloperidol and has been maintained on 5 mg/day. About a month ago, she stopped the antipsychotic agent when her prescription ran out. Shortly afterward, she began to reexperience auditory hallucinations, and she began to feel that someone was coming into her apartment at night to rifle through her belongings. Ten days before admission, she became depressed. She lost her appetite, could not sleep through the night, and cried every day. These symptoms intensified up to the time of admission. The psychotic symptoms remained unchanged.

    A. Is her previous diagnosis correct?
    B. What additional information do you want?
    C. How will you treat her?

Case Answers

22-1 A. ***Learning objective:* Recognize that schizophrenia does not include physical signs.** Although the age of onset, the course, and the content of his hallucinations and delusions are typical for schizophrenia, elevated heart rate and blood pressure and dilated pupils are not typical and must be explained. Ask about physical symptoms, drug use, and past medical conditions. Do a good physical examination including a neurologic examination. A urine toxicology screen may help, especially if the result is positive.

22-1 B. ***Learning objective:* Know the indications for antipsychotic drugs.** Antipsychotic drugs treat most psychotic symptoms regardless of etiology. Choose an appropriate antipsychotic. (An atypical such as risperidone would be a good first-line choice because of mild side effects.) You will relieve his anxiety and may get a better history when the hallucinations and delusions resolve. If he is extremely apprehensive and agitated, you might want to supplement the antipsychotic with a benzodiazepine. It is premature to begin treating his hypertension, which could be the result of intoxication with a central nervous system stimulant such as cocaine.

22-1 C.   *Learning objective:* **Know how schizophrenia is diagnosed.** You can't tell them he has schizophrenia because you don't know. Schizophrenia is a chronic illness with waxing and waning symptoms and cannot be diagnosed on the basis of a single episode. Moreover, the diagnosis requires that you rule out possible medical and drug-related causes. You can explain that he has psychotic symptoms, that they are treatable, and that further investigations and follow-up are necessary to determine the cause.

22-2 A and B.   *Learning objective:* **Distinguish schizophrenia from other psychotic disorders.** The woman currently meets diagnostic criteria for schizoaffective disorder. A diagnosis of schizophrenia will not explain such prominent mood symptoms. If she had experienced mood symptoms and psychotic symptoms together, your differential would include major depression with psychotic features. However, her history clearly describes a period of psychotic symptoms alone followed by psychotic symptoms combined with mood symptoms during the same episode—the very definition of schizoaffective disorder. In addition to ruling out any medical or drug-related factors, it would be helpful to review the records of her previous admissions to see if mood symptoms were present in the past. You will also need to document any prior history of suicidal thoughts or actions. The presence of suicidality does not indicate a diagnosis of depression. Suicide cuts across diagnostic boundaries.

22-2 C.   *Learning objective:* **Plan drug therapy for a person with schizoaffective disorder.** The woman needs antipsychotic medication. If haloperidol was an effective and well-tolerated drug in the past, it is a reasonable place to start. (You must keep in mind, however, the long-term risk of tardive dyskinesia, which will be lower with an atypical drug.) A mood stabilizer is usually included for schizoaffective disorder. However, because the available mood stabilizers are less effective than antidepressants in treating depression, you should start with an antidepressant such as a selective serotonin reuptake inhibitor (SSRI) and then switch to a mood stabilizer when her mood is back to normal.

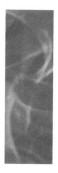

23

Major Depressive Disorder

MICHAEL DULCHIN

What Is Depression?

Sadness, grief, and demoralization are universal human experiences. Psychiatrists mean something different when they speak of depression (more properly, major depression): a medical syndrome of symptoms that includes mood changes but also involves disturbances of sleep, appetite, energy, and libido. Unlike those with sadness and grief, people cannot bounce back from depression. In fact, many depressed people are intensely self-critical for not being able to pull themselves out of it.

Who Becomes Depressed?

Depression is among the more common of psychiatric disorders in the United States. It is estimated that over 13 million people become depressed each year. Major depression has a lifetime prevalence of about 15%. About 5% of men and 10% of women are diagnosed with depression during their life. Up to 40% of patients who come to a primary care clinic have depression. There are no race, ethnic, or class differences; wealthy people become depressed as often as do poor people. Women, as already noted, become depressed at least twice as frequently as men. It is estimated that the cost of depression in terms of lost productivity and medical care is about $45 billion each year.

Do People Typically Become Depressed at a Particular Age?

Depression can happen at any time in someone's life, but there tend to be peak incidences in the late 20s for men and late teens for women. For patients who develop their first episode of depression after the age of 65, this is often the beginning of a dementing illness.

What Causes Depression?

As with many psychiatric disorders, all evidence suggests an inherited vulnerability in combination with some environmental factors. Identical twin studies show that if one twin has a history of a single episode of major depression, the other twin has about a 33% chance of a single episode. The rate is nearly 60% for recurrent depression. In depression, the role of life circumstances seems clearer than that for other conditions. Early childhood losses, especially the loss of a parent, leave an individual vulnerable to later depression. Other major losses in adulthood, such as financial setbacks, the loss of a loved one, or being fired from work, can precipitate episodes of major depression in those who are predisposed. Depression can also occur without any identifiable precipitant. It is diagnosed only on the basis of symptoms and course, not on whether something bad has happened to cause the depression.

Is Depression a Chemical Imbalance?

The neurochemical basis of depression is still not fully understood. The catecholamine theory holds that depression is caused by a dysregulation of the catecholamine neurotransmitters serotonin, norepinephrine, epinephrine, and dopamine. Many antidepressants work by increasing the levels of these neurotransmitters in the synapse, but, clearly, low levels of these neurotransmitters are only part of the problem because the antidepressants increase the levels almost immediately but the antidepressants take weeks to work. Receptor changes such as down-regulation of postsynaptic receptors and desensitization of presynaptic autoreceptors are thought to be involved. The hypothalamic-pituitary axis plays some role in the etiology of depression as cortisol dysregulation is frequently found in depressed patients. Hypothalamic responses to sleep and light may be involved as well: sleep patterns are regulated by the hypothalamic chronobiologic center and disruption in sleep seems to precipitate manic and depressive mood changes in predisposed people. It is hypothesized that this is caused by changes in hormones and neurotransmitters with circadian patterns. Light has been shown to precipitate manic episodes and can also act as an antidepressant. Lack of light is thought to be etiologic in the depressed mood of seasonal affective disorder. The effect of light on mood is thought to be through retinal connections to the hypothalamus. More than likely, depression is a final common pathway with many etiologies.

Can Medical Conditions Cause Depression?

People who receive a serious medical diagnosis sometimes become depressed as a result of hearing the bad news. In addition, depression can be part of the presenting symptomatology of some medical syndromes. When depression is caused by an underlying medical illness, it is called a secondary depression. Common causes of secondary depression include malignancies (especially pancreatic), endocrinopathies (hypothyroidism, Addison's disease), viral infections (hepatitis, human immunodeficiency virus [HIV] infection), and stroke. Chronic fatigue syndrome and fibromyalgia, although still poorly defined, typically include a significant depressive component. Some women experience severe depression in the postpartum period.

Major Depressive Disorder

What Drugs Cause Depression?

A number of drugs, both prescription and recreational, can cause depression, even in people who might not have developed depression otherwise. The use of some medications, such as the antihypertensive agent reserpine and the antiviral agent interferon, may be limited by the severity of the depression they can cause. Other antihypertensive agents, such as methyldopa, the β-blocker propranolol, oral contraceptives, and central nervous system depressants such as the benzodiazepines, can cause depression. Recreational drug use is also a prominent cause of secondary depressions, with withdrawal from cocaine or other stimulants being among the most common (Table 23-1).

EVALUATION

What Are the Symptoms of Depression?

A depressed mood is common, but surprisingly it is not invariably present. Some patients experience only anhedonia (an inability to obtain pleasure from usually pleasurable activities). Depression is a syndrome that includes more than mood changes. Insomnia (especially early morning wakening), loss of appetite, decreased libido, and fatigue are very often

Major Depressive Disorder

Table 23-1
Some Causes of Secondary Depression

I. Medical conditions
  A. Malignancy (especially pancreatic)
  B. Endocrinopathy
    1. Hypothyroidism
    2. Addison's disease
  C. Viral infections
    1. Hepatitis
    2. Human immunodeficiency virus
  D. Stroke
II. Drugs
  A. Central nervous system depressants
    1. Alcohol
    2. Benzodiazepines
  B. Antihypertensive agents
    1. Reserpine
    2. Methyldopa
    3. Propranolol
  C. Oral contraceptives
  D. Interferon
  E. Withdrawal from central nervous system stimulants
    1. Cocaine
    2. Caffeine
    3. Nicotine

present and can be more troublesome to some patients than the depressed mood. Memory problems and trouble concentrating are also common and may be so severe that the individual looks demented. In some depressed patients, psychotic symptoms are part of the course; the content is typically consistent with a depressed mood. For example, a person may hear voices making derisive, derogatory comments. A delusional patient may have unwarranted guilt, such as believing himself to be personally responsible for an earthquake. Somatic delusions ("all my internal organs have rotted away") are also characteristic of major depression with psychotic features. The symptoms of major depression are listed in Table 23-2.

Should I Ask about Precipitating Events?

Yes. Even though a precipitant is not needed to make a diagnosis, knowledge of precipitating events will help you better make the diagnosis, understand your patient, and develop better rapport. Understanding precipitating events may help the patient reduce the risk of further episodes. For some patients the precipitating event is very important, and helping the patient change his or her circumstances can therefore help relieve the depressive symptoms.

What Is a Melancholic Depression?

A melancholic depression can be thought of as the "typical" depression to which an atypical depression is contrasted. Patients with a melancholic depression are likely to have prominent vegetative symptoms (e.g., trouble falling asleep or staying asleep, loss of appetite, and weight loss). They are less likely than patients with other kinds of depression to report a precipitating event, and they are less likely to respond to placebo treatments.

Major Depressive Disorder

Table 23-2

Symptoms of Major Depression

I. Mood
   A. Despondence, hopelessness
   B. Anhedonia
II. Vegetative
   A. Early morning wakening (sometimes hypersomnia)
   B. Loss of appetite (sometimes increased appetite)
   C. Fatigue
   D. Decreased libido
III. Cognitive
   A. Impaired memory and concentration
   B. Slow thinking
IV. Psychotic (not always present)
   A. Derogatory auditory hallucinations
   B. Delusions of guilt
   C. Somatic delusions

The symptoms in atypical depression are variations from those seen in most depressed patients. Instead of insomnia and decreased appetite, the patient experiences hypersomnia and increased appetite with weight gain. Atypical features are more common in children and adolescents. They are also seen in seasonal affective disorder (depression brought on by decreased hours of sunlight during the winter months) and in many people with bipolar disorder who become depressed. Patients with atypical depression also experience the symptom of leaden paralysis (the feeling that the body is very heavy and difficult to move) and rejection sensitivity (sensitivity to interpersonal rejection).

Are There Other Depressive Subtypes?

In the DSM-IV-TR, the depressive disorders include major depression, which can be noted as a single episode or recurrent; dysthymic disorder; and depression not otherwise specified (NOS).

How Should I Interview a Depressed Patient?

Depressed patients often have psychomotor retardation (a slowing down of thinking and activity). It may take more energy on your part to move the interview forward. Such patients seldom do well with open-ended questions and long silences. Because of the possible cognitive disturbance, your questions will need to be very focused and direct. A thorough assessment of suicide potential is essential.

What Is the Relationship between Depression and Suicide?

Suicide is best understood with the stress-diathesis model. A person may have a predilection for suicidal behavior, but this will be acted upon only if there is a severe enough stressor for that particular person's suicidal propensity. Psychiatric disorders in general in this model serve as stressors, and depression can be a significant one. There is about a 10% lifetime prevalence of suicide among patients with major depression, and of people who kill themselves, half to three quarters carry a diagnosis of depression.

What Should I Tell Patients about the Role of Sleep and Anxiety in Depression?

Sleep disturbances and anxiety symptoms are often part of the depressive syndrome. Many times patients see difficulty sleeping and anxiety as causes of depression (which they can be) when they are actually the results of the depression. Helping these patients understand that their anxiety will lessen and sleep improve when the depression remits is crucial to helping them through the episode. Pharmacologic treatment of these symptoms can be very effective.

Aren't Some Depressions Worse than Others?

There certainly is a range of severity from mild to severe, but it is difficult to quantify subjective experience. It is easier to gauge the severity by looking at the indirect effects of depression, such as the extent to which

Major Depressive Disorder

work or school performance is impaired. Dysthymia describes a chronic, low-grade depression in people who are always moody and out of sorts. Major depression is characterized by symptoms that are more severe and that occur in discrete episodes with a clear beginning and ending, followed by normal functioning. When major depression is superimposed on dysthymia, it is called double depression. Often, the more chronic low-level depressions require higher doses of antidepressants than major depressive episodes.

How Do I Distinguish Normal Sadness and Grief from Major Depression?

The clinical course is most helpful. Sadness and grief, although painful, are not lasting. An episode of depression hangs on relentlessly for weeks (always at least 2 weeks and often for months). The presence of persistent vegetative symptoms and cognitive symptoms also indicates depression. The quality of the mood disturbance itself may further help. People who are grieving experience the emotion in waves. A reminder of the lost loved one prompts a surge of emotion that wells up, feels overwhelming, and then subsides. There are moments throughout the day when people who are grieving feel normal and may even laugh and joke. (Some people feel guilty that moments of levity could be interspersed with grieving, but this is normal.) Depression is all-consuming; there are no times during the day when a person feels normal, although the intensity of the depressed mood often diminishes by late afternoon or early evening. Moreover, depressed patients often express a self-contempt that is not seen in uncomplicated bereavement: "I'm no good. I'm worthless. The world would be a better place without me." (Remember that people who are grieving can also become depressed.)

Should I Ask about Depression if My Patient Doesn't Look Sad?

Yes. Depression is sufficiently common that some screening questions must be included in every complete medical and psychiatric evaluation. Patients may pull themselves together and put on their best face for a visit to the physician, leaving a misleading impression of their overall emotional health. Other patients have a mood disturbance that is mild compared with other symptoms. "Are you depressed?" is a poor question. It is so stark that it invites denial, and depression is a diagnosis you must make on the basis of multiple symptoms. Good screening questions include "How has your mood been recently? How are you sleeping? Have you noticed any change in appetite? How's your energy? Any trouble concentrating?"

How Do I Evaluate Suicide?

Suicide must be evaluated carefully. It is helpful to understand that there is a range of suicidal thinking and behavior. Some patients have fleeting thoughts of suicide but no intent to act upon them or plan. Other patients have frequent or even persistent thoughts of suicide but no plan or intent. Passive suicidal ideation describes a thought pattern in which the patient wishes not to be alive but has no thoughts of taking any action to make this happen. It is important to ask about past suicidal thinking or acts, as one of the best predictors of suicide is having made a past attempt. Ask about the intent at the moment and in past attempts and not just the method. Sometimes people do not understand the lethality of taking acetaminophen, for instance, or overestimate the lethality of taking small doses of aspirin or antidepressants. It is important to ask patients what they imagine the effect of their death will be on their families because patients at risk for suicide often feel that their families will be better off without them. It is also important to assess a patient's reasons for living. (Assessment of suicide is discussed more fully in Chapter 17.)

Does Depression Present Differently in Adolescents and Elderly People?

Yes. Elderly patients often present with somatic and vegetative symptoms and not depressed mood. Elderly patients may also present with severe cognitive changes that can appear to be dementia. This is known as pseudodementia and can be difficult to distinguish from dementia. Typically, however, demented patients give incorrect answers to questions and appear to be undisturbed by their cognitive difficulties, whereas patients with pseudodementia give "I don't know" answers and are disturbed by their inabilities. Adolescent depression also often arises without the overt mood symptom of sadness but instead can manifest as irritability, social withdrawal, anxiety, and moodiness.

What Is Included in the Differential Diagnosis of the Chief Complaint "I Am Depressed"?

Patients with other psychiatric diagnoses sometimes present with a chief complaint of "I am depressed." This can be seen in bipolar patients who are in the midst of bipolar depression or mixed bipolar episodes. Sometimes patients with schizophrenia do not feel right because of an exacerbation of psychotic symptoms and describe this as depression. Patients with schizoaffective disorder become depressed. It is also common for patients with personality disorders and borderline personality disorder in particular to have complaints of depression. Patients with all of these diagnoses can in fact be having a major depressive episode, but sometimes the complaint of depression comes from a feeling of unwellness related to the psychotic or personality disorder itself. Patients with primary substance abuse problems also frequently complain of depression. Adjustment disorder with depressed mood is a diagnosis used for patients with mild or brief depressive symptoms with a clear psychosocial cause.

What Are Some Depressive Comorbidities?

Patients with depression frequently have comorbid psychiatric disorders including generalized anxiety disorder, panic disorder, post-traumatic stress disorder, and substance abuse disorders including alcohol and stimulant abuse. Interestingly, patients with a history of depression who attempt to stop smoking cigarettes often become depressed.

Are There Laboratory Tests to Confirm the Diagnosis of Depression?

Not yet, although a number of biologic-physiologic abnormalities have been seen in patients with major depression. For example, when some depressed patients are administered a dose of oral steroid at night, they fail to show the normal suppression of the endogenous cortisol peak early the next morning. Also, many people with depression start rapid eye movement sleep earlier after falling asleep than do nondepressed people, and some degree of immune impairment is common during episodes of major depression. However, none of these observations is sufficiently sensitive or specific to serve as a diagnostic marker. The diagnosis can be made only on the basis of clinical symptoms and course. Laboratory tests are not only helpful but necessary to rule out secondary causes of depression, such as hypothyroidism or HIV infection.

TREATMENT

Is It Necessary to Treat Everybody Who Is Depressed? Don't Most People Pull Out of It Eventually?

If your patient has symptoms of sufficient intensity to justify a diagnosis of major depression, he or she deserves treatment for this illness. It is true that most episodes of depression are self-limited, often resolving, even without treatment, after months or years, but there are compelling reasons to shorten the episode as much as possible. First, it is difficult to comprehend the emotional pain caused by depression. Patients have said that it is like the pain of childbirth or of passing kidney stones except that it seems it will never end. In addition, untreated depression has morbidity and mortality risks. Depressed patients are, of course, at higher risk for suicide, but there are other risks as well. In one study of patients with myocardial infarction, depression was an independent risk factor for mortality equivalent to left ventricular dysfunction. Whether this results from decreased medication compliance or other factors is not known.

What Drugs Are Available for the Treatment of Depression?

An ever-increasing number and variety of antidepressant medications are available (Table 23-3). The older groups, the tricyclic antidepressants (TCAs) and the monoamine oxidase inhibitors (MAOIs), are used less often than the newer drugs despite the fact that they are powerfully effective antidepressants. The TCAs have significant unpleasant side effects for almost everyone who takes them, including sedation, anticholinergic effects (dry mouth, constipation, urinary hesitancy, blurred vision), and orthostatic hypotension. The most serious effect is their cardiotoxicity, with a quinidine-like effect of slowing cardiac conduction; when taken as an overdose, TCAs can be fatal. The MAOIs also cause unpleasant side effects such as weight gain and anorgasmia, but the greatest limitation to their use is the absolute necessity for patients who are taking them to

Table 23-3

Antidepressant Agents

Drug Class	Drug	Trade Name(s)	Typical Doses (per day)	Common Side Effects	Potential Problems
Selective serotonin reuptake inhibitors (SSRIs)	Citalopram	Celexa	20–40 mg	Sexual side effects, gastrointestinal upset, headache, anxiety, insomnia, weight gain	Serotonin syndrome: restlessness, myoclonus, hyperreflexia, diaphoreses, shivering, tremor, and mental status changes
	Escitalopram	Lexapro	10–20 mg		
	Fluoxetine	Prozac, Prozac Weekly	20–60 mg, 90 mg/week		
	Paroxetine	Paxil, Paxil CR	20–50 mg, 25–62.5 mg		
	Sertraline	Zoloft	50–200 mg		
	Fluvoxamine*	Luvox	50–150 mg		
Serotonergic noradrenergic reuptake inhibitors (SNRIs)	Venlafaxine	Effexor, Effexor XR	75–225 mg	Increased blood pressure, sexual side effects, gastrointestinal upset, headache, anxiety, insomnia, weight gain	
	Duloxetine	Cymbalta	40–60 mg		
Tricyclics	Amitriptyline		50–150 mg	Sedation, anticholinergic effects including dry mouth, constipation, blurred vision, and urinary retention; orthostatic hypotension, sexual dysfunction	Cardiotoxic: quinidine-like effect can produce arrhythmia (dangerous in overdose)

(Continued)

Major Depressive Disorder

Major Depressive Disorder

Table 23-3
Antidepressant Agents (Continued)

Drug Class	Drug	Trade Name(s)	Typical Doses (per day)	Common Side Effects	Potential Problems
	Nortriptyline	Pamelor, Aventyl	50–150 mg		
	Imipramine	Tofranil, Tofranil PM	150–300 mg		
	Desipramine	Norpramin	100–200 mg		
Monoamine oxidase inhibitors (MAOIs)	Phenelzine	Nardil	45–90 mg	Sedation, sexual side effects, orthostatic hypotension, serotonin syndrome	Hypertensive crisis: severe headache, diaphoresis, mydriasis, neuromuscular irritability, hypertension, cardiac arrhythmias
	Tranylcypromine	Parnate	10–60 mg		
	Isocarboxazid		20–60 mg		
Others	Bupropion	Wellbutrin, Wellbutrin SR, Wellbutrin XL, Zyban	300–450 mg, 150–400 mg, 150–450 mg	Nausea, anxiety, insomnia	Seizure
	Mirtazapine	Remeron, Remeron Sol Tab	15–45 mg		

*Indicated for obsessive-compulsive disorder only.

maintain a tyramine-free diet to avoid a hypertensive crisis. Because so many foods contain tyramine (beer, wine, aged cheeses, and meats), this dietary restriction can be difficult to follow. It may be impossible for people with cognitive limitations or psychotic symptoms or for children. The selective serotonin reuptake inhibitors (SSRIs) are the most popular antidepressants because of benign side effects and low risk with overdose. Sexual side effects, such as decreased libido, delayed ejaculation, and trouble reaching orgasm, are common with the SSRIs. Other medications such as the venlafaxine, duloxetine, and mirtazapine are called dual-action agents because they affect both serotonin and norepinephrine. Venlafaxine and duloxetine are reuptake inhibitors, and mirtazapine acts as an antagonist at central presynaptic α_2-adrenergic inhibitory autoreceptors and heteroreceptors. Bupropion works on norepinephrine and dopamine and has a very low incidence of sexual side effects.

What Causes Hypertensive Crises with MAOIs and What Foods and Drugs Should Be Avoided?

MAOIs inhibit the enzyme monoamine oxidase. This enzyme metabolizes catecholamines in presynaptic nerve terminals and bioactive amines in the liver and gut. When this enzyme is inhibited in the gastrointestinal tract, foods that are high in tyramine or other vasoactive amines can enter the blood stream and cause a massive release of endogenous catecholamines. This causes sympathetic overactivity including extreme hypertension of the hypertensive crisis. See Table 23-4 for foods, medications, and drugs to avoid. This table is only a general description of the proscribed substances, and patients must be careful to work closely with their doctors to understand the dietary limitations.

How Do I Know Which Is the Right Drug for My Patient?

All antidepressants are effective, but none of them work for all patients. About 60% to 70% of people with major depression respond to any one drug, and about 90% respond after three drugs have been tried. People who have received particular antidepressants in the past and have done well or poorly are likely to have the same response in the future. Unfortunately, for a particular individual who has never received medication for depression, there is no way to predict which of the many available choices will be therapeutic. Consequently, the choice must be based on factors other than anticipated efficacy, such as side effects, dosing complexity, medical status, and cost. It is important to remind your patient that successful treatment may require sequential, empirical drug trials before the drug that works is identified. SSRIs are often chosen as the drug with which to start because of benign and usually well-tolerated side effects, because they are not toxic, and because dosing is usually an easy once-a-day regimen. They are also effective for anxiety disorders including obsessive-compulsive disorder. If a patient's blood relative has responded to a particular drug, it is thought that the patient will have a higher chance of responding to that drug because of shared genes.

Major Depressive Disorder

Major Depressive Disorder

Table 23-4		
To Be Avoided with Monoamine Oxidase Inhibitors		
Foods		
Meats	Preserved poultry, meat, or fish	Smoked fish or meat, salami, mortadella, bologna, pepperoni, pastrami, corned beef, liver, pickled herring
Vegetables	Broad beans	Fava beans, Chinese snow peas, lima beans, black beans, English beans, Italian beans
Dairy	Aged cheeses (strong smell and flavor)	Stilton, cheddar, blue, parmesan, gorgonzola, limburger, romana
Alcohol	Red wine and beer or foods prepared with these forms of alcohol	
Beverages	Excess caffeine	
Other	Excess chocolate and soy sauce, sauerkraut, beef bouillon, marmite, pickles, tofu	
Psychiatric medications	Amphetamines, selective serotonin reuptake inhibitors, tricyclic antidepressants (TCAs)	TCAs and amphetamines can be used in patients with refractory depression but only under very close observation of an experienced clinician.
Medications	Many cough, cold, decongestant, hay fever, and diarrheal medications, diet pills, meperidine, barbiturates	
Drugs	Cocaine	

Is an SSRI Always the First Choice for Treatment?

In addition to prior drug experience, there are specific considerations to be made with individual drugs. Bupropion has been recognized to decrease nicotine craving, so you might want to consider it for your depressed patient who is trying to stop smoking, and it may have some proattentional characteristics. Anecdotal reports suggest that it may be less likely than other antidepressants to induce cycling in bipolar patients. High doses carry a risk of seizure, particularly in patients with eating disorders. The SSRIs are only mildly sedating at best, and you should consider a drug such as mirtazapine for patients with troubling insomnia, although weight gain is common with this medication. Some patients will tell you that the very possibility of sexual side effects is unacceptable, and bupropion or mirtazapine may be a good choice for this reason as well.

During the initial week or so of treatment or after a dose of medication is raised, some patients can feel more anxious with SSRIs, and additional medication such as a benzodiazepine is needed to help the patient through this period.

Do SSRIs Cause Patients to Become Suicidal?

A great amount of attention has been paid to this question lately. It was originally thought that any suicidal thoughts and actions that occurred during a treated depressive episode were due to the underlying depressive illness. Some recent studies have shown, however, that there was an increase in suicidal thoughts (but not behaviors) in a small number of patients who were taking an SSRI as compared with the placebo control group. In general, it is thought that the benefit of treating major depression and thus reducing this suicidal stressor greatly outweighs the very small risk of increasing suicidal thinking. Nevertheless, it is very important to monitor patients who are started on SSRIs for increased suicidality. This most often occurs in the initial weeks of treatment.

Does Treatment Differ in Elderly Patients?

For elderly patients, the general adage of starting at lower doses of medication and raising the dose of the medication slowly also holds for antidepressant treatment. Psychotherapeutic treatment is often cognitive and supportive and less psychodynamic, although this can be beneficial to selected patients. It is not the case that it is "normal" for people to be depressed in the setting of the physical difficulties of old age. Treating the major depressive illness can change the way the patient feels about his or her medical illness, loss of friends and support, or loss of independence.

How about for Adolescents?

As a generalization, psychosocial and psychotherapeutic interventions are more helpful in adolescents than antidepressant medications. Although the antidepressants do have a clear role in the treatment of adolescent depression, studies show that they are less efficacious than in adults. Evaluating stressors and providing support and structure can be particularly helpful. Of the SSRIs, fluoxetine is the only one with Food and Drug Administration (FDA) approval for treating adolescents and children, although the others are used frequently and thought to be equally efficacious. Paroxetine, however, has not been shown to be efficacious and has a greater risk of increasing suicidality—the FDA has recommended against its use in adolescents.

Are Adolescents at Greater Risk for Suicide with SSRIs?

Although SSRIs have been shown to be efficacious in adolescents, there has been a question of SSRIs also increasing suicide risk in this populations. An FDA review of over 2100 patients treated with SSRIs found no suicides but did find an increase in suicidal thinking and behavior, including attempts in 4% of the patients. In the placebo group, this suicidality was found at a rate of 2%. The FDA has thus issued a "black box" warning about this increased risk. More recent studies have corroborated this. On the other hand, there has been increased use of SSRIs in the adolescent population and a concurrent decrease in suicides over the past decade. In sum, it is most likely that a small subset of patients are at greater risk for suicidal thoughts and behaviors when taking SSRIs but the vast majority have their risk of suicide reduced by the effective treatment of depression. As it cannot be determined whether a particular patient falls into this small subset ahead of time, all patients should be monitored closely, particularly during the first 4 weeks of treatment. Changes to watch out for include increased thoughts of suicide, erratic behavior and agitation, sleeplessness, and social withdrawal.

How Long Does It Take for an Antidepressant to Start Working?

It is rare for an individual to feel better right away. Depression begins to lift for most people after 10 days to 4 weeks, and sometimes longer, of continual medication at therapeutic doses. Vegetative symptoms typically improve before mood symptoms do.

How Long Does My Patient Need to Take an Antidepressant?

For a single episode, several months beyond full recovery. Many people think (naturally enough) that they can stop medication once they feel back to normal, but stopping too soon increases the possibility of relapse. Recent thinking in the field holds that patients who have had even a second major depressive episode should take antidepressants for many years if not for life. It is also thought that depressive episodes may have a kindling effect (having an episode makes a patient more likely to have another one). Conversely, therefore, not having episodes makes patients less likely to have future ones.

How Should I Treat a Patient with Depression with Psychotic Symptoms?

Start with the combination of an antipsychotic drug and an antidepressant. When the psychotic symptoms have resolved, the antipsychotic agent can be stopped but the antidepressant is continued for several more months. Patients will need full doses of the antidepressant and full antipsychotic doses of the antipsychotic medication as well. Electroconvulsive therapy (ECT) is also an effective, safe, and quick treatment for a person with depression with psychotic symptoms. In fact, the prognosis for a full recovery from a severe psychotic depression can be better than that for a low-grade chronic depression.

What Is ECT?

ECT (sometimes called "shock therapy") involves the use of a brief pulse of electricity to create a grand mal therapeutic seizure. The seizure, not the electricity, treats depression. Each year between 60,000 and 100,000 people receive ECT. It should be considered for depressed patients with psychotic symptoms and patients who have not responded to medication; other indications are listed in Table 23-5.

Isn't ECT Dangerous?

The morbidity and mortality associated with ECT are less than for all anti-depressants considered collectively (although probably not for the SSRIs considered separately). The primary risk is that associated with general anesthesia, and the main contraindications to ECT are anesthetic contrain-dications, such as cardiac or pulmonary compromise. The major adverse effects of ECT are confusion after the treatment (similar to other types of postictal confusion) and short-term memory loss.

How Is ECT Given?

The procedure is performed in a special suite with adequate resuscitation equipment. The patient receives a general anesthetic agent such as a short-acting intravenous barbiturate, along with a muscle relaxant such as succinylcholine so that the peripheral manifestations of the seizure are blocked. Because of the muscle paralysis, assisted ventilation is required. Electrodes are placed on the two temporal areas (bilateral) or, alternatively, on the forehead and nondominant temporal area (unilateral) (Figs. 23-1 and 23-2). A very brief pulse of electricity is administered to the anesthe-tized patient. Both the voltage and the length of the pulse are calibrated by machine and titrated to induce a brain seizure lasting about 40 to 60 sec-onds. The patient can experience a period of postictal confusion lasting from a few minutes up to 2 hours. If the patient is receiving the treatment as an outpatient, he or she must be accompanied home. Optimally, each patient's seizure threshold is ascertained during the first treatment by finding the lowest electrical dose that induces a seizure. Unilateral treat-ment initiated with an electrical pulse that is 4.5 to 6 times greater than the threshold dose needed to induce a seizure has been shown to be as effec-tive as bilateral treatment. As unilateral treatments result in less short-term memory loss, patients should start with unilateral treatment and proceed to bilateral if this proves ineffective. Bilateral treatment may be the first choice for severely suicidal patients or those who are unable to eat or drink because of their depression. The usual course of treatments is two or three times a week for a total of 6 to 12 treatments.

Table 23-5
Indications for Electroconvulsive Therapy
Previous good response Medication failure Psychotic depression Contraindications to medication Severely suicidal

Major Depressive Disorder

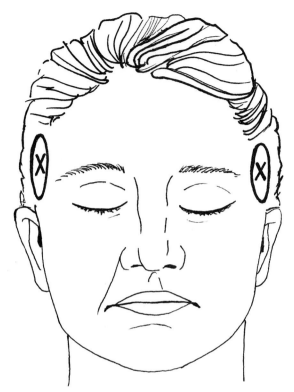

FIGURE 23-1 Electrode placement for bilateral electroconvulsive therapy.

Are There Other Somatic but Nonpharmacologic Treatments besides ECT?

Yes, a great deal of work is being done in this area. Vagal nerve stimulation was initially developed to treat refractory epilepsy but has recently been shown to be effective for refractory depression as well and has received FDA approval. The vagus nerve is connected to areas of the brain involved with mood and sleep. The vagal nerve stimulator is a battery-powered electrical device that is surgically implanted in the chest like a pacemaker and is attached to the vagus nerve. Electrical impulses are then sent to the brain at regular intervals. This stimulation has been effective for some patients in the treatment of depression that has not responded to other means.

Magnetic stimulation therapy is similar to ECT in that a seizure is induced and the patient must be anesthetized and paralyzed. In this case, however, the seizure is induced with a very powerful electromagnetic coil positioned next to the patient's head. The cognitive side effects are minimal, but efficacy is still being studied. Some of the current limitations of this

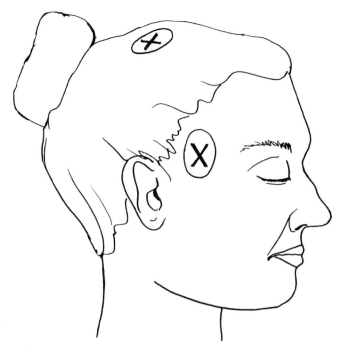

FIGURE 23-2 Electrode placement for unilateral electroconvulsive therapy.

treatment involve the difficulties inducing seizures at deeper areas of the brain that may be more effective seizure induction sites for antidepressant efficacy.

Transcranial magnetic stimulation has been studied in the treatment of depression for over a decade. In this treatment, an electromagnet is used to induce electrical impulses in the brain of an awake patient and no seizure is induced. The electromagnetic coil can deliver pulses to specific areas of the brain involved with mood regulation. The sessions usually take about half an hour and are given 5 days a week for a number of weeks. The side effects are minimal. This treatment is not yet FDA approved.

Does Psychotherapy Work for Depression?

For mild to moderate depression, psychotherapy and medication tend to be equally effective. Many studies have shown, however, that the combination of psychotherapy and medication is more effective than either alone. For severe depressive episodes, pharmacologic intervention is necessary.

Which Psychotherapy Is Best?

This depends on your patient—on his or her previous experience, personality, and interests. The most robust outcome data exist for cognitive psychotherapy and interpersonal psychotherapy, although these modalities are not appropriate for severely depressed or psychotic patients. Psychodynamic psychotherapy is especially useful as a vehicle for understanding the unconscious meaning of events that give rise to depression and the emotional reasons for the patient's maladaptive behavioral patterns. Supportive therapy provides comfort, reassurance, and strategic advice on getting through the day for more seriously depressed patients who are waiting for the medication to take effect. Whereas dynamic therapy tries to help patients understand and then change their intrapsychic defenses against the anxiety caused by underlying internal conflicts, supportive therapy tries to reinforce and shore up these defenses. Inpatient hospitalization may be necessary for patients who are incapacitated by depression or are actively suicidal.

How Do I Treat Dysthymia?

Dysthymia, the milder, more chronic form of depression, responds to the same treatments used for major depression: antidepressant medication and psychotherapy. There are some patients whose symptoms are mild enough that they prefer psychotherapy alone. You should consider, however, the addition of medication for any patient with dysthymia who is not getting better with just psychotherapy. Higher doses of medication than for major depression are sometimes needed.

What Do I Do When My Patient Doesn't Get Better?

When your patient does not get better with a particular medication, you should next try a drug of a different class with a different mechanism, although some patients respond to a different SSRI even if another one has already failed. For the patient who does not improve after trials of several classes of antidepressants, you can try augmenting an antidepressant with lithium, thyroid hormone, or a stimulant such as methylphenidate. Do not overlook the importance of medication combined with psychotherapy. ECT is also an excellent option for refractory depression.

KEY POINTS

- ◆ Depression is not diagnosed on the basis of an identifiable precipitant. Some depressions occur for no discernible reason. Do not ask your patient, "Why are you depressed?"

- ◆ Always ask your depressed patient about suicidal thoughts. However, the presence of suicidal thinking by itself is not diagnostic of depression.

- ◆ If your patient describes persistent early morning wakening, fatigue, and loss of interest in sex, consider depression. Depressed mood is not necessary for the diagnosis.

Major Depressive Disorder

Case 23-1

A 72-year-old woman with no previous psychiatric history is brought to her internist by her concerned son, who reports that she has not been eating well for the past 2 to 3 months and appears to have lost a considerable amount of weight. The woman appears apathetic and answers questions in a flat voice with few words. She complains of profound fatigue and of having no appetite. She falls asleep with no difficulty but wakes after 4 or 5 hours and cannot get back to sleep. Her mother died of colon cancer at age 73, and although the patient has no signs or symptoms, she has become preoccupied with the idea that she also has cancer and has little time left to live. She denies feeling depressed but says she has no interest in anything. Although she was an active gardener, she has not worked in her garden for more than 6 weeks. She said that she no longer reads or watches television because she can't concentrate. Her mental status examination reveals that she is alert and oriented, but recent and remote recall, the ability to perform calculations, and her concentration are all impaired. There are no psychotic symptoms. She is not currently taking any medication, and she does not drink alcohol. Her physical examination (including neurologic examination) is unremarkable.

    A. What work-up should she receive?
    B. What psychiatric diagnoses should be considered?
    C. What treatment do you recommend?

Case 23-2

A 34-year-old woman is admitted to a psychiatric hospital for depression after the birth of her first baby 8 weeks earlier. In the past 10 days, she has developed auditory hallucinations, somatic delusions, and suicidal thoughts. She states that she has the will and the means to take her life and possibly her baby's life as well. A trial of paroxetine and a trial of bupropion had no beneficial effect in the weeks before admission. She had two milder episodes 4 and 6 years earlier, neither of which responded well to a variety of antidepressant medications.

    A. What treatment do you recommend?

Case 23-3

A 51-year-old man comes to his physician complaining of depression for the past 2 months. In addition to the mood disturbance, he has experienced increasing fatigue, hypersomnia, a 15-lb weight gain, trouble thinking clearly, memory impairment, and the feeling of always being cold. He has no prior psychiatric history and no serious medical history. He does not use drugs or alcohol. Physical examination reveals a lethargic and overweight man whose temperature is 36.5 °C. His hair is brittle, and his deep tendon reflexes are sluggish in all extremities.

A. What is the most likely diagnosis?
B. What additional information do you need?
C. How would you treat him?

Case Answers

23-1 A.   *Learning objective:* **Be familiar with the medical differential of depression.** Despite the unremarkable physical examination, the possibility of a medical cause for her symptoms must be considered. It is sensible to start with a general medical screening and then focus on the conditions that can also cause fatigue, anorexia, insomnia, and weight loss. Hypothyroidism would more likely cause weight gain and hypersomnia. A stroke would be unlikely to arise without neurologic findings. A viral infection is possible, and cancer is of particular concern because there is a family history of cancer.

23-1 B.   *Learning objective:* **Understand how depression is diagnosed.** A diagnosis of depression requires *either* a depressed mood *or* the presence of anhedonia (loss of enjoyment in previously pleasurable activities). Although she denies feeling depressed, her loss of interest, fatigue, and appetite and sleep disturbances all strongly suggest the possibility of an episode of major depression. The fact that she has no prior psychiatric history does not rule it out. The beginning of a dementia such as Alzheimer's disease should also be considered. She demonstrates some cognitive abnormalities, although they are not typical of Alzheimer's disease: she has impaired long-term memory, which is often spared for several years in Alzheimer's.

23-1 C.   *Learning objective* **Understand the use of antidepressants in major depression.** It is reasonable to recommend a trial of antidepressant medication, even while the medical work-up is under way. All antidepressants have a delayed onset of action. An SSRI such as paroxetine or fluoxetine is a good first choice because of their benign side effect properties. These SSRIs are extremely unlikely to cause harm and may well provide relief.

23-2 A.   *Learning objective:* **Understand the rationale for various treatments of depression.** The presence of psychotic symptoms means that she would need an antipsychotic medication in addition to an antidepressant medication. However, because of her current and past medication nonresponsiveness, because of the urgency of the current situation created by her suicidal and possibly homicidal thoughts, and because of the need for fast treatment in order to reunite mother and baby safely, a better treatment recommendation is ECT, which is faster, safer, and more likely to be effective than medication.

23-3 A. *Learning objective:* **Recognize medical conditions arising with depressed mood.** Although his symptoms are consistent with an episode of major depression, the presence of physical signs—sluggish deep tendon muscle reflexes, brittle hair—is not. Although there is not enough information to establish the diagnosis, his symptoms (including cold intolerance) and physical findings all suggest hypothyroidism.

23-3 B. *Learning objective:* **Learn how to evaluate depression secondary to an underlying medical condition.** Although hypothyroidism may be at the top of your differential diagnosis, other causes of secondary depression must be ruled out. Thyroid studies may confirm the diagnosis, but other tests such as cortisol levels, complete blood cell count, sedimentation rate, and viral antibodies may also be necessary.

23-3 C. *Learning objective:* **Understand the rationale for treatment of depression.** The appropriate treatment of a secondary depression is treatment of the underlying medical condition. If the final diagnosis is in fact hypothyroidism, your treatment will consist of replacement thyroid hormone. There is no advantage in adding an antidepressant. Antidepressants have a delayed onset of therapeutic action, by which time the thyroid replacement will already have worked.

Major Depressive Disorder

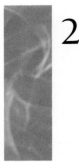

24

Bipolar Disorder

MICHAEL DULCHIN

What Is Bipolar Disorder?

Bipolar disorder is the DSM-IV-TR term used to describe a chronic relapsing mood disturbance that includes manic and depressive episodes. Manic-depression is the term that was previously used. Both terms are misleading, however: a single manic episode (with no episodes of depression) is sufficient to justify the diagnosis of bipolar disorder. A distinction is made between bipolar I and bipolar II on the basis of the severity of the manic episode (Box 24-1).

How Common Is Bipolar Disorder?

Depression is one of the most prevalent psychiatric disorders. About 5% to 10% of the population in the United States are diagnosed with major depression at some time during their life. The rate for bipolar disorder is about 1%, roughly comparable to that of schizophrenia. If bipolar II disorder is included, the prevalence rises to over 3% and may be as high as 6.5% if all bipolar spectrum disorders are included.

What Are the Bipolar Spectrum Disorders?

The bipolar disorders listed in the DSM-IV-TR include bipolar I, bipolar II, cyclothymic disorder, and bipolar disorder not otherwise specified (NOS). Bipolar I involves manic and depressive episodes. Bipolar II involves hypomanic and depressive episodes. Cyclothymia refers to having mood symptoms vary between hypomania and dysthymia. Bipolar disorder NOS describes patients with bipolar symptoms but who do not fall clearly into one of the other diagnostic categories often involving hypomania without clear depressive episodes. Some psychiatrists include the unofficial diagnoses of bipolar III, bipolar IV, and hyperthymic temperament in the bipolar spectrum. Hyperthymic temperament describes people who are unusually ebullient, gregarious, energetic, and extroverted but who do not suffer distress or disability. Bipolar III

BOX 24-1

CLASSIFYING BIPOLAR DISORDER

Bipolar I	Bipolar II
Always one or more manic episodes	Always hypomanic episodes, never manic episodes
May or may not have episodes of depression	Always major depressive episodes

Manic and hypomanic episodes have similar symptoms and differ in severity. In manic episodes, there is always social or vocational impairment; in hypomanic episodes, there never is. Psychotic symptoms may or may not occur in manic episodes; they never occur in hypomanic episodes.

describes a patient with depressive episodes but who has had only manic or hypomanic episodes when receiving antidepressants. Bipolar IV is also an unofficial term that refers to depression superimposed on a hyperthymic temperament.

Who Gets Bipolar Disorder?

People who have a relative with bipolar disorder are more likely than people in the general population to be diagnosed with bipolar disorder. In fact, monozygotic twins have an eightfold greater risk of having bipolar disorder among affected co-twins compared with dizygotic twins. The concordance rate in monozygotic twins is about 75%. There are no sex differences and no differences among racial or ethnic groups or socioeconomic classes.

When Does Bipolar Disorder Tend to Present?

Bipolar disorder is most often diagnosed after a manic episode that characteristically occurs between the ages of 20 and 40. Interestingly, it often takes 8 or so years from the time of first symptoms until the time of diagnosis. Patients often initially present with depressive symptoms and carry a diagnosis of major depression until their first manic or hypomanic episode. These depressive episodes are called pseudo-unipolar episodes. Nearly 70% of bipolar patients have been misdiagnosed before receiving a bipolar diagnosis. Bipolar disorder can arise in childhood and adolescence. It is often difficult to distinguish from attention deficit hyperactivity disorder at this time.

What Causes Bipolar Disorder?

The causes remain elusive, and the underlying pathophysiology is still unclear. This is a bit of a paradox because bipolar disorder is one of the most neurologic appearing of psychiatric disorders. There is a clear genetic component. What is inherited is a vulnerability for the disorder, but the genetic contribution for bipolar I is greater than that for schizophrenia and is much greater than that for major depression. (Bipolar II more closely resembles major depression in etiology, course, and epidemiology.) Moreover, bipolar I is often effectively treated with maintenance medication alone; psychosocial interventions focus on medication compliance. For people with the disorder or the predisposition, it is recognized that certain events may precipitate an episode: periods of sleeplessness (e.g., during a medical internship or while caring for a newborn), travel across time zones, and heavy alcohol consumption. There even is some evidence that the euphoria brought about by happy life events—getting married, winning a prize, getting a big raise—may progress to become an autonomous manic episode in people with the disorder. Women with bipolar disorder are at risk for postpartum depression or mania. In fact, postpartum depressions and particularly postpartum psychoses are frequently a manifestation of bipolar disorder.

EVALUATION

What Should I Look for in the History or Mental Status Examination to Make a Diagnosis of Bipolar Disorder?

Evidence of a manic or hypomanic episode is essential, whether in the current episode or in the past. A single manic episode at any time is sufficient to make the diagnosis of bipolar I. Conversely, the diagnosis cannot be made if a manic episode has never occurred.

The symptoms of a manic episode can be clustered into four groups: mood symptoms, physical symptoms, behavioral symptoms, and (not always present) psychotic symptoms (Table 24-1). The mood during a manic episode is typically euphoric. Patients describe feeling on top of the world, as good as it is possible to feel, or better than anyone in the history of the world has ever felt. Some unlucky manic patients, however, feel no euphoria at all, only irritability, and many people are both irritable and euphoric. Mood lability is also very common. For little or no reason, a person in the middle of a manic episode suddenly and sometimes violently switches from feelings of extreme well-being to furious anger. As a manic episode begins to unfold and throughout its duration, most patients experience great energy in addition to the mood changes. They describe being able to undertake multiple projects and may find that they need very little sleep. The ability to continue functioning and even to be doing more than normal with very little sleep can reach truly impressive proportions. Some patients get by with only 1 or 2 hours of sleep at night; some stop sleeping altogether. Increased libido and a pervasive hypersexuality are common features. Patients are often grandiose and show little insight into their change in mental state. Speech can be rapid and without pauses—pressured speech. The ideas being expressed may move rapidly from one to the next to the next as if there were a superabundance of associations with each idea expressed, a condition commonly described as flight of ideas. Clang associations (a thought disorder in which thoughts are linked by

Table 24-1

Common Symptoms of a Manic Episode

Mood
Euphoria
Irritability
Lability

Physical
Decreased need for sleep
Increased energy
Hypersexuality

Psychotic (May Be Present but Do Not Have to Be)
Grandiose hallucinations
Grandiose and paranoid delusions
Flight of ideas
Clang associations

Behavioral
Increased goal-directed activity
Gregariousness
Increased telephone time
Careless spending
Poor judgment

the sounds of words rather than their meaning) and word salad (incoherent, fragmented speech) can also be manifested.

How Do I Know if My Patient Has Had Prior Manic Episodes?

Your patient may have been diagnosed or treated in the past, but that is not always the case. The average number of misdiagnoses before a patient receives a bipolar diagnosis is 3.5, with the most common being major depression. Because the report of a sustained, elevated mood is so subjective, it may not serve as a reliable indicator of previous episodes. Many people who have had past episodes of depression feel so relieved when the depression has lifted that they describe a normal mood as one of extreme well-being or euphoria. (Conversely, many patients with bipolar disorder describe as a normal mood a state that is actually hypomanic and describe a normal mood as depressed.) Associated symptoms such as a decreased need for sleep, increased energy, undertaking multiple projects, and hypersexuality should be present for a diagnosis of a manic episode. Some striking behavioral abnormalities are seen in many patients who are manic; these may be helpful in making a diagnosis for present and past episodes. Manic patients tend to be gregarious, to talk on the telephone more than usual (typically much more than usual), and to be careless and extravagant with money, spending wildly or even giving away money. Seriously impaired judgment may result in bad business deals, risky sexual involvement, and other superficially pleasurable activities that result in painful consequences. Look for periods of little sleep with lack of tiredness the following day. Periods of extreme irritability and anger can also be part of a manic episode. It can also be helpful to ask if a patient generally has more energy than most people, needs less sleep than most people, is the life of the party, or generally has more "life force" than other people, as some patients are chronically hypomanic prior to a depressive or full-blown manic episode.

Are Manic Patients Psychotic?

Psychotic features may be present, but they are not necessary to make the diagnosis. Psychotic symptoms occur in about one third of manic patients. When they do occur, they are very often consistent with the mood and are likely to include grandiose delusions or hallucinations. Paranoid delusions are also common in psychotic manic persons, and clang associations may also occur. Psychotic symptoms are never seen in hypomanic episodes. Some patients become so thought disordered and agitated that they enter a state called manic delirium.

Are Bipolar Depressive Episodes Different from Unipolar?

When they occur, they are, for the most part, indistinguishable from episodes of major depression, with mood, vegetative, cognitive, and possibly psychotic symptoms. Depressive episodes in bipolar disorder may not last as long as those in major depression, and there is some evidence that atypical depression (increased appetite, hypersomnia) is more common in bipolar disorder. The length of a depressive episode and the presence of atypical features are not, however, diagnostic. There is some thought that a very rapid response to antidepressants or electroconvulsive therapy may be indicative of a bipolar depression, but this also is not diagnostic.

How Common Are Depressive Episodes in Patients with Bipolar Disorder?

Bipolar patients spend much more time in a depressed than a manic state. Approximately 67% of the time that bipolar patients are experiencing symptoms they are of a depressive nature, 20% manic or hypomanic, and 13% mixed.

What Is a "Mixed Episode"?

Occasionally, patients with bipolar I disorder have episodes of serious and debilitating mood disorder that are not clearly manic or depressive but have features of both. They may, for example, experience tearfulness, suicidality, irritability, increased energy, decreased appetite, and decreased need for sleep, all at the same time. A mixed episode can be described as containing the misery of depression and the energy of mania. Patients with mixed episodes are at particularly high risk for suicide.

What's the Usual Long-Term Course in Bipolar Disorder?

Bipolar I is a chronic, episodic mood disorder. People who have a single manic episode have a 90% chance of recurrence, and most patients are at risk for repeated episodes of mania and depression throughout their life. The episodes are usually self-limited, typically lasting a few months. Patterns of recurrence vary enormously from individual to individual, but commonly patients have an episode every few years with periods of normal mood and functioning between episodes. (About a fourth of bipolar I patients have some residual symptoms or impairment between episodes.) There is no predictable relationship between episodes of mania and episodes of depression; one does not invariably follow the other. The risk of a mood episode for women after childbirth is higher than for any other period during life for either men or women with bipolar disorder. This course of illness can make it hard for patients to understand why they need to continue mood-stabilizing medication despite extended periods of euthymia (normal mood) when not taking medication.

Does Bipolar Disorder Go Away as People Get Older?

No, it usually gets worse. As patients grow older, there is a tendency for more frequent and longer lasting episodes. The episodes may also become more refractory to medication.

What Does "Rapid Cycling" Mean?

Rapid cycling is defined by DSM-IV-TR as four or more mood switches in a single year—that is, from manic to depressed or vice versa—regardless of whether there is an intervening period of normal mood. Some patients have even more frequent mood switches. Ultrarapid cycling is sometimes used to describe this situation. Some patients describe mood changes during a single day. This can sometimes be confused with the mood lability of patients with borderline personality disorder. Rapid cycling often happens after many bipolar episodes. It can be caused by antidepressant use and is more common in women. Some patients cycle continuously. Ultrarapid cycling, or ultradian (mood cycles within the course of a day) cycling, can be difficult to distinguish from mixed states.

How Do I Interview a Manic Patient?

Interviewing someone who is in the middle of a full-blown manic episode can be a challenge. The flight of ideas, pressured speech, heightened energy, and emotional intensity may make you feel that you cannot get a word in edgewise. You will need to interrupt, redirect, and continually refocus. Sitting back and letting the patient run with the interview is easy and tempting, but this is unlikely to provide the detailed information you need for an adequate assessment. You may find yourself laughing and caught up in the riotous good spirits of a manic patient, but you must remember that the mood is labile and can quickly turn to irritability and even hostility. Manic patients are potentially dangerous because of the increased energy, the paranoia, the mood lability, and the hypersexuality. You will need to provide a steadiness and clarity that your patient cannot provide. The risk

Bipolar Disorder

is increased for manic patients who have psychotic symptoms. If a patient is too disorganized to provide an accurate history, the interview time is best spent fostering an alliance (as best you can) and taking a mental status, knowing that you can get the history from collateral sources.

Are There Medical Conditions That Need to Be Ruled Out in Evaluating a Patient with Mania?

Hyperthyroidism, Cushing's disease, and multiple sclerosis can all include some features that are similar to a manic episode, but they are unlikely to include the full complement of signs and symptoms needed for a bipolar diagnosis. Obvious physical findings also make a misdiagnosis extremely unlikely. Frontal lobe dysfunction caused by trauma, stroke, degenerative disorders, or tumors can cause intensification of emotions and mood lability. Drug-related states must be given serious consideration in your differential diagnosis. They may be more difficult to distinguish from bipolar disorder than are the medical conditions just mentioned. Central nervous system stimulant intoxication (e.g., cocaine, amphetamines) can cause psychotic symptoms, increased energy, hypersexuality, and a decreased need for sleep. Exogenous steroids, both corticosteroids and androgenic steroids, when taken in excess can lead to a state that may be difficult to distinguish from an acute manic episode. Signs and symptoms of steroid intoxication can include euphoria and mood lability, irritability, paranoia, hypersexuality, and hallucinations and delusions. Table 24-2 lists some causes of secondary mania.

How Can I Distinguish a Drug-Related State from a Real Manic Episode?

There is no substitute for a good history and physical examination. Past medical and psychiatric histories, previous episodes and their treatments,

Table 24-2
Some Causes of Secondary Mania
Medical
Hyperthyroidism
Cushing's disease
Multiple sclerosis
Frontal lobe damage
Trauma
Degenerative disorders
Tumor
Stroke
Drugs
Steroids
Corticosteroids
Anabolic steroids
Central nervous system stimulants

Bipolar Disorder

and known drug use are of obvious importance. Bipolar disorder does not include physical signs. Dilated pupils, increased deep tendon reflexes, tachycardia, and hypertension all suggest an underlying medical or drug-related state. There also may be secondary evidence of prolonged drug use. Men who use anabolic steroids have increased muscle mass, acne and other skin problems, and testicular atrophy; laboratory tests may reveal liver abnormalities. People with heavy prolonged corticosteroid use begin to show typical cushingoid features such as a round moonlike face and truncal obesity. Treatment with mood stabilizers and antipsychotics is often started before the etiology of the mania is known.

What Medical Evaluation Is Necessary for Patients with Bipolar I Disorder?

The medical evaluation serves two purposes: to rule out secondary causes of mania and to screen for medical contraindications to medication. The medical history, review of systems, and physical examination may raise the likelihood of underlying medical illness that can be confirmed with appropriate laboratory studies such as thyroid function tests or cortisol levels. There are no laboratory tests or imaging studies that establish a diagnosis of bipolar disorder; this can be made only on clinical grounds. Because all of the major medications used to treat bipolar disorder are potentially toxic, the examination and laboratory studies must establish the baseline health of the patient's kidneys, thyroid, heart, and liver and the patient's blood counts (discussed more fully later). All three major mood stabilizers are teratogenic, so you must establish pregnancy status for female patients.

What Psychiatric Disorders Are Often Comorbid with Bipolar Disorder or Confused with Bipolar Disorder?

Substance abuse disorders, particularly marijuana, alcohol, and cocaine, are frequently comorbid with bipolar disorder, perhaps up to 60%. Bipolar patients use alcohol and marijuana to "slow down" and use cocaine to enhance euphoria. Attention deficit hyperactivity disorder, bulimia nervosa, borderline personality disorder, and impulse control disorders such as gambling are also often frequently comorbid.

Does a Postpartum Manic Episode Mean That the Patient Has Bipolar Disorder?

It is likely that an initial psychiatric presentation of postpartum mania will require future treatment of or at least monitoring for bipolar disorder. More than 50% of women with a postpartum mania have future manic or depressive episodes.

Are Bipolar Patients at Risk for Suicide?

Bipolar patients are at the highest risk for suicide of patients with all the major psychiatric disorders. The lifetime rate for suicide attempts in bipolar patients is 20% to 25%, and 10% to 15% succeed. Patients who suffer from mixed episodes are at particularly high risk because, unlike patients with major depression, they may have the energy to act on suicidal impulses. Attempts are most likely during mixed or depressed episodes.

What Factors Affect the Prognosis?

The presence of mixed episodes, rapid cycling, and multiple prior episodes makes for a more guarded prognosis in bipolar I disorder.

TREATMENT

What Happens When a Person with Bipolar I Disorder Is Not Treated?

The results of no or inadequate treatment can be disastrous. As many as 25% of bipolar patients make suicide attempts. Impulsivity and grandiose disregard for danger lead patients into dangerous behavior with potentially catastrophic consequences for themselves and for other people. For example, an acutely manic airline passenger may believe himself more capable of flying the airplane than the pilot. Another patient may enter a series of unsafe sexual encounters. Reckless behavior and bad judgment can ruin businesses, disrupt friendships, and seriously jeopardize family relationships. Divorce and unemployment are substantially higher in bipolar populations compared with controls.

What Drugs Are Used to Treat Bipolar Disorder?

The mainstays of pharmacotherapy are the mood stabilizers: lithium, valproate, and to some extent carbamazepine (Table 24-3). The most data are available for these three traditional mood stabilizers—experts favor lithium and valproate because of their greater efficacy and side effect/risk profile. Other drugs that are used but for which there are less convincing data on efficacy include the anticonvulsants oxcarbazepine, lamotrigine, gabapentin, and topiramate. The atypical antipsychotics play a role in treating psychotic symptoms, sedating agitated patients, treating mania, and preventing future episodes. Benzodiazepines are often used to treat agitation, insomnia, and anxiety.

How Do I Choose a Mood Stabilizer for My Patient?

Lithium has been used to treat bipolar I disorder in the United States since 1970, and there is a wealth of research data and clinical experience regarding its use. It remains the medication treatment of choice for acute manic episodes and for long-term maintenance therapy. Lithium is somewhat less effective than valproate in treating mixed episodes and rapid cycling, but these are generalizations to which there are many individual exceptions. Carbamazepine has also been extensively studied and is considered along with lithium and valproate to be a traditional mood stabilizer, although it is usually used by experts as the first of the second-line medications. Sometimes patients need more than one mood-stabilizing agent.

Table 24-3

Mood Stabilizers

Drug	Indications	Typical Doses*	Common Side Effects	Main Toxicities	Teratogenic
Lithium	Acute manic episode Long-term prophylaxis	900–1500 mg/day	Thirst Increased urination Tremor Weight gain	Kidney Thyroid	Yes but infrequent
Valproate	Rapid cycling Mixed episodes Long-term prophylaxis	750–2500 mg/day	Sedation Weight gain Nausea Hair loss	Liver Hematologic	Yes
Carbamazepine	Failure to respond to lithium or valproate Previous good experience	600–1200 mg/day	Fatigue Sedation Dizziness Blurred vision Nausea	Liver Pancreas Hematologic	Yes

*Doses for individual patients may vary considerably.

Bipolar Disorder

What Medical Screening Is Necessary before Starting My Patient on Lithium?

It is most important for you to know the functional health of your patient's kidneys for two reasons. First, lithium is excreted almost completely by the kidneys. (Negligible amounts are lost through sweat, saliva, and feces.) People with impaired renal function have difficulty getting rid of lithium and are at risk for toxic effects. The second reason is that lithium can damage the kidneys, both at high levels and with prolonged use at therapeutic levels. You need to determine baseline blood urea nitrogen and creatinine levels so that the effects of lithium over time can be monitored. You must also obtain thyroid function tests results (thyroid-stimulating hormone (TSH), thyroxine [T_4], and triiodothyronine resin uptake [T_3RU]) to screen for preexisting thyroid disease. TSH alone can be followed for long-term monitoring. Lithium is known to have effects on cardiac conduction, and you should establish a baseline electrocardiogram before starting therapy. Adverse cardiac events, however, are rare in clinical practice, and preexisting heart disease is not an absolute contraindication to using lithium.

How Does Lithium Work?

Lithium affects the second-messenger system in the postsynaptic neuron, but it is not known whether this or another effect results in mood stabilization.

How Do Valproate and Carbamazepine Work?

Both drugs are anticonvulsants that enhance gamma-aminobutyric acid (GABA) neuroinhibition. The GABAergic properties are probably related to their anticonvulsant effect, but it is not yet established whether this is what makes them good mood stabilizers.

Can Lithium Be Used during Pregnancy?

Lithium does pose some risk to the baby developing in utero and can cause abnormalities of the heart and great vessels, especially when the mother takes lithium during the first trimester. The degree of risk, 0.1%, is actually rather small and must be weighed against the risk to mother and baby of not being treated with lithium. Lithium gets into breast milk and may cause side effects such as stomach upset in nursing infants. The long-term consequences of lithium ingestion by newborns are unknown.

How Do I Know What Is the Right Dose of Lithium for My Patient?

The correct dose of lithium is the one that gives a therapeutic blood level, 0.6 to 1.2 mEq/L. Use a higher level to treat acute episodes and a lower level for maintenance. The dose needed to obtain these levels varies considerably and will need to be titrated for your individual patient. A typical starting dose is 300 mg two or three times a day. Watch closely for side effects and for signs and symptoms of toxicity. After 4 or 5 days, obtain a blood sample to check the lithium level and adjust the dose up or down to hit the desired range. The blood sample should be drawn roughly 12 hours after the last dose.

What Happens if the Lithium Level Is Too High?

Lithium toxicity is serious and can be a medical emergency. Early signs of toxicity include nausea, vomiting, and diarrhea. Patients develop dysarthria (slurred speech) and ataxia. At higher blood levels, patients become obtunded or comatose. There are increased deep tendon reflexes, and seizures may develop. Lithium levels above 2.0 mEq/L are toxic, and levels above 3.0 mEq/L are life threatening. Patients can have permanent brain damage. Sudden hypotension and cardiac arrhythmias may signal cardiovascular collapse, which can be fatal.

How Do I Keep My Patient from Becoming Toxic?

Lithium has a narrow therapeutic index, and it is not difficult for the dosage to slip from therapeutic levels into the toxic range. Every person taking lithium should be thoroughly familiar with side effects and early symptoms of toxicity and must understand the circumstances that can increase blood levels. All patients taking lithium should have periodic blood tests to monitor lithium levels—once every 6 months for stable patients on maintenance and more frequently when dosages are being adjusted. Medications that affect renal clearance, such as nonsteroidal anti-inflammatory drugs and thiazide diuretics, must be taken with caution and careful monitoring.

What Side Effects Should I Tell My Patient to Expect?

Almost everyone taking lithium experiences some side effects that range from mild to intolerable. Among the most common are mild tremor, increased thirst (polydipsia), increased urination (polyuria), and weight gain. Polyuria can be a particular nuisance at night. Many people also experience mild gastrointestinal upset and loose stools. More serious gastrointestinal symptoms such as vomiting and diarrhea or neurologic symptoms should arouse your suspicion of toxic levels. If the tremor is significant, you can control it with the addition of a β-blocker. The side effects and toxicities of lithium are summarized in Table 24-4.

Does Lithium Work for Both Depression and Mania?

Lithium prevents the recurrence of both manic and depressive episodes. It is less effective in treating acute depressions than acute manic episodes. In mania, it is not usually effective until the patient has been taking it for 1 to 2 weeks.

Is Valproate Less Toxic than Lithium?

The spectrum of toxic effects is different. The lithium ion is excreted by the kidneys. It is not metabolized and it is unaffected by liver functioning. Valproate, however, is hepatically metabolized and in turn can damage the liver. Elevation of serum transaminase levels is common and usually benign. Serious hepatotoxicity is less common and can be fatal. Other rare but potentially life-threatening effects of valproate are acute pancreatitis and thrombocytopenia. Patients who are taking valproate and who develop either bruising or symptoms of hepatic dysfunction (malaise, lethargy,

Table 24-4
Side Effects and Toxicities of Lithium
Common side effects at therapeutic levels (0.6–1.2 mEq/L)
Polyuria (increased urination)
Polydipsia (thirst)
Weight gain
Tremor
Signs and symptoms of toxic levels (greater than 2.0 mEq/L)
Dysarthria (slurred speech)
Ataxia (unsteady gait)
Increased deep tendon reflexes
Nausea, vomiting, diarrhea
Mental obtundation
Long-term effects at therapeutic levels
Hypothyroidism
Impaired renal function

anorexia, vomiting) should stop taking the drug and be assessed. Women are at risk for developing polycystic ovary disease, and this must be taken into account when prescribing for young female patients.

What Are Common Side Effects of Valproate Therapy?

Alopecia (hair loss), gastrointestinal upset, sedation, and weight gain are all common. These effects are benign, but the ability to tolerate them varies among individuals.

How Do I Decide on a Dose of Valproate for My Patient?

As is true with lithium, the dose must be titrated to a therapeutic blood level, which for valproate is 50 to 100 mg/mL. The usual starting dose is 250 mg three or four times a day. The blood level can be checked after 4 days, and the appropriate dosage adjustments can be made.

Does Maintenance Valproate Therapy Require Laboratory Monitoring?

Yes. You should periodically check blood counts, including platelets, liver functions, and blood levels of valproate. However, these investigations do not replace your regular personal evaluation of a patient receiving maintenance medication. Valproate can also increase ammonia levels.

What Side Effects and Toxicities Are Associated with Carbamazepine?

Common side effects are sedation, fatigue, dizziness, blurred vision, and nausea; these effects tend to diminish with time. More serious reactions include an allergic hepatitis, in which the future use of carbamazepine is proscribed, and blood dyscrasias (aplastic anemia, agranulocytosis,

Bipolar Disorder

and thrombocytopenia). Hepatitis and blood dyscrasias are rare but serious reactions and must be kept in mind. Blood counts should be checked in people who experience bruising or bleeding or in whom an infection develops.

Can I Use Valproate or Carbamazepine for Pregnant Patients?

No. Both agents are teratogenic and more risky than lithium. Valproate is associated with neural tube defects, and carbamazepine is associated with craniofacial abnormalities such as cleft palate. Other abnormalities have been reported. Both drugs get into breast milk in significant concentrations, and they should not be used by nursing mothers.

How Are Atypical Antipsychotic Medications Used in Treatment of Acute Episodes and Maintenance in Bipolar Disorder?

Currently, lithium and valproate are considered the first-line medications and carbamazepine second line. The atypical antipsychotics are playing a large and emerging role, however. Many have been shown to have efficacy in acute mania and some in maintenance and depression. Because of the long-term side effects of these medications and the low but real risk of tardive dyskinesia, the American Psychiatric Association guidelines consider most of the atypicals as second line and best used for psychotic or refractory patients. The Food and Drug Administration–approved agents for manic, mixed, and maintenance therapy include aripiprazole and olanzapine. Risperidone and ziprasidone are approved for manic and mixed episodes, and quetiapine is approved for manic episodes. Expert consensus, however, recommends the use of olanzapine, risperidone, and quetiapine for manic, mixed, and maintenance therapy. As new evidence comes to light, however, the atypicals may be used more often.

If Antidepressants Induce Mania, How Do I Treat Bipolar Depression?

Antidepressants carry the risk of precipitating manic episodes in bipolar patients or of increasing mood cycling. The risk is decreased but not eliminated when the patient is also taking a mood stabilizer. This makes bipolar depression difficult and delicate to treat. There is some controversy in the field about the role of antidepressants. It is generally thought that it is best to try to maximize mood stabilizers to treat depression without the use of an antidepressant if this is possible. Lithium and lamotrigine are the mood stabilizers with the most antidepressant efficacy. It is also generally agreed, if not always practiced, that if an antidepressant is used, a mood stabilizer must be used as well.

Some clinicians are more comfortable using antidepressants, as they feel that because bipolar patients spend much of their ill time depressed and studies have shown depressive relapse with the discontinuation of antidepressants, the benefits of treatment outweigh the risks. Other clinicians are more convinced by studies which have shown that antidepressant use precipitates mania and cycling and feel that the risk of treating the current depression with an antidepressant is offset by the long-term sequelae of increased cycling and possibly worsening the course of illness. These decisions must be made on an individual basis. Tricyclic antidepressants are thought to cause switching and rapid cycling more than bupropion and selective serotonin reuptake inhibitors (SSRIs).

What Dose of Lamotrigine Should I Use?

Lamotrigine has the potential to cause Stevens-Johnson syndrome, a serious and potentially lethal skin condition. For this reason, it must be titrated slowly to an effective dose. It is started at 25 mg per day for 2 weeks, then increased to 50 mg for 2 weeks and then increased to 100 mg. If the patient is also taking valproate, this dosage level is halved and the patient starts at 12.5 mg per day or 25 mg every other day.

What Are Some Other Common Drug Interactions in the Pharmacotherapy of Bipolar Disorder?

The most common drug interactions in the treatment of bipolar disorder involve the anticonvulsant medications. As noted previously, the lamotrigine level is essentially doubled by even small doses of valproate. Lamotrigine lowers the valproate level as well. Carbamazepine has the opposite effect on lamotrigine level, so that a patient receiving carbamazepine will need double the lamotrigine dose. Valproate and carbamazepine are both hepatic enzyme inducers and often reduce the effect of other hepatically cleared medications. Carbamazepine can reduce the levels of valproate, haloperidol, and benzodiazepines and can have its own levels reduced by phenobarbital and phenytoin (Dilantin) and increased by erythromycin and cimetidine. As carbamazepine can also cause agranulocytosis, it should be given with clozapine only in very rare circumstances. Medications that affect renal clearance must be monitored when lithium is being used, as they can affect lithium level. Both valproate and carbamazepine can decrease the effectiveness of oral contraceptives.

How Long Does My Patient Need to Take Medication?

Most patients with an established diagnosis of bipolar I disorder, certainly after three episodes, need lifelong maintenance medication. The situation after a single episode is less clear. Although 90% of people go on to have recurrent episodes, 10% do not. To avoid the unnecessary burden of lifelong medication with potentially toxic drugs, most physicians do not prescribe maintenance therapy after one episode and choose instead to monitor their patients closely in the following months and years. Whether long-term medication should be started after two episodes depends on the severity of the episodes, the length of time between them, and the family history of mood disorders and treatment.

Why Do Patients Stop Taking Medication?

The single greatest cause of relapse is medication noncompliance, and the causes of noncompliance are multiple. Some patients simply do not understand the need for long-term medication and stop taking it when they feel well. Many people stop because they do not like the side effects, and some women who want to become pregnant and are aware of the risks of mood stabilizers during pregnancy stop on their own. Cost is a factor for some people, but lithium, valproate, and carbamazepine are all available in generic form and the expense is relatively modest. Some people simply do not like the nuisance of taking medication on a long-term basis or believe that it implies disability or deficiency. There also are some patients who like being high. They enjoy the energy, exuberance, good feelings, increased productivity, and heightened sexuality. Unfortunately, there is no way to adjust medication to allow for hypomania without risking a full-blown, possibly psychotic episode or an equally devastating episode of depression. Some patients see a hyperthymic or hypomanic mood state as normal and do not feel that medication is needed. In addition, relapse is usually not immediate after the discontinuation of medication and can happen months or even years later. Patients often have difficulty seeing cause and effect when this happens. Compliance is enhanced in an established, trusting therapeutic relationship with free exchange of ideas in both directions. A wise psychiatrist will want to learn the reasons for noncompliance and then make adjustments rather than blame the patient for being uncooperative. Judgment and insight are often the first things to go when a patient's mood becomes elevated, which also contributes to noncompliance.

Is Bipolar II Disorder Treated in the Same Way as Bipolar I Disorder?

The treatment for hypomania is similar to that for mania including mood stabilizers and atypical antipsychotic medication, although there are very few studies looking at hypomania in bipolar II patients exclusively. There is little clear evidence about the treatment of bipolar II patients, particularly with regard to the likelihood of inducing switching to hypomania and cycling. Given this lack of evidence, it is most likely advisable to treat bipolar II depression like bipolar I depression and use mood stabilizers, particularly lamotrigine as first line with the judicious use of antidepressants in addition. Lamotrigine is particularly favored in patients in the depressed phase of bipolar II disorder because it is an effective antidepressant that has a low risk of inducing hypomania or mania.

Does Electroconvulsive Therapy Have a Role in the Treatment of Bipolar Disorder?

Electroconvulsive therapy (ECT) is a safe, effective treatment for both manic and depressive episodes. It works more quickly than medication and should be considered the preferred treatment for patients who are extremely combative, homicidal, or suicidal. It is safe to use during pregnancy and with elderly patients, who may have reduced tolerance for medication side effects. There is some evidence that ECT administered to people who are taking lithium increases the post-treatment confusion. People who are taking lithium should discontinue it for 24 hours before receiving ECT.

Bipolar Disorder

Does Psychotherapy Work for the Treatment of Bipolar Disorder?

Psychotherapy without medication does not work, and it is harmful if it gives your patient the impression that the disorder is being treated. When psychotherapy is used in conjunction with good pharmacotherapy, the focus is often on psychoeducation and compliance. It is helpful in long-term management for patients to be thoroughly familiar with the disorder and to become reliable reporters of their own emotional states. Supportive, cognitive, and behavioral therapies all help patients devise specific coping strategies for the consequences of the disorder. For example, a patient may recognize growing irritability as one of the symptoms of an incipient manic episode and learn to avoid temper flare-ups and confrontations until better medication control is effected.

There are no data to support the effectiveness of psychodynamic therapies in controlling bipolar mood swings. However, the increased self-understanding and the resolution of earlier conflicts that result from these therapies may prevent or repair the loss of self-esteem that sometimes accompanies a serious chronic illness. Group therapy can be an extremely valuable forum for patients with mood disorders to learn about the experiences and coping strategies of others with the same condition. Groups are especially helpful in destigmatizing disorders. Self-help groups organized by and for patients without physician involvement are growing in popularity in large cities across the country. Studies of their effectiveness are lacking, but anecdotal evidence suggests that for at least some patients they can be of considerable benefit when combined with good medication management. Group therapy is contraindicated during an acute episode; patients are too disordered to participate in any meaningful way and will be disruptive to other members of the group.

KEY POINTS

- ◆ The major cause of relapse in bipolar patients is medication noncompliance.
- ◆ Ninety percent of people who have a single manic episode have future episodes.
- ◆ Bipolar I disorder can be diagnosed on the basis of a single manic episode, even in the absence of any episodes of depression.
- ◆ Bipolar depression can be difficult to treat; the use of antidepressants should be evaluated carefully in each patient and a mood stabilizer should always be used concomitantly.
- ◆ A common long-term course for patients with bipolar I disorder is more frequent, more severe, and more treatment-resistant episodes over time.
- ◆ The appropriate treatment for bipolar disorder is medication. Psychotherapy alone does not work.

Case 24-1

A 32-year-old man with a long-standing history of major depression treated with the selective serotonin reuptake inhibitor fluoxetine develops, over a 2-week period, greatly increased energy and libido and the ability to feel refreshed after only 2 to 3 hours of sleep at night. He is in unusually good spirits and has started a number of projects, including teaching himself classical Greek, building hand-crafted wood furniture, and repainting his house inside and out. When he wanted to invest his family's life savings of over $400,000 in a suspicious copper mining venture proposed by a stranger in a restaurant, his wife insisted that he undergo a medical evaluation. His physician finds him to be loud and talking so fast that it is difficult to understand him.

A. What should his medical work-up consist of?
B. What is the most likely psychiatric diagnosis?
C. What treatment is appropriate?

Case 24-2

A 26-year-old woman has an 8-year history of bipolar disorder. During her first pregnancy 4 years ago, she developed preeclampsia with some residual damage to her kidneys. (Typically, her blood urea nitrogen level is 30 mg/dL and her creatinine level is 2.5 mg/dL.) Since that time she has been well controlled with valproate. Three months ago, she stopped taking the valproate on the advice of her physician because she wanted to try to become pregnant again. Six weeks into her pregnancy, she developed signs and symptoms of a manic episode: decreased need for sleep, increased energy, extreme irritability, and the belief that someone was trying to hurt her baby by poisoning the drinking water. Her symptoms are not due to drug use or an underlying medical condition.

A. What medication options are there to treat the manic episode?
B. What nonmedication options are available?

Case 24-3

A 42-year-old woman with recurrent major depressive episodes is well maintained with fluoxetine. During one of her monthly meetings with her psychiatrist for medication management, she appears unusually cheerful and bright. She talks rapidly and describes having had unusual energy during the past 2 weeks. She has been sleeping only 4 to 5 hours at night instead of her usual 7 to 8, but she feels well rested during the day. She is finishing several projects that had gone untouched for months and states that this is the best she has felt in years. She describes one period similar to this one that occurred just after her first depressive episode and resolved after 1 month with no treatment. She has had no trouble at work or in her social relationships. She denies any recent drug or alcohol use and is taking no medications other than the prescribed fluoxetine. She does not have psychotic symptoms, and she has never had a manic episode.

A. What is the most likely diagnosis?
B. Do you recommend a change of treatment?

Case Answers

24-1 A.   *Learning objective:* **Be familiar with the medical differential for a manic episode.** It appears that the man has developed a fairly typical manic episode. The medical work-up will focus on ruling out secondary causes of mania from an underlying medical condition or drug use. His physician will review all drugs the man is taking, both prescription and recreational. A good history, review of symptoms, and physical examination will look for additional evidence of drug use (e.g., dilated pupils, acne with testicular atrophy) or previously undetected medical illness such as hyperthyroidism or endogenous hypercortisolism. A family history of bipolar disorder will be helpful but by itself is not diagnostic. Laboratory tests will extend the search for medical causes and will also prepare for the selection of a mood-stabilizing drug by looking at kidney, thyroid, and liver function tests and blood counts.

24-1 B.   *Learning objective:* **Understand the way in which bipolar disorder is diagnosed.** If the history, physical examination, and laboratory studies do not suggest a medical or drug condition, we can focus on psychiatric diagnoses. The severity of the man's symptoms qualify him as manic rather than hypomanic (especially the foolish and risky investment he is about to make). Although he has a standing diagnosis of recurrent major depression, the occurrence of a single manic episode warrants a change to bipolar I disorder.

24-1 C.   *Learning objective:* **Know the basics of how bipolar disorder is treated.** The SSRI he has been taking for depression may exacerbate symptoms of mania and should be stopped. He will need to take a mood-stabilizing drug. For an acute manic episode, lithium is a good choice if his kidneys are healthy. The dose should be titrated to result in a blood level of about 1.0 mEq/L for the acute episode and should be lowered to around 0.6 mEq/L for maintenance. Whether to begin long-term maintenance lithium therapy is a decision the physician and patient must make together, taking into consideration the unique circumstances of the patient. If the patient is reliable and has a trustworthy network of family and friends who could recognize the early emergence of future manic symptoms, you may wish to withhold maintenance treatment following a single episode and to observe him closely in the months and years after resolution of the episode. Good psychoeducation is essential. He will need to know both the circumstances (such as irregular sleep patterns) that put him at risk and the earliest signs and symptoms of future episodes. If he does receive maintenance medication, an antidepressant can be withheld until proved necessary because lithium is effective in preventing both recurrent manic and depression episodes. Although the man has pressured speech, the case does not clearly describe the presence of psychotic symptoms. If he has hallucinations or delusions, an antipsychotic should be added to the lithium until the psychotic symptoms resolve.

24-2 A.   *Learning objective:* **Understand the indications and contraindications for mood-stabilizing drugs.** Valproate and carbamazepine pose serious risks to the developing baby and should not be used. Lithium has the risk of teratogenicity and could further harm her kidneys; at worst it could lead to a renal failure. A useful alternative may be the atypical antipsychotic olanzapine, which is recognized to have mood-stabilizing properties. Because she appears to have a psychotic symptom (the belief about the drinking water being poisoned sounds delusional), she would probably need the addition of an antipsychotic anyway.

24-2 B.   *Learning objective:* **Be familiar with nonpharmacologic ways of managing bipolar disorder.** With close medical supervision, a pregnant woman is sometimes able to ride through a mild episode of mania with no medications other than occasional treatment for insomnia. The presence of psychotic symptoms makes this much less likely. ECT is an effective treatment for acute manic states and poses minimal risk to mother or baby.

24-3 A.   *Learning objective:* **Be familiar with the different classifications of bipolar disorder.** Her current episode is one of hypomania. She has had major depressive episodes in the past but has never experienced a manic episode. This defines a diagnosis of bipolar II.

24-3 B.   *Learning objective:* **Understand the different treatment approaches to bipolar I and bipolar II.** It is not at all clear that this woman needs the addition of a mood stabilizer to her antidepressant. Her current hypomanic state does not appear to be destructive or intolerable, and she had a previous episode that resolved without treatment. It would be acceptable to continue fluoxetine alone and to observe her closely for the emergence of more troublesome manic symptoms. An alternative approach would be to suspend the fluoxetine and observe her closely, planning to restart the antidepressant when the hypomanic episode subsides. Frequent cycling or more serious symptoms may indicate the need for a mood stabilizer in the future.

Bipolar Disorder

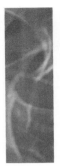

25

Anxiety Disorders

MOLLY E. POAG

Part I. Overview

ETIOLOGY

How Common Are Anxiety Disorders?

Anxiety disorders are the most common of all psychiatric disorders. Studies indicate that about one in four people develop an anxiety disorder at some point in their life. Anxiety disorders often begin in childhood, and women are at a higher risk than men.

EVALUATION

Do I Need to Be Concerned about Looking for Anxiety Disorders If I'm Not a Psychiatrist?

Absolutely. Anxiety disorders are extremely common in a general medical practice and are often missed. One recent study found that over 75% of patients with panic disorder initially seek treatment from a primary care practitioner or emergency department. Other studies have shown that only about 25% of patients with an active disorder have received any treatment. Ask patients directly if they or anyone in their family has ever had anxiety. Reports of headaches, muscle tension, insomnia, worrying, "nervous habits," or patterns of avoidance raise suspicion and should prompt very detailed questioning about criteria for the specific disorder.

Do I Need to Screen for Other Psychiatric Disorders?

Yes. Most anxiety disorders are associated with high rates of comorbidity. For example, up to 90% of patients with generalized anxiety disorder (GAD) have another mental disorder, and up to 70% develop major depression at some point in their life. Most patients with panic disorder also have an additional anxiety or mood disorder at some point in their illness. Conversely, over half of all depressed patients also suffer from at least one comorbid anxiety disorder. Alcohol abuse is also common.

TREATMENT

What Drugs Should I Use to Treat Anxiety Disorders?

Antidepressant medications and high-potency benzodiazepines are the most effective classes of psychotropic agents for anxiety disorders. Because of their equal efficacy and superior side effect profile, selective serotonin reuptake inhibitors (SSRIs) are the first-line treatment for panic disorder, social anxiety disorder, obsessive-compulsive disorder (OCD), and post-traumatic stress disorder (PTSD). The first antidepressants that were shown to be effective were the tricyclic antidepressants (TCAs), and they should be considered depending on comorbidity or failure of the SSRIs (related to side effects or lack of efficacy). Although the side effects of TCAs are numerous, they can sometimes be used to advantage, such as for insomnia or pain. Monoamine oxidase inhibitors (MAOIs) are effective for panic disorder and social phobia but necessitate a strict low-tyramine diet to minimize the risk of hypertensive crisis. High-potency benzodiazepines (alprazolam or clonazepam) are also efficacious but carry the risk of dependence and withdrawal if used on a long-term basis. Buspirone, a 5-hydroxytryptamine (serotonin)1A partial agonist, is sometimes useful for GAD but cannot treat panic or other anxiety disorders. Agents that selectively target GABA systems, such as tiagabine and other anticonvulsants, represent an exciting future direction for anxiolytics, with the goal of improved efficacy and fewer adverse side effects. The medications used to treat anxiety are outlined in Tables 25-1 and 25-2.

Are Antidepressants Used in the Same Way for Anxiety as for Depression?

As a rule, "start low and go slow." Patients with anxiety disorders are more susceptible to the activating effects of antidepressants, including agitation and anxiety. Although antidepressant dosages of the medication should be reached, the starting dose should be lower and rate of rise slower. Also, all of the antidepressants take 3 to 6 weeks to have effect, so initially patients may require combined treatment with a benzodiazepine, which can be tapered after 1 to 2 months.

Are Psychological Treatments Useful for Anxiety Disorders?

Many anxiety disorders tend to be chronic, with relapse rates of up to 50% or greater when medications are discontinued. Some studies have shown that treatment with cognitive-behavioral psychotherapy (CBT) is better tolerated and more durable than treatment with medication and of equal efficacy in some of the disorders. CBT has also been shown to treat comorbid anxiety disorders in patients being treated specifically for panic disorder. Behavioral therapy is particularly effective for specific phobias and OCD.

Table 25-1

Major Medications Used for Anxiety Disorders

Medication	Typical Daily Doses* (mg/day)	Starting Dose
Selective Serotonin Reuptake Inhibitors		
Paroxetine (Paxil)	10–60	10 mg/day
Sertraline (Zoloft)	50–200	12.5–25 mg/day
Fluoxetine (Prozac)	20–80	5–10 mg/day
Fluvoxamine (Luvox)	50–300	25-50 mg/day
Citalopram (Celexa)	20–60	10 mg/day
Escitalopram (Lexapro)	20–60	10 mg/day
Tricyclic Antidepressants		
Clomipramine (Anafranil)	150–250	12.5 mg/day
Imipramine	150–300	10–25 mg/day
Nortriptyline (Pamelor)	50–150	10–20 mg/day
Desipramine (Norpramin)	150–300	10–25 mg/day
Monoamine Oxidase Inhibitors		
Phenelzine (Nardil)	45–90	15 mg/day
Tranylcypromine (Parnate)	30–60	10–20 mg/day
Benzodiazepines		
Alprazolam (Xanax)	1–8	0.25 mg qid
Clonazepam (Klonopin)	1–4	0.25 mg bid
Lorazepam (Ativan)	2–12	1.0 mg bid
Azaspirones		
Buspirone	10–60	10 mg bid

*Doses for individual patients may vary considerably. bid, two times daily; qid, four times daily.

Table 25-2

Anticonvulsants: Potential GABA Enhancing Agents for Anxiety Treatment

Medication	Typical Daily Dose* (mg)	Starting Dose (mg)
Valproic acid (Depakote)	750–2000	250–500
Carbamazepine (Tegretol)	600–1600	200–400
Lamotrigine (Lamictal)	200–400	25
Gabapentin (Neurontin)	600–3600	300–600

*Doses for individual patients may vary considerably.

Is Education of Patients Important in Treating Anxiety Disorders?

Definitely. Patients need to be educated about the basis for their symptoms, naming of the condition, and the rationale for treatments. Education about the importance of adequate sleep, stress management, caffeine reduction, and adverse effects of substance use is critical. Lifestyle counseling including exercise and planning pleasurable activities is also useful.

Part II. Specific Disorders

What Are the Specific Anxiety Disorders?

Although anxiety is a common feature, the specific disorders differ significantly in their severity and prognosis and in the events or settings that trigger anxiety (Table 25-3). Treatment (and education of patients) is most effective when a specific diagnosis has been made.

PANIC DISORDER

ETIOLOGY

How Common Is Panic Disorder?

The lifetime prevalence is 1% to 3%, but in primary care settings, about 1 in 10 patients meets the criteria for panic disorder. Even higher rates have been found among patients in specialty practices such as cardiology. Patients with panic disorder use medical services five times as often as the general population. The onset of panic disorder is commonly between

Table 25-3	
The Major Anxiety Disorders	
Panic disorder with or without agoraphobia	Sudden paroxysmal bouts of intense fear with physical symptoms (agoraphobia is the fear and avoidance of situations in which the patient might be trapped in open spaces without help)
Social phobia (social anxiety disorder)	Intense anxiety about scrutiny by others resulting in embarrassment or humiliation
Specific phobia	Unrealistic fear and avoidance of a specific thing or situation
Generalized anxiety disorder (GAD)	Feeling anxious all the time without reason
Obsessive-compulsive disorder (OCD)	Presence of obsessions (unwanted, intrusive thoughts) or compulsions (the urgent need to perform needless ritualistic acts) or both
Acute stress disorder (ASD)	Emotional numbing and reexperiencing the traumatic event through nightmares or daytime flashbacks; symptoms last less than 4 weeks
Post-traumatic stress disorder (PTSD)	Reexperiencing a traumatic event through nightmares and daytime flashbacks; symptoms last more than 4 weeks after the trauma

the ages of 15 and 25 years and is often preceded by a stressful life event within the year before the initial attack.

What Causes Panic Disorder?

Numerous theories exist, but no complete pathophysiologic mechanism has been determined. Central biologic theories involve a hypersensitized "alarm response" or a defective inhibitory system—the "fight or flight" system gone awry. Panic disorder runs in families. First-degree relatives of a person with panic disorder are up to eight times more likely to develop panic disorder. Twin studies support a genetic contribution. Psychological theories involve psychologically meaningful triggers for the attack, perhaps through the neuroendocrine impact of an extremely stressful life event leading to the development of panic disorder. A primarily biologic basis is supported by the fact that the initial panic attack (and often subsequent attacks) is spontaneous or occurs without a cue. In addition, attacks can be triggered in patients with panic disorder (although not in normal subjects) by the administration of lactate, yohimbine, or flumazenil and by manipulations of CO_2. Patients with panic disorder also have decreased heart rate variability, which may be linked to cardiovascular problems and malignant arrhythmias.

EVALUATION

How Does Panic Disorder Usually Present?

Patients are likely to appear in general medical settings, often emergency departments. The initial attack occurs "out of the blue" and has a rapid escalation within about 10 minutes. The intense anxiety rarely lasts beyond 30 minutes. Typically, a patient has both physical and cognitive symptoms (Box 25-1); fear of dying is common. Results of the medical work-up are typically negative. The Panic Disorder Severity Scale is a seven-item scale that may be useful diagnostically and after treatment.

When Should I Suspect That an Organic Factor Is Causing Symptoms of Panic Disorder?

Numerous medical and substance use disorders can cause panic attacks and can mimic panic disorder. For example, more than half of adult

BOX 25-1	
COMMON SYMPTOMS OF PANIC ATTACKS	
Physical Symptoms	**Mental Symptoms**
Palpitations	Fear of dying
Shortness of breath	Fear of losing control
Chest pains	Fear of going crazy
Lightheadedness	

Anxiety Disorders

male patients with alcoholism have panic attacks at some point. Hyperthyroidism is one of many medical disorders that can present with panic symptoms. In general, patients who have physical symptoms but no cognitive panic symptoms are more likely to have a medical or drug-related cause. Onset of the symptoms in the 30s or later is also suggestive. A careful history, physical examination, and laboratory studies are necessary to make the distinction.

When Should I Suspect Depression?

Patients with panic disorder are at significant risk for depression, especially if the disorder goes untreated. In fact, approximately two thirds of patients with panic disorder develop a depression at some point, and one in four patients with major depressive disorder has panic symptoms. If your patient appears sad or hopeless or has suicidal thoughts, a diagnosis of depression should be suspected. Decreased sleep and appetite should be asked about, but anxiety disorders alone often impair sleep and are associated with decreased appetite and weight loss. Suicide risk is significantly greater in panic disorder patients with comorbid depression.

If This Is My Patient's First Panic Attack, Does He Have Panic Disorder?

No. Isolated panic attacks are not uncommon and can occur in the context of numerous medical and psychiatric conditions. In panic disorder, attacks are recurrent and are followed by fear of another attack, worry about the consequences or meaning of the attack, and behavioral change (often, avoidance or frank agoraphobia).

TREATMENT

What Are the Essential Goals of Treatment?

Regardless of the type of treatment chosen, there are essentially four major goals: to resolve or reduce the panic attacks, to resolve or reduce anticipatory anxiety, to minimize avoidance, and to treat comorbidities.

Should I Start Treatment with Medication?

If there are no relative contraindications to pharmacotherapy, medications have the advantage of producing faster relief (within 2 to 6 weeks) than psychotherapy. Numerous antidepressants are effective. SSRIs are considered first-line treatment given their favorable side effect profile (few anticholinergic side effects, safe cardiovascular profile, and low lethality in overdose) and related superior compliance. TCAs (imipramine and clomipramine) are well studied and work well, but side effects are burdensome. MAOIs are also effective. There have also been some small studies supporting the effectiveness of venlafaxine (a serotonergic noradrenergic reuptake inhibitor) and selected anticonvulsants (although not carbamazepine) for panic disorder. Bupropion was deemed ineffective, but new data are confounding. In sum, the choice of antidepressant should be based on symptoms and side effects. (For example, a patient with insomnia may benefit from a sedating antidepressant such as amitriptyline.) High-potency benzodiazepines are also effective for panic attacks; they have an immediate onset of action, giving a patient relief within the same day. They may not, however, be a good choice if there is a history of substance abuse.

How Long Should I Continue an Effective Medication?

To reduce the risk of relapse, the medication should be taken for 12 to 18 months. When it is time to discontinue the medication, taper slowly. CBT can facilitate the medication taper. If relapse occurs, resume medication treatment.

Is Psychotherapy Effective for Panic Disorder?

Yes. Some studies indicate that CBT is as effective as pharmacotherapy and possibly more enduring. Most patients' symptoms recur when they stop taking medication; CBT results in more permanent change. Psychoeducation—about the illness, treatments, and other relaxation or lifestyle strategies—is also a powerful element of the therapy for this disorder. Family education or treatment is sometimes appropriate.

What if My Patient Is an Alcoholic or a Drug Abuser?

It is critical to explain to the patient the relationship between substance use (even caffeine) and panic attacks and that initial treatment must be of the substance use disorder. This may involve detoxification or rehabilitation if the patient has a dependence disorder. Once the substance use is in remission, the patient may or may not require pharmacologic treatment for panic disorder. If so, antidepressants are the best choice. GABAergic agents hold future promise for anxiety in general and may be especially helpful for this population.

Will the Presence of Depression Change My Treatment Strategy?

Comorbid depression increases the risk of suicide. Benzodiazepines alone are not adequate and in fact can worsen the depression. Because SSRIs, TCAs, and MAOIs are all effective treatments for panic disorder and depression, the class and specific agent may be chosen on the basis of the type of depressive symptoms (e.g., insomnia versus hypersomnia) and the side effect profile of the antidepressant.

What If My Patient Does Not Respond to Medications or CBT?

Consider an undiagnosed medical condition, a personality disorder, substance abuse, undiagnosed comorbidities, and noncompliance.

SOCIAL PHOBIA

ETIOLOGY

How Common Is Social Phobia?

The primary fear for a patient with social phobia is intense anxiety about scrutiny by others resulting in embarrassment or humiliation. This disorder is actually quite common and accounts for about 10% to 20% of all patients with anxiety disorders seen in psychiatry outpatient settings. Community samples estimate a lifetime prevalence of more than 10%.

How Do People Develop Social Phobias?

No one really knows. Social phobia begins early, usually in the teens, although even in childhood it can arise as excessive shyness in a toddler or as extreme difficulty in starting school. Children display heightened sensitivity to rejection and show general social avoidance. Adolescents who develop social phobia may have intense anxiety about dating or participation in group sports or may worry for weeks about an upcoming social event. There is probably a strong biologic vulnerability, but negative developmental, social, or interpersonal experiences with authority figures or groups appear to be important.

EVALUATION

What Should I Look for to Make a Diagnosis of Social Phobia?

Patients with social phobias typically fear scrutiny by others and worry that they will be embarrassed or humiliated. Sometimes they worry that they will throw up or pass out; sometimes they worry simply that others will see their anxiety. Although they recognize their fears as excessive, they avoid the social situations that trigger symptoms, which often leads to isolation, loneliness, and depression. If they cannot avoid the situation, they are likely to endure it with great distress.

Does Fear of Public Speaking Mean My Patient Has Social Phobia?

Yes. This is a particularly common type of social phobia, essentially limited to performance situations. It usually causes much less impairment than generalized social phobia, and the treatments differ. In generalized social phobia, the fears and limitations are more pervasive and the prognosis is poorer; patients experience intense anxiety about most social situations outside the family or home (e.g., parties, dating, school). Without treatment, generalized social phobia, especially when accompanied by mood and substance use disorders, often leads to decreased school and work achievement.

How Do I Ask My Patient About Possible Social Phobia?

Patients with social phobia rarely spontaneously report their fears and symptoms; the encounter with the physician often re-creates a feared

Anxiety Disorders

"social" situation with an authority figure. Patients may seem extremely self-conscious during the interview, appearing tongue-tied or embarrassed, and their palms may be sweaty. Asking patients how they feel on the job, what they do for fun (including social events), and to whom they are close is useful for screening. The physician should listen for discrepancies in social versus solitary activities. Asking about physical symptoms of anxiety, especially a problem with blushing, can help pick up social phobia. Finally, ask directly if the patient ever feels uncomfortable with unfamiliar people or in particular social situations.

What Other Psychiatric Conditions Are Common in Patients with Social Phobia?

As with all anxiety disorders, depression and alcohol and drug abuse are common.

How Can I Distinguish Social Phobia from Other Anxiety Disorders?

Agoraphobia can appear to be social phobia, but in agoraphobia the patient's anxiety is reduced if she is with someone regardless of whether she is in a social situation. Having a companion does not usually help a person with social phobia. Patients with GAD report global anxiety, which is often somewhat better in social situations, perhaps because of distraction.

There are also many useful rating scales for assessing social phobia. The Social Interaction Anxiety Scale (SIAS) and the Social Phobia Scale (SPS) are companion self-report measures, are easy to administer, and have also been shown to separate social phobia from other anxiety disorders.

Can a Panic Attack Be Part of Social Phobia?

Yes, but in social phobia the history of social anxiety and avoidance should precede the panic attack, and the attack will have occurred in the setting of anticipating or enduring a social situation. In panic disorder, the panic attack occurs out of the blue.

Is Social Anxiety the Same in All Cultures?

No. Social fears appear to be affected by cultural beliefs. For example, in Asian cultures the fear is often of offending others rather than of personal humiliation or embarrassment. In Japan, taijin kyofushos ("fear that one's bodily odor is offensive to others") is common.

TREATMENT

Isn't a Diagnosis of "Social Phobia" Just an Attempt to Medicalize Shyness?

Probably not. Social phobia has been an underrecognized condition associated with significant morbidity. In children, school refusal and inability to play with others can increase the risk of significant psychiatric illness with lasting consequences into adulthood. Teens and adults with social phobia are likely to have poorer school and job performance, are less likely to date or marry, and are at risk for suicide, especially with coexisting depression or drug abuse.

Is Medication Helpful for Social Phobia?

Yes, but the response is often partial. SSRIs are now considered the first-line treatment for social phobia. MAOIs are also well studied and effective but require strict adherence to a low-tyramine diet and can cause hypotension and hypertensive crisis. However, about 50% of patients do not have an adequate response to the first SSRI trial. If an increased dose is not fully effective, switching to or augmenting with clonazepam is a reasonable next step. Some data support a role for the anticonvulsant gabapentin and possibly glutamate antagonists, but more research is needed. β-Blockers (propranolol or atenolol) can be useful for social phobia restricted to performance situations with prominent autonomic symptoms such as tachycardia and hand tremor. Taken 1 hour before the performance, β-blockers are effective in diminishing or eliminating such symptoms. They are not effective for generalized social phobia and should be avoided in patients with asthma or cardiovascular illness.

Won't I Cause My Patient to Become Addicted if I Treat Her with Benzodiazepines?

Except in patients who have a history of substance abuse, benzodiazepine addiction or abuse is extremely uncommon (especially with clonazepam), although those who have taken benzodiazepines for 3 or 4 weeks have a withdrawal syndrome on discontinuation. A slow taper (a decrease of 0.25 mg of clonazepam or its equivalent every 2 weeks) is necessary when the drug is to be stopped. With a mean daily dose of about 2.5 mg, this can take 4 to 5 months.

Are Psychological Treatments Effective?

Yes, and they are particularly useful because medication response may be partial and relapse rates after medication-only treatments are high. CBT helps decrease anxiety and avoidance. Some studies suggest that CBT group therapy is most effective. The use of psychological treatments may be a first choice during pregnancy and breastfeeding and in patients with various medical problems.

Will Medication for Social Phobia Interfere with the Psychotherapy?

On the contrary, decreasing anxiety with medication may help a patient make behavioral changes with psychotherapy. The combination of medication and CBT is the treatment of choice.

SPECIFIC PHOBIAS

ETIOLOGY

What Causes Specific Phobias?

Specific (or simple) phobias are syndromes of intense acute fear and apprehension triggered by specific objects or situations, such as spiders or heights. They may originate in part through hyperactivity of pathways involving the amygdala, an area of the brain that alerts to danger. There may also be failure of habituation to innate fears or a lack of congruence between cortical and emotional memories. The development of specific phobias runs in families, although affected family members often have different subtypes (or foci) of the disorder. A blood phobia seems to have a strong genetic component. Some specific phobias follow a traumatic event associated with the focus of the phobia, such as a hurricane or dog bite, suggesting an environmental trigger activating the phobia in a biologically vulnerable individual.

How Common Are Specific Phobias?

Specific phobias are extremely common, especially in childhood. In fact, before the age of 18 years, the phobia must persist for at least 6 months to qualify as a disorder. As a group, specific phobias are the most common of all the anxiety disorders. Overall, about 1 in 10 people have a specific phobia at some time in their life. Women are affected to a greater degree than men, but sex differences vary depending on the subtype (Table 25-4).

When Do Specific Phobias Develop?

Generally between childhood and young adult life, with peaks that occur depending on the subtype (Table 25-5). Periods of stress may trigger a specific phobia that had previously been more of a vague fear or aversion.

Table 25-4

Specific Phobia Prevalence

Phobia	Lifetime Prevalence (% of General Population)	
	Female	**Male**
Spiders, bugs, mice, snakes	6.63	2.44
Heights	4.57	3.36
Transportation (airplane, bus, elevator)	3.80	1.33
Being in water	3.58	1.28
Storms	2.95	0.83
Being in closed spaces	2.67	1.36
Other harmless animals	1.42	0.33

Anxiety Disorders

Table 25-5	
Phobias and Age of Onset	
Phobia	**Peak Age of Onset**
Animals/insects	Early childhood
Storms/weather	Early childhood
Heights	Teens
Situational	Young adulthood

EVALUATION

What's the Difference between an Everyday Fear and a Phobia?

Specific phobias involve intense fear of a specific object or situation, but the diagnosis of "phobia" includes avoidance and functional impairment based on the fear and avoidance, respectively. A nanny with a fear of spiders who is fired because she cannot take the children outside for fear of encountering a spider has a specific phobia of the animal subtype.

How Do I Ask about Phobias?

Very often patients do not describe their phobias without being asked; men especially tend to underestimate their fear. Patients often avoid bringing the problem up during a general medical visit because just talking about the phobic stimulus creates tremendous anxiety or even a panic attack. A useful screening question is, "Have you noticed any fears that keep you from doing what you want to do? A fear of dogs? Riding in an elevator?" Screening tools such as symptom checklists or self-report measures that include questions about circumscribed fears of common objects or situations also may be useful.

If My Patient Has Panic Attacks, How Can I Decide if They Are Related to a Specific Phobia versus Panic Disorder?

Patients with specific phobias often experience anxiety in the form of a panic attack when exposed to the phobic stimulus. This is especially true with the situational subtype.

Determine whether the focus of the fear is an object or a situation (as in specific phobia) versus the fear of having another panic attack (as in panic disorder). In a patient with a specific phobia, fear of the particular object (e.g., spiders) often precedes by years the full phobic syndrome, with avoidance and dysfunction.

TREATMENT

How Treatable Are Specific Phobias?

Specific phobias are among the most treatable of all psychiatric disorders. About 90% of patients obtain relief, often quickly, with behavioral psychotherapy, sometimes with only a few sessions. Exposure-based behavioral therapy is the treatment of choice. It involves confrontation by the patient of the phobic stimulus. Features of a behavioral psychotherapy that seem helpful in the treatment of specific phobias are outlined in Table 25-6.

Are Medications Effective for Specific Phobias?

No; in general, behavioral psychotherapy with some cognitive techniques is the indicated treatment for specific phobias. Benzodiazepines are sometimes appropriate for certain situational phobias, such as flying. If common comorbid conditions such as depression exist, appropriate medication such as an SSRI should be considered.

GENERALIZED ANXIETY DISORDER

ETIOLOGY

How Common Is Generalized Anxiety Disorder?

About 1 in 20 people have GAD, and, like panic disorder, GAD is more common in women (about 2:1 ratio). These patients are chronic worriers and experience a number of chronic physical symptoms of anxiety.

When Do People Develop Generalized Anxiety Disorder?

As with social phobia, GAD often begins in childhood or adolescence, although some studies have shown a peak age of onset around 21 years, similar to that in panic disorder. Once present, the disorder is fluctuating but chronic, with exacerbations at times of stress.

What Causes Generalized Anxiety Disorder?

The specific biologic and psychological mechanisms are not fully known. One theory is that GAD is associated with abnormalities at the gamma-aminobutyric acid (GABA)–benzodiazepine receptor complex, but a long list of neurochemical and neurotransmitter system abnormalities have been described. Studies of patients with GAD and comorbid cardiac disease implicate impaired autonomic flexibility in patients with GAD. Neuroimaging studies suggest abnormalities of the basal ganglia and limbic system.

Table 25-6
Behavioral Psychotherapy Features Associated with Successful Treatment of Specific Phobias
Short intervals between sessions Longer sessions (1 to 2 hours) Real-life exposure to the phobic stimulus (not just imagery) Therapist involvement in the real-life exposure Use of family members (e.g., parent) as coaches for homework between sessions

Anxiety Disorders

Psychologically, worry can serve the function of avoiding other more specific and noxious emotions (e.g., anger). Cognitively, these patients selectively attend to threatening or personally relevant stimuli or thoughts. A hallmark of GAD is its high rate of comorbidity with other psychiatric disorders, in some studies up to 90%.

Who Gets Generalized Anxiety Disorder?

Lower socioeconomic status, recent stressful life events, family history of generalized anxiety or depression, and being female are some risk factors for GAD. Comorbid medical illness can also put a patient at risk. For example, a study of poststroke patients revealed that one in four met criteria for GAD. Common comorbid psychiatric disorders are depression, dysthymia, panic disorder, agoraphobia, and alcoholism.

EVALUATION

How Do Patients with Generalized Anxiety Disorder Usually Present?

Patients usually present in the primary care setting, often with physical complaints of headaches, fatigue, muscle aches, and other physical symptoms. Unlike those in panic disorder, however, the symptoms are not paroxysmal but are chronic and fluctuate over a long period of time. Worry is the cornerstone of this disorder, but the worries are excessive and unrealistic.

What's the Difference between Generalized Anxiety Disorder and Normal Worrying?

In GAD, anxiety is present regardless of whether there are worrisome events, and there is general worry about the future. In addition, when presented with the regular problems of daily living, patients with GAD tend to view them as catastrophes. For example, informing such a patient that you would like to recheck some laboratory results can be experienced by the patient as a probability that she has cancer. Common fears are shown in Box 25-2.

How Should I Ask My Patient about Generalized Anxiety?

Although palpable anxiety and general somatic complaints may manifest during an initial office visit, primary care physicians need time-efficient

---

BOX 25-2

SOME COMMON FEARS IN GENERALIZED ANXIETY DISORDER

Fear of poverty (despite adequate resources)
Fear of becoming medically ill
Fear that one's child will become ill
Fear of losing a job

Anxiety Disorders

techniques to elicit psychosocial data to diagnose disorders such as GAD. Stuart and Lieberman proposed a set of questions with the acronym BATHE (Box 25-3.). A patient with GAD answers these basic questions in a way that makes clear the excessive and unrealistic worry and the inability to control or manage that worry.

TREATMENT

What's the Best Treatment for Generalized Anxiety Disorder?

Medication treatment, cognitive psychotherapy, relaxation techniques, and anxiety management techniques (e.g., time management) all appear to be helpful in treating generalized anxiety. Acute phase treatment of anxiety is most responsive to medications, but relapse rates with discontinuation are again high.

What Medication Should Be Used?

Antidepressants, benzodiazepines, and buspirone are all effective. Given the rule of comorbidity with GAD, the choice should include the consideration of depression, any history of substance abuse, onset of action, and any medical conditions. Antidepressant dosage is generally the same as that used to treat depression. Benzodiazepines are effective but have the risk of exacerbating depression or inducing dependence. With buspirone, there is a delay of 2 to 4 weeks between start of the medication and therapeutic benefit.

BOX 25-3

SOME SCREENING QUESTIONS FOR GENERALIZED ANXIETY DISORDER ("BATHE")

Background:
"What is going on in your life?"

Affect:
"How do you feel about that?"

Trouble:
"What troubles you the most?"

Handling:
"How are you handling that?"

Empathy:
An empathic or supportive statement, when appropriate, to conclude.

From Hidalgo RB, Davidson JR. Generalized anxiety disorder. An important clinical concern. Med Clin North Am 2001;85:711–733 with permission from Elsevier.

OBSESSIVE-COMPULSIVE DISORDER

ETIOLOGY

How Common Is Obsessive-Compulsive Disorder?

OCD is best understood as a group of heterogeneous conditions primarily defined by the presence of obsessions and compulsions. It is quite a common disorder and underreported, in part because patients are secretive about their symptoms. Patients usually recognize that their thoughts (obsessions) and behaviors (compulsions) are abnormal and experience a great deal of shame about their condition. Even latency-age children see their symptoms as odd or "crazy" and try to conceal them from friends and family. Patients with OCD have distressing symptoms on average for 5 to 10 years before presentation. Lifetime prevalence appears to be close to 2.5%. Onset of the illness is usually in adolescence, and it becomes fully manifest by the early 20s. Presentation in childhood is more common in boys, but lifetime rates are equal for men and women. Pediatric autoimmune neuropsychiatric disorder associated with streptococcal infection (PANDAS) is an interesting variant of OCD that occurs in some children who have had a streptococcal infection. These children may have neuroreceptor vulnerability, in the basal ganglia, to streptococcal antibodies. PANDAS often includes tics and other motor abnormalities.

What's the Difference between Obsessions and Compulsions?

Obsessions are unwanted thoughts or impulses that create intense anxiety. Compulsions are behaviors that temporarily reduce or neutralize the anxiety. Pure obsessions without compulsions are rare. Compulsions can be physical (e.g., hand washing) or mental (e.g., counting) ritualized behaviors.

Is Obsessive-Compulsive Disorder Biologic, or Is It Caused by the Way People Are Raised?

Numerous findings support a biologic basis for the development of OCD. Concordance in monozygotic twin studies ranges from about 50% to 85%, compared with 20% to 50% for dizygotic twins. First-degree relatives of people with OCD are five times as likely as the general population to have OCD. In other words, if a parent has OCD, his child has about a 1 in 10 chance of developing the disorder. Environmental factors combined with genetic loading probably lead to expression of the illness. Positron emission tomography studies in persons with OCD show increased glucose metabolism in the orbitofrontal cortex and caudate nucleus. Recent functional imaging studies suggest abnormalities in the brain pathway involving the prefrontal cortex, the corpus striatum, and the thalamus in people with OCD. Early parenting styles were once thought to be important but probably have little to do with the development of OCD.

Anxiety Disorders

How Are Obsessions and Compulsions Related?

Intrusive and typically unwanted thoughts (obsessions) lead to increasing anxiety. The anxiety leads to a compulsive repetitive behavior that temporarily decreases anxiety. With time, the obsessions again intensify, and the cycle of obsessions alternating with compulsions is perpetuated, often with shortened periods of relief. A number of common subtypes of obsession-compulsion pairs are listed in Box 25-4.

EVALUATION

When Should I Suspect That a Patient Has Obsessive-Compulsive Disorder?

Because patients are often ashamed of their obsessive thoughts and compulsive behaviors or fear they are going crazy, they rarely complain about these symptoms until they are causing severe distress. It is therefore important to ask directly about the presence of obsessive thoughts or ritualized behaviors. Rates of OCD are increased in the postpartum period and also following miscarriage. Asking by giving common examples (e.g., hand washing, checking, getting things "just right") is helpful. Telling the patient that these thoughts and behaviors are not uncommon and that good treatment is available also helps. Patients who avoid common activities (e.g., cooking or driving) should be asked if specific worries get in the way. If the patient endorses some of these symptoms, use of rating scales such as the Yale-Brown Obsessive Compulsive Scale are helpful for monitoring treatment.

Is the Physical Examination Helpful in Diagnosing Obsessive-Compulsive Disorder?

It can be, at least in raising the suspicion. For example, patients with OCD who have hand-washing rituals—among the most common rituals—often develop dermatitis of the backs of their hands. (Early OCD researchers would sometimes recruit subjects by screening patients at dermatology clinics.) The presence of motor tics would also prompt questions for OCD, as they are often comorbid conditions.

BOX 25-4	
SOME COMMON SUBTYPES OF OBSESSIONS AND COMPULSIONS	
Obsession	**Compulsion**
Contamination	Washing
Doubt	Checking
Aggressive thoughts	Confessing or checking
Symmetry	Rituals

Anxiety Disorders

Do Patients with Obsessive-Compulsive Disorder Always Think That Their Thoughts or Rituals Are Senseless?

Generally, a patient's insight into the senseless nature of the symptoms helps distinguish OCD from psychotic disorders such as delusional disorder or schizophrenia. Although most patients with OCD view their symptoms as senseless or excessive, a minority of patients with OCD experience their symptoms as reasonable or plausible. This variant of OCD has sometimes been termed OCD without insight, or schizo-obsessive disorder, and may indicate treatment with an SSRI and an antipsychotic agent. Surprisingly, some studies have indicated that a patient's degree of insight does not predict response to medication or behavioral treatments.

How Can I Differentiate Obsessive-Compulsive Disorder from Obsessive-Compulsive Personality Disorder?

Patients with OCD always have obsessions or compulsions or both. Patients with obsessive-compulsive personality disorder have neither obsessions nor compulsions. They are individuals who tend to be perfectionists and inflexible and who see nothing wrong with themselves. (Obsessive-compulsive personality disorder is discussed more fully in Chapter 28.)

TREATMENT

Is Medication or Psychotherapy the Best Treatment for Obsessive-Compulsive Disorder?

Treatment with serotonergic agents and treatment with behavioral therapy have both been shown to decrease OCD symptoms. In fact, each treatment alone was shown to decrease metabolic activity in the caudate nucleus (Fig. 25-1). A combination of pharmacotherapy and behavioral therapy yields the best results. Analytic psychotherapy is not usually helpful in this disorder and sometimes makes the condition worse. It is important to educate patients that the natural history of OCD is a waxing and waning course and that although treatment is likely to diminish symptoms, fluctuating increases are common. Stress appears to increase symptoms.

What Medications Are Most Effective in Obsessive-Compulsive Disorder?

SSRIs and clomipramine (a TCA with a prominent serotonin effect) work best. Antidepressant doses of clomipramine (150 to 250 mg) should be used, but patients with OCD may require SSRI doses that are much higher than those used to treat depression (e.g., fluoxetine at 80 mg rather than 20 mg). The choice of drug will be based on side effects. Because there is a high degree of comorbidity with OCD, the need for augmentation strategies is common. Severe depression or bipolar disorder may require the addition of lithium. The presence of near delusions or tics may be helped by a low-dose antipsychotic. Refractory OCD with severe disability may respond to a trial of intravenous clomipramine or stereotactic neurosurgical procedures.

MEDICATION THERAPY   BEHAVIOR THERAPY

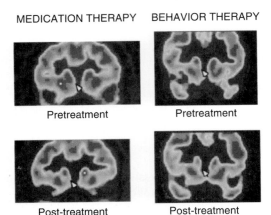

FIGURE 25-1 Positron emission tomography scans with [^{18}F] fluorodeoxyglucose in obsessive-compulsive disorder. Decreased right ventral-medial head of caudate nucleus (arrows) glucose metabolism in patients with obsessive-compulsive disorder who were successfully treated with either medication or behavioral therapy alone. These findings were the first documentation of specific biologic brain changes in response to nonsomatic psychiatric therapy. (From Baxter L Jr, Schwartz JM, Bergman KS, et al. Caudate glucose metabolic rate changes with both drug and behavior therapy for obsessive-compulsive disorder. Arch Gen Psychiatry 1992;49:681–689.)

What Type of Behavioral Therapy Is Useful?

The main technique that is used is exposure and response prevention. This involves helping the patient expose herself to gradually increasing amounts of the feared situation or thoughts while preventing her from responding with the usual compulsive behavior. For example, a patient who has contamination fears will slowly increase contact with dirty feared objects and will resist washing her hands ritualistically. Flooding imagery (often with a videotape) is sometimes helpful, and thought stopping (using a wrist rubber band to interrupt obsessive thoughts) has also been tried with some success.

Should I Encourage My Patient to Talk About His Obsession?

No. When the presence of obsessions is clear, your job is to get your patient to stop thinking about them. Talking about them can make them worse.

Do Obsessive-Compulsive Disorder Symptoms Return When Treatment Is Stopped?

Yes. Although 85% of patients achieve some reduction in symptoms with medication and behavioral therapy, 90% of people treated with medication relapse with discontinuation, and 25% of those treated with behavioral therapy relapse when therapy is stopped. Treatment with pharmacotherapy is usually chronic; behavioral treatment is more enduring.

Anxiety Disorders

DSM-IV: POSTTRAUMATIC STRESS DISORDER

ETIOLOGY

How Common Is DSM-IV: Posttraumatic Stress Disorder?

Stress is ubiquitous, and many people experience or witness life-threatening trauma at some point in their lives, yet PTSD was thought to be relatively uncommon and often synonymous with combat syndromes. Some studies, however, indicate a lifetime prevalence of about 9%, or 1 in 12 people. Common traumatic events that can trigger PTSD in vulnerable individuals are listed in Table 25-7.

Why Do Some People Develop DSM-IV: Posttraumatic Stress Disorder and Others Not?

Ninety percent of people who experience severe trauma do not develop PTSD. Risk factors include early separation from parents, prior history of depression or anxiety disorders, a family history of anxiety or depression, prior history of exposure to severe trauma, severity or "dose" of trauma, and lack of social support. Biologic vulnerability probably also plays a role. Protective factors, such as specific cultural rituals, may decrease risk for some.

EVALUATION

When Does DSM-IV: Posttraumatic Stress Disorder Develop?

Technically, a trauma-related stress disorder should not be called PTSD until symptoms have lasted for 1 month after the traumatic event, but in most cases PTSD symptoms begin within days or a few weeks. When symptoms have lasted for more than 3 months, PTSD is termed chronic. The duration is extremely variable and severity can fluctuate. With treatment, most patients recover in months to 1 to 2 years, but a sizable minority have

Table 25-7

Common Traumas Associated with Development of DSM-IV: Posttraumatic Stress Disorder

Sudden unexpected death of a loved one
Violent crime
Domestic violence
Sexual assault
Natural disaster
Combat
Terrorism or manmade disaster
Traumatic childbirth/complicated pregnancy

Anxiety Disorders

persistent symptoms. For example, some survivors of the Nazi concentration camps with PTSD have had severe symptoms 50 years later.

What Is Acute Stress Disorder?

Acute stress disorder (ASD) is very similar to PTSD but refers to symptoms that appear within days of the trauma and that can last up to 1 month. If the symptoms last longer than 1 month, the individual is diagnosed with PTSD. There is some evidence that treatment of ASD with CBT is effective for decreasing symptoms of ASD and prevention of PTSD.

What Symptoms Should I Be Looking For?

The cardinal symptoms are reliving the traumatic event through daytime flashbacks and nightmares. In addition, many individuals avoid reminders of the trauma and demonstrate symptoms of hyperarousal such as insomnia or an exaggerated startle response.

What Else Should I Look for in My Patient with DSM-IV: Posttraumatic Stress Disorder?

Substance abuse, especially alcohol abuse and dependence, is an extremely common complication in patients with PTSD. Patients who present with PTSD symptoms should be asked detailed, nonjudgmental questions about their substance use patterns and any change in these patterns since the traumatic event. Depression is present in about 50% of patients with PTSD, and suicidal ideation should be asked about. Fear, paranoia, and dissociation as well as delusions or hallucinations may all be part of the clinical picture of PTSD. Continued trauma should also be considered.

Do Patients Usually Seek Treatment for DSM-IV: Posttraumatic Stress Disorder?

No. Retelling of the trauma is feared and avoided, and the avoidance symptoms often extend to health care workers. Patients may present complaining of sleep problems, panic attacks, or intense anxiety but do not spontaneously disclose a traumatic event. You should ask gently about other PTSD symptoms but allow the patient to titrate the degree to which he feels comfortable discussing the trauma. PTSD symptoms should be explored following traumatic childbirth or a complicated pregnancy.

TREATMENT

How Soon Should I Treat a Patient with DSM-IV: Posttraumatic Stress Disorder?

Intervention after trauma and support for ASD symptoms should be offered as soon as possible. Educate patients that it is normal to have some stress symptoms after severe trauma. Encourage patients to use existing social

Anxiety Disorders

supports such as staying and talking with family and friends. A patient's religious community can offer very helpful support. Help patients let go of irrational guilt (often "survivor guilt"). Patients with hyperarousal symptoms of ASD may require the short-term use of hypnotic agents. The brief use of benzodiazepines for intense anxiety can be helpful, but they must be used cautiously, given the high comorbidity of substance abuse. Referrals for trauma counseling and to support groups are often helpful in the early stage.

When Is Medication Indicated?

When symptoms are severe and impair daily functioning. Insomnia, depression, panic, and suicidal thoughts are also reasons to start medication. If patients have ongoing stress related to the trauma, such as job loss or financial hardship, medication may help prevent increasing severity of PTSD symptoms and depression.

What Medications Are Most Useful?

All SSRIs at regular antidepressant doses are effective for many individuals and are the first-line pharmacologic treatment for PTSD. If not, venlafaxine, a tricyclic, or mirtazapine can be tried. Insomnia is often a core symptom of PTSD, and trazodone is a first-line treatment at low doses (50 to 200 mg). If nightmares are prominent, α-adrenergic antagonists (such as prazosin), low-dose TCAs, or atypical antipsychotics are alternatives. Short-term use of benzodiazepines for intense anxiety may be appropriate if substance abuse is not an issue, although, again, benzodiazepines are controversial for PTSD symptoms. Buspirone can also be used but takes a number of weeks to be effective. Future directions for somatic treatments other than medication include repetitive transcranial magnetic stimulation (rTMS). (See Chapter 23 for a fuller discussion of rTMS.)

How Long Should Pharmacotherapy Be Continued after Response?

Pharmacotherapy should be continued at least 1 year to reduce the risk of relapse.

What Psychotherapies Are Most Useful in DSM-IV: Posttraumatic Stress Disorder?

CBT has proved to be most useful. Exposure therapy consists of desensitization through progressive exposure to reminders of the trauma but without avoidance. Cognitive therapy may help correct irrational beliefs and guilt. Anxiety management techniques such as muscle relaxation, breathing retraining, visual imagery, reframing, assertiveness training, and thought stopping have all been used with benefit. Support groups and group psychotherapy are also helpful for certain patients.

Anxiety Disorders

KEY POINTS

Overview

◆ Anxiety disorders are the most common of all psychiatric disorders.

◆ Patients with anxiety disorders usually present to their primary care physician.

◆ First-line treatments for anxiety disorders include the following:

   SSRIs and high-potency benzodiazepines

   Cognitive-behavioral psychotherapy (CBT)

KEY POINTS

Panic Disorder

◆ Patients with panic disorder usually present to a medical setting fearing a severe medical illness.

◆ Panic disorder is chronic and fluctuating, but patients respond well to antidepressants and CBT.

KEY POINTS

Social Phobia

◆ Social phobia has an early onset, often in childhood.

◆ The treatment of choice for social phobia is antidepressant medication and CBT.

◆ Untreated social phobia increases the risk for drug abuse and depression.

KEY POINTS

Specific Phobias

◆ Specific phobias are the most treatable of all psychiatric disorders.

◆ The treatment of choice for specific phobias is exposure.

Anxiety Disorders

KEY POINTS

Generalized Anxiety Disorder

◆ Generalized anxiety disorder (GAD) is characterized by chronic worry and anxiety symptoms.

KEY POINTS

Obsessive Compulsive Disorder

◆ Obsessive-compulsive disorder (OCD) has a biologic and probably a genetic basis.

◆ OCD has high comorbidity (depression and other anxiety disorders).

◆ The treatment of choice for OCD is serotonergic medication combined with behavioral therapy.

KEY POINTS

DSM-IV: Posttraumatic Stress Disorder

◆ Posttraumatic stress disorder (PTSD) is more common than previously recognized.

◆ Early support and even pharmacologic treatment may prevent the development of full PTSD.

◆ SSRIs, CBT techniques, and group therapy are first-line treatments for PTSD.

Case 25-1

A 24-year-old woman presents to your office 2 months after experiencing a sudden onset of tachycardia, shortness of breath, weakness, and fear that she was about to drown while swimming in the ocean in front of her family summer home. The experience came on "out of the blue" and persisted intensely for close to 15 minutes, requiring her best friend to swim in with her to shore. Since that time, she has had bouts of similar symptoms nearly once a week. Despite enjoying the ocean and her long-time summer home, she returned to a city apartment but is fearful of staying there alone. She has stopped driving and takes only showers rather than her usual bath because baths have triggered episodes. The patient graduated from college the previous spring and has been debating between applying to graduate school and getting a "meaningful job." About 6 months ago, her college boyfriend broke up with her. Overall, however, she had been well and busy before the swimming incident.

A. What laboratory tests, if any, are indicated?
B. If the medical work-up is unremarkable, what should you tell the patient?
C. What is your initial treatment plan?
D. Would you refer this patient for psychotherapy?

Case 25-2

A 19-year-old art student presents to your office with fears that his lungs and brain are being contaminated by various environmental toxins. He fears toxins in bus and car fumes as well as in all prepared foods. He is 5 feet 9 inches and weighs 125 lb. He describes pervasive anxiety about the route he took to your office today because he inadvertently passed a doorman using polish on decorative brass and he cannot stop thinking that the fumes may have harmed his brain.

A. What is your initial diagnostic impression?
B. What other diagnoses should you be concerned about?
C. If the physical examination and laboratory test results are normal, how will you treat this patient?

Case 25-3

A 42-year-old businessman who has been a patient of yours for many years with no known psychiatric history comes to your office complaining of insomnia, intense anxiety, and a wish to move to a small country town after his escape from a fire in his office building 3 weeks earlier. He describes nightmares and periods when he can see flames and smell smoke engulfing the office and corridors. He tearfully describes guilty feelings and intrusive thoughts of colleagues trapped on the floors above him. He has been staying in the suburbs with his family and has avoided returning to the city except for this appointment. To keep the appointment, he drank a six-pack of beer earlier in the day.

A. What is your diagnosis?
B. What other questions should you ask?
C. How will you treat this patient?

Case Answers

25-1 A. *Learning objective:* **Recognize that the initial evaluation of patients with panic disorder with or without agoraphobia should include laboratory work to rule out a medical cause of the attacks.** Although this young healthy female, like most patients with panic disorder (especially because she has symptoms of agoraphobia), will have normal laboratory work, initial evaluation should include urine toxicology, a metabolic profile, thyroid-stimulating hormone (TSH), complete blood cell count, human chorionic gonadotropin , and, given her tachycardia, an electrocardiogram.

25-1 B. *Learning objective:* **Medical education about panic disorder and treatment options is the first treatment intervention.** In many cases, explaining that panic disorder is a common and treatable physiologic condition itself often decreases anxiety and even the frequency and duration of the panic attacks.

25-1 C. *Learning objective:* **Consider the risk/benefit ratio of initial treatment with medication versus psychotherapy for a particular patient.** Pharmacologic treatment of panic disorder is fastest if there are no relative contraindications and the patient is open to the use of medication. Initial treatment with an SSRI would be a good choice. If the panic attacks are occurring multiple times per week, initial augmentation with a benzodiazepine would give fast symptomatic relief. If the patient is reluctant to take medication, initial treatment with cognitive-behavioral psychotherapy (CBT) and relaxation techniques is a reasonable approach. In a pregnant patient, an initial CBT trial would probably be preferable.

25-1 D. *Learning objective:* **Be familiar with the indications for psychotherapy in a patient with panic disorder.** This patient has developed fear of staying alone, of bathing, and of driving over a period of months. These behavioral patterns are unlikely to respond to medication alone. Gradual exposure, relaxation, and cognitive reframing techniques are useful to target the agoraphobia. In addition, the effects of the psychotherapy may be more enduring and decrease the rate of relapse.

25-2 A. *Learning objective:* **Understand the main differences between OCD and delusional disorders.** You need to determine whether this patient thinks his fears are senseless or exaggerated. Typically, patients with the anxiety disorder OCD have insight about their fears. Patients whose fears are part of a primary psychotic disorder, such as schizophrenia or delusional disorder, are certain their fears are legitimate. Occasionally, patients seem to fall between these two poles, making the distinction on the basis of insight alone more difficult.

25-2 B. *Learning objective:* **Recognize the high comorbidity associated with anxiety disorders.** This patient is significantly underweight. Although this may be secondary to obsessive fears of toxins in foods, he may also have decreased appetite and weight loss because of a major depressive episode. A complete physical and neurologic examination and basic laboratory work should also be done to rule out medical illness, which might account for weight loss and emergent OCD symptoms.

25-2 C. *Learning objective:* **Be familiar with treatment for OCD.** Any SSRI is a good first-line treatment. Start at 25% to 50% of the antidepressant dose to avoid initial activation or panic, but increase to higher than antidepressant dose (e.g., 60 to 80 mg of fluoxetine) for OCD. Full response may take longer (2 to 3 months) than for depression symptoms.

25-3 A. *Learning objective:* **Understand the relationship between acute stress disorder (ASD) and post-traumatic stress disorder (PTSD).** Technically this man is suffering from ASD because his symptoms have not persisted for more than 1 month, at which point the syndrome would be termed acute PTSD. Clinically, however, the syndromes are very similar, consisting of hyperarousal symptoms, reexperiencing, and avoiding.

25-3 B. *Learning objective:* **Recognize the high comorbidity associated with stress disorders.** This man is tearful and expresses feelings of guilt. Although these symptoms can be accounted for by ASD or PTSD, they should also prompt a review of symptoms of major depression, including suicidal ideation. This patient also illustrates the use of alcohol to cope with anxiety. A history of prior substance use, family history of substance use or abuse, and post-trauma use should be obtained to assess for a current substance abuse disorder.

25-3 C. *Learning objective:* **Be familiar with treatment for PTSD.** SSRIs at normal antidepressant doses are often effective in decreasing PTSD symptoms. Hypnotics and short-term use of benzodiazepines may be helpful for insomnia if there is no history of substance abuse. This man should also be referred for behavioral psychotherapy because of his prominent avoidance symptoms. Support groups and group psychotherapy with patients who have experienced similar trauma can also be very helpful.

Anxiety Disorders

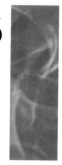

26

Substance Use Disorders

MARIANNE T. GUSCHWANN

What Are Substance Use Disorders?

They are behavioral syndromes caused by the use of drugs or alcohol ("substances"), and they exist on a spectrum of severity from misuse to abuse and finally to dependence. A particular drug may cause intoxication, withdrawal, abuse, and dependence as well as psychiatric symptoms. (*Intoxication* is what happens when a person *takes* the drug; *withdrawal* is what happens when he *stops* taking it.)

What's the Difference between Abuse and Dependence?

A diagnosis of substance *abuse* is made when a person repeatedly experiences a bad consequence from the use of a drug—a failure to meet expectations at school or work or a legal problem. Examples include driving while drunk, getting into fights after drinking, and using a drug despite worsening health problems (e.g., using alcohol with liver disease). *Dependence* describes all of the problems of abuse *plus* tolerance, withdrawal, or compulsive use. A physical withdrawal syndrome is not required for dependence if there is a pattern of compulsive drug use. This makes possible a diagnosis of dependence for drugs such as marijuana that do not cause marked physiologic withdrawal.

What Is Tolerance?

Tolerance is the phenomenon whereby prolonged exposure to a substance causes decreased effects (or larger amounts of the substance are needed for the same effect). A nontolerant individual may feel her muscles relax and mood lift after one alcoholic drink, whereas a tolerant individual may require several drinks to achieve the same effects.

What Is Drug Addiction?

"Addiction" is not a medical term. Its use in lay conversations is roughly equivalent to "dependence" with an emphasis on the person's not being able to stop using the drug.

249

Isn't Addiction a Matter of Control?

Yes and no. DSM-IV-TR criteria for dependence include symptoms of out-of-control use (more substance is taken than intended, unsuccessful efforts to control use). However, even though environmental and social factors contribute to the development of a substance use disorder, genes have an influences as well. In addition, the brain is altered with prolonged drug and alcohol use, and these changes may contribute to the development of an addiction.

Who Develops Problems with Drugs and Alcohol?

People of all ages, socioeconomic levels, and ethnicities. People who begin using alcohol or drugs in their early teens greatly increase their chance of developing a substance use disorder.

What's the Difference between a Social Drinker and an Alcoholic?

Most people (80%) drink alcohol at some point in their lives. Approximately 50% of the general population are current drinkers. Many of those people experience a problem related to alcohol such as drinking too much and getting sick or experiencing a hangover. Most of those who experience a problem try to cut down or stop using alcohol. Many succeed; if they are able to sustain this reduction or elimination of use, they are probably not alcoholics. It is those who have difficulty stopping alcohol use who are alcoholics. Although the use of illicit drugs is much less common, the same principles apply. Many more people try an illicit drug than actually develop a problem.

How Common Are Substance Use Disorders?

The lifetime prevalence is almost 15% for alcohol abuse or dependence and roughly 6% for drugs. Twice as many men as women develop alcohol abuse or dependence. The sex difference is even greater with other drugs (more men than women are affected).

What Drugs Are We Talking About?

There are dozens, but it's easier to talk about *classes* of drugs that have similar effects. Four major categories are stimulants, depressants, opioids, and a heterogeneous class of "others" that includes cannabinoids, inhalants, and club drugs. Common drugs of abuse are listed in Table 26-1.

Aren't Nicotine and Caffeine Addictive?

Absolutely. Once you start using them, it's hard to stop.

Why Aren't They Listed in Your Table on Drugs of Abuse?

Maybe they should be. DSM-IV-TR describes a caffeine intoxication syndrome (the most prominent symptom is anxiety) and a nicotine dependence and withdrawal syndrome (symptoms are depression, insomnia, and

Table 26-1

Classes of Common Drugs of Abuse

Central nervous system stimulants
    Amphetamines
    Cocaine
Central nervous system depressants
    Alcohol
    Benzodiazepines
    Barbiturates
Opioids
    Heroin
    Morphine
    Codeine
    Meperidine
    Hydrocodone
    Oxycodone
Others
    Cannabinoids
      Marijuana
      Hashish
    Hallucinogens
      PCP (phencyclidine)
      LSD (lysergic acid diethylamide)
      Ketamine (special K)
      Methylenedioxymethamphetamine (MDMA) (ecstasy, X)
    Inhalants
      Toluene
      Acetone
      Butane

irritability). One difference between caffeine and nicotine and the other drugs of abuse is that despite very widespread use, impaired judgment and specific *behavioral* problems are exceedingly rare. It is very unlikely that a person will miss work or have an automobile accident because of caffeine or nicotine. (Cynics argue that this is because they are so easy to get: if caffeine and nicotine were as unavailable as heroin, behavioral problems would increase.) Nevertheless, caffeine and nicotine use must be considered in any comprehensive health assessment.

Is Marijuana Addictive?

Yes. In fact, more people are dependent on cannabis than any other illicit substance. A withdrawal syndrome has been described, although it is not yet included in the diagnostic manuals because there has not been a consensus about the full syndrome. Symptoms of withdrawal are likely to include irritability, anxiety, decreased appetite, and insomnia. There has been an increasing demand for treatment of cannabis use disorders. This may be due to the fact that marijuana has become more potent over the past 30 years. In the 1960s, the average potency of marijuana as measured by tetrahydrocannabinol (THC) level increased from 0.05% to 5%, with some more potent forms of cannabis containing as much as 22% THC.

EVALUATION

How Do I Ask My Patient About Drug and Alcohol Use?

Asking about drugs and alcohol can be awkward, but the questions should be asked routinely. Start by asking, "How much do you drink?" If the patient says none, ask why. This can yield a great deal of information. For example, the patient may be in recovery from an alcohol or a drug problem, his religion may prohibit the use of drugs, or there may be a family history of alcohol and drug problems. If a person reports that he does drink alcohol, the clinician should ask how much and how often. Follow-up questions could include, "Do you sometimes drink more than you want?" "Has drinking ever gotten you into trouble?" Several instruments have been developed to screen for alcohol problems. The four-item CAGE questionnaire is one of the simplest and most commonly used screening tools for substance use disorders (Box 26-1). Although quantity and frequency of alcohol use are not diagnostic of an alcohol use disorder, a positive answer to the question of whether someone has had five or more drinks on one occasion in the last month is a good indication to probe further about an alcohol use disorder.

How Do I Ask About Other Drugs of Abuse?

Gently probe. Never assume that a person does not use drugs. Although it is not necessary (or desirable) to mention every conceivable drug of abuse, suggest some common possibilities. A friendly, respectful, nonjudgmental tone will help get more accurate information. "Have you ever tried other drugs (than alcohol)?" "Did you ever smoke marijuana? Did you smoke in college?" "Have you ever tried cocaine?"

Can My Patient Be an Alcoholic if She Drinks Only at Night?

Yes. The quantity and frequency of use do not define a substance use disorder. If a patient drinks only at night or uses cocaine only on weekends but

---

BOX 26-1

CAGE QUESTIONS

C "Have you ever felt you ought to **Cut** down on your drinking or drug use?"

A "Have people **Annoyed** you by criticizing your drinking or drug use?"

G "Have you felt bad or **Guilty** about your drinking or drug use?"

E "Have you ever had a drink or used drugs first thing in the morning to steady your nerves or to get rid of a hangover (**Eye-opener**)?"

has consequences from its use (e.g., driving while intoxicated, arriving to work late the next day), she may still qualify for a diagnosis of substance abuse or dependence.

Can My Patient Be an Alcoholic if He Only Drinks Beer?

Yes, of course. A can of beer (12 oz), a glass of wine (5 oz), and a jigger of 80 proof liquor (1.5 oz) all contain the same amount of alcohol.

What Am I Supposed to Assess Besides How Much and How Often a Person Drinks or Gets High?

Intoxication or withdrawal. Information on patterns of abuse comes mostly from the history. Information on intoxication and withdrawal comes from the review of systems, mental status examination, and physical examination.

What Signs and Symptoms Do I Look For?

They vary with the drug. In general, the signs and symptoms of intoxication are the opposite of those of withdrawal (e.g., constricted versus dilated pupils [Figs. 26-1 and 26-2]), but there are many exceptions to this generalization. Table 26-2 gives a description of intoxication and withdrawal syndromes seen with commonly abused drugs.

When Does Withdrawal from Alcohol Occur?

It begins 8 hours after the last drink. Symptoms include tremulousness, flushing, nausea, diarrhea, vomiting, anxiety, and insomnia. Tachycardia and hypertension are usually found. These signs and symptoms peak at 48 hours and diminish significantly within 5 days. Rarely, alcohol withdrawal progresses to delirium tremens (DTs).

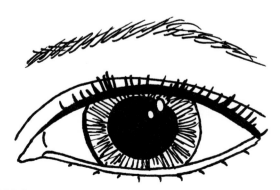

FIGURE 26-1 Dilated pupil, characteristic of central nervous system stimulant intoxication and opioid withdrawal.

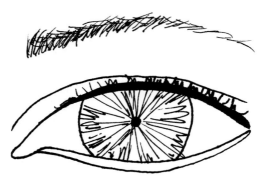

FIGURE 26-2 Pinpoint pupil, characteristic of opioid intoxication.

How Can I Tell if My Patient Is at Risk for DTs?

The risk is always there in a long-time heavy drinker, and detoxification is usually necessary for patients who are intoxicated at admission. Patients are particularly at risk if they have a history of DTs in the past or have comorbid medical conditions. DTs are a late-occurring phenomenon—occurrence 3 to 5 days after the last drink is not unusual—and the early withdrawal signs and symptoms may be minor and overlooked. Autonomic instability (increased temperature, heart rate, and blood pressure, all with fluctuations) is a critical early signal of impending DTs.

What Do the DTs Look Like?

As the name suggests, delirium tremens is a delirium with marked tremulousness. The individual is typically confused, disoriented, and fearful. Auditory, tactile, and visual hallucinations are all common. The person with DTs is usually sweating heavily. Heart rate and blood pressure are elevated. Seizures may or may not occur. The risk of death related to cardiovascular collapse is 10% of *treated* patients.

Are There Long-Term Alcohol Problems I Should Be Alert To?

Yes. Alcohol has toxic effects on almost every organ system in the body. Gastrointestinal effects range from gastritis, pancreatitis, peptic ulcer disease, and esophageal varices to gastric and pancreatic cancers. Heavy alcohol use (more than eight drinks a day over 10 years) puts patients at risk for the development of cirrhosis, which can lead to hepatocellular carcinoma. Cardiovascular complications from alcohol include hypertension, stroke, and cardiomyopathy (alcohol is directly toxic to the heart muscle). Vitamin deficiencies put alcoholics at risk for anemia and peripheral neuropathy. Alcoholics are at risk for an acute thiamine deficiency state called Wernicke's encephalopathy; this is delirium accompanied by a gait ataxia and abnormal eye movements. The administration of intravenous thiamine prevents Wernicke's encephalopathy from progressing to Korsakoff's

Table 26-2

Intoxication and Withdrawal Syndromes of Commonly Abused Drugs

Drug Class (Examples)	Syndrome	Symptoms	Signs	Dangers
Central nervous system sedatives (alcohol, benzodiazepines)	Intoxication	Decreased anxiety. Disinhibition	Slurred speech. Ataxia Decreased deep tendon reflexes	Respiratory depression
	Withdrawal	Anxiety. Irritability, headache, psychotic symptoms (when extreme)	Tremulousness. Increased heart rate and blood pressure. Increased deep tendon reflexes	Seizures. Withdrawal delirium (10% mortality)
Central nervous system stimulants (cocaine, amphetamines)	Intoxication	Excitability Increased libido Paranoid delusions. Auditory and tactile hallucinations	Increased heart rate and blood pressure Cardiac arrhythmias Dilated pupils (see Fig. 25-1)	Heart attack Stroke Seizures Suicide
	Withdrawal	Depression		
Opioids	Intoxication	Euphoria Anesthesia Calm Drowsiness Nausea Projectile vomiting	Pinpoint pupils (see Fig. 25-2) Decreased blood pressure	Respiratory depression
	Withdrawal	Multiple aches and pains Drug craving Anxiety	Dilated pupils Piloerection Runny nose and eyes Diarrhea Yawning	

(Continued)

Table 26-2
Intoxication and Withdrawal Syndromes of Commonly Abused Drugs (Continued)

Drug Class (Examples)	Syndrome	Symptoms	Signs	Dangers
Marijuana	Intoxication	Altered time sense Carbohydrate craving Increased intensity of sensory impressions Paranoid thoughts Hallucinations and delirium (extreme cases)	Bloodshot eyes Increased blood pressure Increased heart rate	
	Withdrawal	Irritability Drug craving		
Phencyclidine (PCP)	Intoxication	Heightened emotions Floating feeling Euphoria	Increased heart rate Runny eyes Sweating Nystagmus	Coma Severe hypertension Delirium
	Withdrawal	Irritability Lethargy		
Ecstasy	Intoxication	Euphoria Feeling of closeness	Increased heart rate Increased blood pressure Sweating Jaw clenching	Hyperthermia Hyponatremia Hepatic failure Seizures
	Withdrawal	Depression Insomnia Memory impairment		

Impaired judgment is a feature of both intoxication and withdrawal for all classes.

disorder, a permanent anterograde amnesia. Korsakoff's disorder is a disastrous condition in which the individual loses the ability to transfer recent memories into long-term memory storage. In addition (and unrelated to Wernicke's encephalopathy or Korsakoff's disorder), some alcoholics experience persistent auditory hallucinations (often threatening) in a clear sensorium, a condition called alcohol-induced hallucinations.

Is the Physical Examination Helpful in Assessing Substance Use Disorders?

It is essential in diagnosing intoxication and withdrawal states. The signs listed in Table 26-2 may be the most prominent and definitive findings. Other aspects of the physical examination may alert you to the presence of a serious drug or alcohol problem. Track marks (usually on the forearms but potentially anywhere, including the genitals) indicate intravenous drug use. Burns on the lips and fingers can result from crack cocaine use. The stigmata of chronic, heavy alcohol use are palmar erythema, spider angiomata, and liver findings (early on, an enlarged liver; late, a small liver).

Are Laboratory Findings Helpful?

Diagnosis of a substance use disorder is made only on the basis of history and mental status and physical findings. Laboratory studies can provide useful ancillary information. Alcohol use disorders often cause abnormalities of liver function tests. A finding of aspartate transaminase (AST [SGOT]) twice the level of alanine transaminase (ALT [SGPT]) may indicate acute alcoholic hepatitis. Gamma-glutamyl transferase (GGT) may also be elevated in alcoholic patients and may be more specific to alcohol-induced damage. These enzymes are followed to monitor the development of cirrhosis, but they may not be increased if there has already been a significant amount of liver damage. Poor nutrition and perhaps the direct toxic effects of alcohol affect the complete blood cell count, in particular by decreasing the white blood cell count and by causing anemia. The mean corpuscular volume of red blood cells is often increased because of vitamin B_{12} deficiency. The stimulants have cardiac effects, and an electrocardiogram is needed to evaluate for arrhythmias.

All drug-using patients are at risk for sexually transmitted diseases. Testing for syphilis, human immunodeficiency virus, and gonorrhea may be indicated.

Isn't a Urine Toxicology Screen the Most Important Test?

Surprisingly, no. If the test is positive, it tells you that the person has that drug in her system but not much more. A negative test *does not* rule out a drug-related cause of psychiatric symptoms. Some symptoms of intoxication persist after the drug has been cleared (e.g., hallucinations caused by cocaine intoxication), and for symptoms caused by withdrawal states, you would expect the toxicology screen to be negative. Similarly, a positive toxicology screen does not rule out psychiatric causes. A patient with schizophrenia may have smoked marijuana just before coming into the emergency department. Also, a urine drug test may not pick up all of the substances that a patient might abuse.

How Can I Tell if My Patient's Psychiatric Symptoms Are Caused by Drug Use?

It is often difficult and sometimes impossible. A careful history will document preexisting psychiatric disorders. Establishing the temporal relationship between symptoms and drug use will help. It may be necessary to wait until the patient has been abstinent for an extended period of time to establish a diagnosis with reasonable certainty. In the meantime, significant symptoms such as depression or hallucinations can still be treated. Table 26-3 lists some psychiatric symptoms commonly caused by different drug classes.

TREATMENT

What Is the Difference between Rehab and Detox?

The goal of detoxification ("detox") is to help a patient become drug free while limiting the morbidity and mortality associated with withdrawal. A rehabilitation ("rehab") program's main goal is to help a patient remain abstinent and may begin with a detoxification stage. In a rehabilitation program, a combination of group and individual therapy is used to help a person identify triggers to drug or alcohol use, cope with painful emotional states, and use coping mechanisms to prevent relapse. Programs can last from 1 to 12 months or more. Treatment can be provided on both inpatient and outpatient bases. Choice of the proper treatment depends on the status of the addiction, the patient's living situation, and other resources. The patient should play an active role in choosing treatment.

Table 26-3

Psychiatric Symptoms Commonly Caused by Different Drug Classes

Substances that cause psychotic symptoms
   Cocaine intoxication
   Amphetamine intoxication
   Alcohol hallucinosis or withdrawal
   Central nervous system depressant withdrawal
   Phencyclidine (PCP) or ketamine intoxication
Substances that can cause depression
   Cocaine withdrawal
   Alcohol intoxication
Substances that can cause anxiety
   Caffeine intoxication
   Nicotine intoxication
   Cocaine intoxication
   Amphetamine intoxication
   Central nervous system sedative withdrawal

When Is Detoxification Indicated?

Detoxification is used in alcohol (and other sedative) withdrawal to prevent morbidity and mortality and in opioid withdrawal to ease withdrawal symptoms and prevent relapse.

How Do I Detoxify My Patients from Alcohol?

Alcohol withdrawal can be life threatening. Benzodiazepines are cross-tolerant with alcohol and can be used to minimize the symptoms of withdrawal in a patient who is alcohol dependent. The most common detoxification protocols use tapering doses of a benzodiazepine. When starting the taper, the patient should be given enough of the benzodiazepine to cause sedation, typically 25 to 50 mg chlordiazepoxide or 1 to 2 mg lorazepam. Some patients require higher doses: if the person is still awake and tremulous 1 hour after an oral dose of medication, a second dose should be given and the patient reevaluated. Once sedation is achieved, the individual should be given the same dose every 6 hours for the next 24 hours. The dose is then decreased daily for the next several days. One rule is to decrease the dose of benzodiazepine by no more than 20% per day. In a hospital setting, however, medication can be decreased more rapidly because the patient is observed more closely. If the person shows signs or symptoms of withdrawal between scheduled doses, such as an elevation of blood pressure or temperature, he should be given a dose on an as-needed basis, and the schedule of tapering should be reevaluated.

An important component of detoxification is adequate nutrition and hydration, including the prescription of thiamine (100 mg/day) and folic acid (1 mg/day). Thiamine deficiency is associated with the development of Wernicke's encephalopathy and Korsakoff's disorder in alcohol dependence, and folic acid deficiency can result in macrocytic anemia.

If DTs Are Caused by Alcohol Withdrawal, Why Can't I Give Alcohol to Treat the DTs?

Many hospitals have ethanol on their formularies; however, there are no data to support its efficacy in treating DTs over more researched treatments such as benzodiazepines. Furthermore, alcohol has direct toxicity to the body, as mentioned earlier, that makes it a less desirable treatment. One effect includes water retention, which in the hospitalized patient should be avoided.

How Do I Detoxify My Patients from Opioids?

Withdrawal from opioids, although not life threatening, can be very uncomfortable. Vomiting during withdrawal can result in dehydration and electrolyte imbalances. Detoxification is best accomplished using a longer acting opioid such as methadone. A starting dose of 20 to 40 mg of methadone is usually sufficient to blunt the initial withdrawal symptoms. Although a general rule of detoxification protocols is to taper by no more than 20% per day, decreasing by 5 mg/day is a common practice. The Drug Enforcement Administration has strict regulations regarding the use of narcotics (opioids) in treating addiction. Methadone for maintenance or detoxification can be distributed only in a clinic with a special license or on inpatient units. An outpatient physician is allowed to prescribe narcotics to treat an opioid addiction for only up to 3 days, after which the patient must be treated in a specialized clinic or inpatient unit or by a physician with a special license to prescribe buprenorphine, a partial opioid agonist. Physicians must complete specialized training in order to prescribe buprenorphine and can treat only up to 30 patients with this treatment in their practices.

Is There a Way to Detoxify Someone that Doesn't Use Such Restricted Drugs?

Yes. Detoxification protocols using nonopioid medications have been studied. One uses a taper of clonidine (an α_2-agonist) and lorazepam, supplemented by as-needed medications to treat other symptoms. Clonidine decreases symptoms caused by adrenergic output, and lorazepam treats the anxiety and muscle cramping that are associated with opioid withdrawal. Adjunctive medications include antiemetics for nausea and vomiting and nonsteroidal anti-inflammatory agents to treat pain. Although the studies looked promising, in practice the protocol is not as effective as using methadone for withdrawal, particularly in controlling drug craving.

Can I Treat Dependence with Medications?

Yes, depending on the drug and the disorder. Disulfiram is sometimes used to treat alcoholism and is being studied in the treatment of cocaine addiction. The medication works by inhibiting the enzyme aldehyde dehydrogenase, which leads to a buildup of acetaldehyde. When a person who has been taking disulfiram drinks alcohol, the metabolism of alcohol is blocked, resulting in a buildup of acetaldehyde (Box 26-2) that causes flushing, nausea, tachycardia, and hypotension. This unpleasant reaction is intended to put the brakes on impulse drinking. (It does not stop *planned* drinking by the alcoholic who discontinues disulfiram in anticipation of having a drink later.) Disulfiram should probably be avoided in patients with comorbid medical illnesses.

There are also medications to treat cravings for alcohol. Those medications include naltrexone and acamprosate. Currently, there are no good treatments for stimulant cravings, although a number of medications have been tested.

BOX 26-2

ALCOHOL METABOLISM

Alcohol $\longrightarrow$ Acetaldehyde $\longrightarrow$ Acetate
     Alcohol   *Aldehyde*
   dehydrogenase   *dehydrogenase*
Aldehyde dehydrogenase is usually not rate limiting.

What About Medications for Opioid Dependence?

The treatment of choice for opioid dependence is opioid substitution therapy, of which methadone is the best studied. Because it is has a longer half-life than heroin, methadone does not provide the same reinforcing high. Methadone can be prescribed *only* in a licensed methadone clinic. A usual starting dose is about 40 mg. The medication is then increased weekly until sufficient blockade of the opioid receptor is achieved to diminish cravings. A patient is required to go daily to pick up the dose.

Buprenorphine is also being used for maintenance treatment at doses ranging from 8 to 24 mg. Like methadone, it has a longer half-life than heroin and does not cause patients to become high. One difference is that buprenorphine precipitates withdrawal in patients who have opioids in their system. Also, at higher doses, it becomes an antagonist, making it more difficult for patients to overdose on it.

Isn't Giving Methadone Just Substituting Addictions?

Yes and no. A methadone patient is still physically dependent on the opioid, but the goal of methadone treatment is to reduce the other symptoms of the addiction, such as job problems, legal problems, physical problems, relationship problems, and psychological problems. (Methadone intoxication does not cause the euphoria, drowsiness, and impaired judgment seen in heroin addiction.) Methadone treatment has been shown to decrease morbidity associated with intravenous drug use as well as to decrease criminal behavior.

Isn't This Called Harm Reduction?

Yes. The idea of harm reduction is to minimize the risks while an addicted person is using drugs. However, the ultimate goal should be to stop the drugs or alcohol if use is causing harm because we know that controlled use of a substance in a dependent person is unlikely to be achieved.

What if a Person on Methadone Maintenance Needs Pain Medication?

A temporary increase in dose may be sufficient to achieve analgesia. If not, other additional opioid analgesics may be needed. This is best done in consultation with an addiction or a pain management specialist.

Does Alcoholics Anonymous Help?

Very much. Alcoholics Anonymous is a self-help recovery group. The individual meets regularly in a group with other addicts and, with the group support, commits himself to following the 12-step program (Table 26-4). Other 12-step groups have developed from the basic model of AA, including Narcotics Anonymous, Cocaine Anonymous, Marijuana Anonymous, and Methadone Anonymous. Studies have shown that the best outcomes for the treatment of substance use disorders occur when patients receive professional treatment combined with 12-step groups.

Table 26-4

Twelve Steps

Steps 1 through 3
Admit powerlessness over alcohol.
Belief in a "power greater than ourselves."
Turn will over to the care of God "as we understand Him."

Steps 4 through 7
Take a moral inventory.
Admit to God, to ourselves, and to another human being the exact nature of our wrongs.
Be ready to have God remove all these defects of character.
Ask Him to remove our shortcomings.

Steps 8 through 10
Make a list of all persons harmed and become willing to make amends to them all.
Make direct amends wherever possible.
Keep an ongoing personal inventory and promptly admit when we are wrong.

Steps 11 and 12
Through prayer and meditation, improve our conscious contact with God, "as we understand Him."
Carry this message to other alcoholics, and "practice these principles in all our affairs."

What If My Patient Doesn't Believe in God?

Although the language of 12-step programs uses the word "God," this is meant to be personalized to the individual's own beliefs. Patients should be encouraged to go to meetings and to share their reservations with others. An alternative to the 12-step groups is Rational Recovery, also a self-help group, in which the emphasis is on personal responsibility rather than on a "higher power." Other options are self-help groups called Women for Sobriety and Men for Sobriety.

What Is Dual Diagnosis?

A patient is considered to have a dual diagnosis when she has both a substance use disorder and a psychiatric disorder. Another term is mentally ill and chemically abusing (MICA).

What if My Patient Is Not Interested in Treatment?

A great deal can be done for a patient who has a substance use disorder but is not interested in treatment at this time. A key to success in treatment is motivation, and this can be worked on using motivational enhancement techniques. These are outlined in Table 26-5.

Table 26-5

Principles of Motivational Enhancement Therapy (MET)

There are five stages of change:
  Precontemplation: No awareness of problem
  Contemplation: Considering treatment for a problem
  Preparation: Making arrangements to make a change to correct the problem
  Action: Actively engaged in changing the problem
  Maintenance: Continuing with the change that was made
Goal is to move the patient from one stage to another.
Emphasize self-efficacy; it is up to the patient to decide what he or she wants to do.
Avoid a punitive stance.
Roll with the patient's resistance.

KEY POINTS

◆ A substance use history should be part of the evaluation of all patients.

◆ A diagnosis of dependence does not require the presence of tolerance or physiologic withdrawal.

◆ Detoxification is indicated for alcohol and opioid withdrawal. Alcohol withdrawal is medically serious; opioid withdrawal is not.

◆ The best treatment for a substance use disorder combines professional treatment with a 12-step self-help program.

◆ Anticraving medications can be a useful adjunct to treatment for alcoholism.

◆ Substitution therapy is the best treatment for opioid addiction.

Case 26-1

A 45-year-old man 2 days after surgical repair of a right femoral fracture becomes acutely agitated and uncooperative, refusing to lie in bed and threatening to pull out all intravenous lines. The man is lucid one moment and preoccupied with a mouse he saw running across the floor the next. He is disoriented to time and place. He is diaphoretic and mildly tremulous. His heart rate is 105 beats per minute, and blood pressure is 140/90 mm Hg. The patient complained of being anxious earlier in the day. He was given a dose of lorazepam without much relief. On admission, his AST and ALT were moderately elevated.

A. What is the diagnosis?
B. What treatment should you order?
C. Should the man be transferred to a psychiatry service?

Substance Use Disorders

Case 26-2

A 24-year-old man comes to a first appointment with an internist complaining of back pain. His is the last appointment of the day. He reports having injured his back in a pick-up game of basketball 1 week earlier. He is in a hurry and wants to be able to catch the last train home. He has tried ibuprofen but says it has not helped. He states that he had taken oxycodone (a narcotic analgesic) in the past and it seemed to work well.

A. What other information do you want?
B. If he had been dependent on opioids in the past but is now abstinent, is it all right to give him opioid analgesics?

Case Answers

26-1 A. *Learning objective:* **Be familiar with the signs and symptoms of the major intoxication and withdrawal syndromes.** The man is suffering from a delirium; the cause of the delirium is less clear. Elevated liver transaminases on admission suggest the possibility of heavy alcohol use, and his current signs and symptoms are completely consistent with the major withdrawal syndrome of alcohol. His work-up at this point must consider other possible causes of delirium such as hepatic encephalopathy or infection. Impending DTs will be high on the differential.

26-1 B. *Learning objective:* **Be familiar with detoxification strategies.** Because DTs are a medical emergency, it is safe to treat him presumptively while the evaluation continues. Benzodiazepines are the treatment of choice for alcohol withdrawal. They are cross-tolerant with alcohol, and an individual who has been abusing alcohol for a long time needs higher than normal doses. If the man is in alcohol withdrawal, a benzodiazepine such as lorazepam in adequate doses will calm his agitation, stop the psychotic symptoms, and medically stabilize him.

26-1 C. *Learning objective:* **Understand the basic approaches to detoxification.** There are at least two reasons the man should not be transferred to a psychiatry service. One is management of his surgical recovery, but at least as important is the need for close medical supervision during the detoxification period, which may span 5 days or longer. During detoxification, he is still at risk for developing DTs.

26-2 A. *Learning objective:* **Recognize the potential for abuse of prescription pain medications.** The fact that it is late in the day, that the man is in a hurry, and that he seems to know exactly what will work should not stop you from doing a thoughtful assessment of the presenting complaint. If anything, you want to be mindful of the possibility for narcotic abuse and take the time to get enough information about him and his condition to feel confident in your prescription.

26-2 B.   *Learning objective:* **Understand the risks in prescribing addictive medications.** There is no absolute contraindication to the use of opioid analgesics in a former addict who is now abstinent, but caution is warranted. It makes sense to explore other options, and it may be advisable to consult with a pain or addiction specialist. None of this is easy at the end of the day. It will help to discuss your concerns with the man honestly and openly.

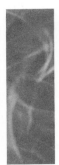

27

Delirium and Dementia

MICHELLE IZMERLY

 DELIRIUM

ETIOLOGY

What Is Delirium?

Delirium, sometimes called toxic metabolic encephalopathy, is an acute confusional state with sudden onset. It always includes a disruption in the level of consciousness, and the symptoms tend to fluctuate.

What Causes Delirium?

There are many causes, but delirium tends to result from either central nervous system infections or systemic processes outside the central nervous system such as fever, hypertension, metabolic abnormalities, and drug intoxication and withdrawal states. A list of common causes is presented in Table 27-1.

What Are the Risk Factors for Delirium?

There are many, including very young and very old age, previous brain injury, medical comorbidities, sleep deprivation, and preexisting cognitive impairment. Many people, especially elderly people, are at risk for delirium following surgery or when hospitalized on an intensive care service.

How Common Is Delirium?

It is very common, especially on medical and surgical services. About 10% to 15% of general medical inpatients, 30% to 50% of hospitalized geriatric patients, and up to 51% of postoperative patients develop delirium. Up to 60% of nursing home residents older than 75 have been delirious at some time.

Table 27-1

Some Common Causes of Delirium

Drug intoxication
  Amphetamines
  Anticholinergics
Drug withdrawal
  Alcohol
Medical conditions
  Infections: Sepsis, pneumonia
  Metabolic: Fluid or electrolyte imbalance
    Renal failure
    Liver failure
  Low-perfusion states: Shock, heart failure
  Hypertension
  Fever
  Nutritional: Thiamine deficiency
  Cancer, metastases or primary
Neurologic
  Infections
    Encephalitis (human immunodeficiency virus, herpes)
    Meningitis

EVALUATION

How Can I Tell if My Patient Has Delirium?

Delirium is a common illness but it is often misdiagnosed. It has a high level of morbidity and mortality, and prompt diagnosis is essential. The diagnosis of delirium is made on the basis of symptoms and clinical course. The onset of symptoms is typically acute or subacute, often occurring over the course of a few hours. Delirium always includes an altered level of consciousness. Other symptoms—altered attention, disorientation, and decreased memory—are commonly present. Associated features such as thought disorganization, hallucinations, and delusions may lead to the misdiagnosis of a psychotic disorder.

What Does "Altered Level of Consciousness" Mean?

The degree of wakefulness, the ability to concentrate, and the ability to attend to and accurately interpret environmental stimuli are altered.

What Mental Status Findings Help with the Diagnosis?

The mental status of a patient with delirium may be described as *hyperactive*, *hypoactive*, or fluctuating from one to the other and displaying features of both. In hyperactive delirium, the patient is disoriented to time, place, or person and is often easily distracted and unable to concentrate. Increased psychomotor activity with agitation, disorganization, delusions, and hallucinations are prominent. A patient's mood is often irritable and labile.

In hypoactive delirium, the person is drowsy, inattentive, and difficult to arouse. He appears depressed with psychomotor slowing, and it is only with a careful clinical assessment of his level of consciousness that depression can be distinguished from this type of delirium.

How Can I Distinguish Delirium from Other Disorders with Psychotic Symptoms?

The level of consciousness is often not affected in other psychotic disorders. Hallucinations, delusions, or disorganized behavior and speech are present, but the patient remains alert and responsive to the environment. However, severe psychotic states with catatonia or very disorganized behavior may be difficult to distinguish from delirium, and if orientation cannot be assessed because of mutism, catatonia, or disorganization, you should consider the possibility of a delirium to ensure that no treatable medical condition is overlooked.

Does the Physical Examination Help in Diagnosing Delirium?

Yes, the physical examination helps to identify the presence of an underlying medical condition or drug-related state. For example, in alcohol withdrawal delirium, the vital signs are unstable because of autonomic instability, and there may be diaphoresis, facial flushing, and dilated pupils. Deep tendon reflexes are usually hyperactive. The neurologic examination may reveal cortical signs such as dysgraphia (trouble writing), apraxia (trouble with motor tasks), and dysnomia (difficulty naming objects) and motor signs such as tremor, asterixis, or myoclonus.

Are Laboratory Tests or Imaging Studies Helpful?

A full set of laboratory studies is essential in any patient suspected of being delirious (Table 27-2). If there are meningeal signs, cerebrospinal fluid analysis should be performed. An electroencephalogram (EEG) is sometimes helpful. In delirium, the EEG typically shows diffuse slowing, but this is also seen in many patients who are taking psychiatric drugs and who are not delirious. In alcohol and other sedative withdrawal states, the EEG shows low-voltage fast activity. Neuroimaging studies such as computed tomography (CT) scanning or magnetic resonance imaging (MRI) are usually indicated unless the cause of the delirium has already been established.

TREATMENT

How Should I Treat My Patient with Delirium?

First, you must identify and treat the underlying condition. Symptomatic and supportive treatment is next, and it is also important to restore any fluid or electrolyte imbalance that is present. Early recognition and treatment of an infection or electrolyte imbalance can readily reverse the delirium. A delirious patient who becomes agitated may require medication. Haloperidol (0.5 to 5 mg orally or intramuscularly, not to exceed 20 mg over a period of 24 hours) is usually recommended. It is a safe, rapid, and

Table 27-2

Suggested Medical Screening for New-Onset Delirium and Dementia

Thorough history, physical examination, and mental status examination
Blood tests
    Complete blood cell count
    Electrolytes
    Glucose
    Thyroid function tests
    Liver function tests
    Renal function tests
    Tests for human immunodeficiency virus
    Tests for syphilis
    Vitamin B_{12}
    Folate
    Thiamine
    Niacin
    Erythrocyte sedimentation rate
Neuroimaging studies
    Head computed tomography scan
    Brain magnetic resonance imaging
Urine
    Toxicology
    Urinalysis
    Heavy metals
Additional tests that may be necessary for delirium evaluation
    Lumbar puncture for meningitis
    Ammonia level for hepatic encephalopathy
    Arterial blood gas for hypoxia, acid-base abnormalities

effective medication for behavioral control in an agitated, dangerous, or disruptive patient. Lorazepam 0.5 to 2 mg intravenously or intramuscularly every 2 to 4 hours may also help, but its use is limited by its potential to cause sedation, respiratory depression, and behavioral disinhibition. There have been a limited number of published studies on the use of atypical antipsychotics (risperidone, olanzapine) in patients with delirium. Initial studies showed an increased rate of cardiovascular accidents (CVAs), but the risk of CVA from atypicals has been found to be the same as that from typicals (e.g., haloperidol.)

You want the environment to minimize the disorientation. It should be filled with familiar objects. Clocks and calendars help to provide some structure and helpful orienting cues. Ideally, the room should be well lit, quiet, and with minimal extraneous stimulation such as mechanical noises and sounds from the nursing station.

What Happens if Delirium Is Not Treated?

It depends on the underlying cause. Because some causes of delirium are life-threatening emergencies (delirium tremens [DTs], for example), the diagnosis and management of delirium should always be considered urgent. The majority of patients have full recovery; however, delirium may progress to more serious conditions, including coma, seizures, and even death, if the underlying cause is not treated. In elderly persons, rates of full recovery are less and some symptoms may persist for up to 6 months after discharge from the hospital.

DEMENTIA

ETIOLOGY

What Is Dementia?

Dementia is a clinical syndrome of decreased cognitive functioning in the setting of a stable level of consciousness. It is characterized by memory impairment and other cognitive deficits such as language disturbances (*aphasias*), difficulty performing common motor tasks such as using a fork or buttoning a button (*apraxias*), failure to recognize familiar objects (*agnosia*), or trouble in planning and organizing tasks with a decline in the functional level of the patient.

How Common Is Dementia?

Very. About 5% of adults older than 65 have moderate to severe dementia, and the prevalence increases with age, affecting about 20% of people aged 85 to 90.

What Causes Dementia?

There are many possible causes. The most common type of dementia in the United States is dementia of the Alzheimer's type. In contrast to those of delirium, the causes of dementia tend to be processes inside the central nervous system. For example, dementia in Alzheimer's disease results from degeneration of neurons in the brain, notably in the areas responsible for memory functions. A list of common causes of dementia is given in Table 27-3.

Are All Degenerative Dementias Related to Alzheimer's Disease?

No, although Alzheimer's is by far the most common. Other degenerative dementias include Huntington's disease and frontotemporal dementia.

What Is Frontotemporal Dementia?

Frontotemporal dementia or FTD is a progressive, idiopathic dementia that affects the frontal and temporal lobes. Pick's disease is the most studied of this type of dementia. It often begins with personality changes and behavioral disturbances (such as poor hygiene and decreased social awareness) rather than memory loss. Common symptoms include disinhibition, mood disturbances (depression or apathy), speech disturbances, and frontal

Table 27-3

Some Common Causes of Dementia

Neurodegenerative diseases
  Alzheimer's disease
  Pick's disease
  Huntington's disease
  Parkinson's disease
  Wilson's disease
  Chronic heavy alcohol use
Brain structural abnormalities
  Tumors
  Subdural hematoma
  Normal-pressure hydrocephalus
Metabolic and endocrine abnormalities
  Hypothyroidism
  Hypercalcemia
Nutritional deficiencies
  Niacin
  Vitamin B_{12}
  Folate
Toxic exposure
  Heavy metals
  Inhalants
  Organophosphates

Delirium and Dementia

release signs (discussed under "Evaluation"). CT or MRI scans show atrophy of the frontal and temporal lobes; CT or MRI scans of patients with Alzheimer's show generalized atrophy. Neuroimaging studies, however, are not diagnostic for either Alzheimer's disease or FTD.

EVALUATION

What Mental Status Findings Help Make the Diagnosis of Dementia?

The essential finding is memory impairment in a patient who is alert, oriented, and cooperative. Typically, short-term memory is most affected and long-term memory remains relatively intact. A person is unable to describe the events of that morning (or to recall three objects after 5 minutes) but retains vivid and detailed recall of childhood events. Other areas of cognitive functioning, such as abstract reasoning, fund of knowledge, and the ability to perform calculations, are often impaired, especially if the dementia is progressive. Difficulty in naming common objects (a pen or comb) and difficulty in finding the right word or misuse of familiar words are common. As the illness progresses there may be psychiatric symptoms such as mood lability, psychotic features, and poor judgment.

What Physical Findings Should I Look for in Dementia?

You must perform a full physical examination with special attention to the neurologic examination when looking for signs of the underlying cause of the dementia. The neurologic examination may, for example, reveal evidence of upper motor neuron lesions through the Babinski reflex. This is elicited by stroking the lateral aspect of the plantar surface of the foot from back to front. A normal response consists of plantar flexion of the great toe; the abnormal response (Babinski's sign) is dorsiflexion of the great toe with or without fanning of the other toes (Fig. 27-1A and B). Other physical signs may include hyperreflexia and increased muscle tone. Ataxia, evidence of a peripheral neuropathy, myoclonus, and abnormal involuntary movements all may suggest a particular diagnosis. Frontal release signs are evidence of frontal lobe impairment. Signs and symptoms associated with specific causes of dementia are outlined in Table 27-4.

What Are Frontal Release Signs?

We are born with a number of reflexes that help us survive when we are infants. For example, light touch around the mouth stimulates a sucking reflex. As the frontal lobes mature, these reflexes are gradually suppressed. Later on in life, if the frontal lobes are damaged, these reflexes may reemerge or be "released" (Table 27-5 and Fig. 27-2).

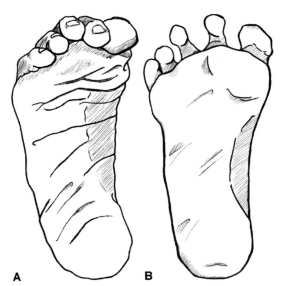

FIGURE 27-1 A positive Babinski response: (**A**) plantar flexion—normal response and (**B**) dorsiflexion—the Babinski sign.

Table 27-4

Signs and Symptoms Associated with Some Different Dementias

Dementia	Signs and Symptoms
Alzheimer's dementia	Aphasia, apraxia, agnosia, loss of executive functions
Creutzfeldt-Jakob disease	Myoclonus and electroencephalographic changes
Human immunodeficiency virus–related dementia	Psychomotor retardation, apathy, ataxia, apraxia, hypertonia, hyperactive reflexes, clonus
Huntington's disease	Choreiform movements, lurching gait
Lewy body dementia	Parkinson's features, hallucinations and delusions
Multi-infarct dementia	Stepwise intellectual deterioration, focal or lateralizing signs
Normal-pressure hydrocephalus	Urinary incontinence, gait ataxia
Pick's disease	Frontal lobe syndrome, gait ataxia, slowed speech

Table 27-5

Some Frontal Release Signs

Suck reflex	A light tap on the lips produces a puckering movement.
Grasp reflex	Gently stroking the patient's palm causes her to grab hold of your finger.
Glabellar reflex	Lightly tap the forehead. A normal response is to blink once or twice and then keep eyes open despite the tapping. An abnormal response is to continue to blink with each tap (see Fig. 27-2).

How Can I Distinguish Dementia from Delirium?

Both are disorders of global cognitive impairment but with different presentations. In delirium there is always an altered level of consciousness; in dementia there is not (except sometimes in the late stages of a progressive dementia such as Alzheimer's disease). Memory impairment is always prominent in dementia. Memory is often difficult to assess in delirium because of the patient's confusion and disorientation. Delirium typically occurs acutely (occurring over hours to days); dementia is more commonly slow and insidious (occurring over weeks to months). Table 27-6 summarizes some of the key differences between delirium and dementia.

Can the Physical Examination and Mental Status Findings Tell Me the Cause of My Patient's Dementia?

They can help. Sometimes your findings will establish the diagnosis, such as with the characteristic neurologic signs of Parkinson's disease (bradykinesia, broad-based gait, resting tremor). More generally, the mental status examination and physical examination will help you classify the dementia as *cortical* or *subcortical*, each of which has different etiologic implications.

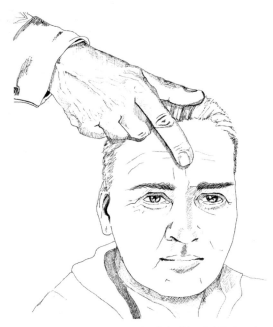

FIGURE 27-2 The glabellar response is elicited by lightly tapping a patient's forehead. Failure to stop blinking with repeated taps is a positive test suggesting frontal lobe dysfunction.

Table 27-6

Differences between Delirium and Dementia

Feature	Delirium	Dementia
Level of consciousness	Always impaired	Never impaired
Thinking	Fragmented, incoherent (memory is difficult to assess)	Coherent, but always marked by memory impairment
Disorientation	Common	Less common but possible
Hallucinations/illusions	Common	Less common but possible
Sleep/wake cycle	Fragmented	Preserved
Emotional features	Fear, anxiety, and apprehension common	Usually stable, but may have apathy or disinhibition and lability
Course	Acute-subacute onset (hours to a few days)	Usually slow and insidious; about 15% are reversible
Causes	Generally outside the central nervous system or brain infection	Commonly inside the central nervous system

What's the Difference between Cortical and Subcortical Dementias?

In cortical dementia, cognitive decline is prominent but apraxias and ataxias are minimal. The reverse is true for subcortical dementias, in which memory impairment may be slight (there is usually an overall sense of thinking being slowed or dulled) but subcortical signs such as ataxias and apraxias are prominent (Table 27-7).

Are Laboratory Tests and Imaging Studies Helpful?

Yes. A head CT scan or MRI should be routinely performed on all patients with dementia. A head CT scan can identify structural abnormalities such as a tumor or hematoma as well as generalized atrophy in Alzheimer's disease and other degenerative dementias. An MRI can identify multiple infarcts, demyelinating diseases, and small lesions, as well as a reduction in brain size, which is characteristic but not diagnostic of Alzheimer's disease. Blood and urine tests are essential in anyone with newly diagnosed dementia. The suggested medical screening for new-onset dementia is outlined in Table 27-2.

How Do I Diagnose Alzheimer's Disease?

Alzheimer's disease is a diagnosis of exclusion made in people who have characteristic signs and symptoms and the usual progressive clinical course and for whom no other cause can be determined. The definitive diagnosis is made by a biopsy and histologic examination of brain, which is rarely, if ever, performed. Histopathologic features such as neuritic plaques and neurofibrillary tangles help to confirm the diagnosis at autopsy, but these findings are not limited to Alzheimer's disease. CT scan and MRI often show brain atrophy (enlarged ventricles, widened sulci), but they are not diagnostic (Figs. 27-3 and 27-4).

How Can I Diagnose Dementia Caused by Human Immunodeficiency Virus?

HIV causes dementia in two different ways. The virus has an affinity for both nerve cells and lymphocytes. When the virus infects lymphocytes,

Table 27-7

Cortical versus Subcortical Dementia

Cortical:
    Marked cognitive impairment, few neurologic signs or apraxias
    Example: Alzheimer's disease
Subcortical:
    Prominent neurologic signs, apraxia, gait abnormalities; milder cognitive deficits
    Examples:
        Huntington's disease
        Parkinson's disease
        Human immunodeficiency virus encephalitis

Delirium and Dementia

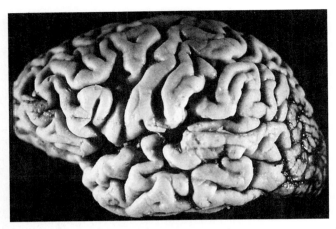

FIGURE 27-3 Brain from a woman who died of Alzheimer's disease at age 67. The loss of brain volume is evident in the widened fissures and sulci. (From the collection of the editor.)

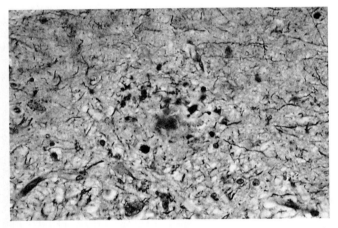

FIGURE 27-4 A section of the hippocampus from the same patient as shown in Figure 27-3. At the center is a neuritic plaque surrounded by darkened cell bodies, the neurofibrillary tangles, in various stages of degeneration. (From the collection of the editor.)

acquired immunodeficiency syndrome (AIDS) can develop and lead to opportunistic brain infections such as toxoplasmosis or cryptococcosis or to brain lymphomas. However, even without immune impairment, the virus itself can infect the brain. HIV encephalitis can cause a subcortical dementia. In HIV encephalitis, spinal fluid shows an elevated protein level and a mild lymphocytosis, and the virus can usually be isolated from the cerebrospinal fluid. MRI shows multifocal lesions of white matter and the basal ganglia.

Is Dementia Always Caused by Medical Disease?

Drugs such as alcohol and inhalants and exposure to toxins such as lead or mercury, organophosphate pesticides, and industrial solvents can all cause dementia. "Pseudodementia," caused by depression, is a treatable dementia, but these patients can present with significant cognitive impairment. Dementia is also sometimes mistakenly diagnosed in patients with hearing impairment.

Does It Matter Whether I Know the Cause of My Patient's Dementia?

Absolutely. Approximately 15% of all dementias are wholly or partially reversible. A main thrust of your evaluation is to rule out treatable causes. Some common reversible causes of dementia are listed in Table 27-8.

TREATMENT

Can Dementia Be Treated?

Cure is rarely achieved, but amelioration of some of the more devastating consequences is almost always possible. When feasible, treatment is directed to the underlying cause. Removal of the offending drug, treatment of the depression with antidepressants, or correction of the endocrine or metabolic abnormality may totally reverse the dementia. Dementia related to alcohol improves with abstinence. Normal-pressure hydrocephalus is treated by the surgical placement of a drainage shunt.

What About Irreversible Dementias Such as Alzheimer's Disease?

The cholinesterase inhibitors such as tacrine and donepezil, which are long acting and orally administered, have been shown to retard cognitive decline and preserve functional capacity for about 6 to 12 months in patients with Alzheimer's dementia. (The use of these medications in other dementias has

Table 27-8
Some (Potentially) Treatable Causes of Dementia
Hypothyroidism
Normal-pressure hydrocephalus
Central nervous system tumors
Subdural hematoma
Pernicious anemia
Pellagra
Depression

Delirium and Dementia

Table 27-9

Medications Used in the Treatment of Alzheimer's Dementia

Drug	Dose	Side Effects	Cautions
Donepezil* (Aricept)	Initial dose is 5 mg once daily; if necessary, dose can be increased to 10 mg once daily after 4 to 6 weeks.	Well tolerated, mild side effects, including nausea, vomiting, and diarrhea	Conflicting evidence about possible interactions with cimetidine (Tagamet), theophylline, warfarin (Coumadin), and digoxin (Lanoxin)
Galantamine* (Reminyl)	Initial dose is 4 mg twice daily (8 mg per day) taken with the morning and evening meals for 4 weeks; dose is then increased to 8 mg twice daily (16 mg per day) for at least 4 weeks. An increase to 12 mg twice daily (24 mg per day) should be considered on an individual basis, depending on clinical benefit and tolerability.	Mild side effects, including nausea, vomiting, and diarrhea	Contraindicated for use in patients with hepatic or renal impairment
Rivastigmine* (Exelon)	Initial dosage of 1.5 mg twice daily (3 mg per day) is generally well tolerated; dosage can be increased as tolerated but no more quickly than by 1.5 mg twice daily (3 mg per day) every 4 weeks to maximum of 6 mg twice daily (12 mg per day).	Nausea, vomiting, diarrhea, headaches, dizziness, abdominal pain, fatigue, malaise, anxiety, and agitation; these effects can be reduced by taking rivastigmine with food.	Some weight loss has been observed; monitor carefully.

Tacrine* (Cognex)	Initial dosage is 10 mg four times daily (40 mg per day) for 4 weeks; dosage is increased to 20 mg four times daily (80 mg per day) for 4 weeks, then to 30 mg four times daily (120 mg per day) for 4 weeks, etc., until maximum tolerated dosage is achieved. Maximum dosage is 40 mg four times daily (160 mg per day).	High incidence of side effects, including gastrointestinal problems	Hepatotoxicity is a problem; liver tests should be performed every other week for 16 weeks and every 3 months thereafter.
Memantine† HCl (Namenda)	Start 5 mg daily, increase by 5 mg weekly. Maximum 20 mg daily. For moderate to severe Alzheimer's dementia in combination with Donepezil	Mild; dizziness, confusion, and headache	

*There are four cholinesterase inhibitors available: donepezil (Aricept), rivastigmine (Exelon), galantamine (Reminyl), and tacrine (Cognex). These agents work by raising acetylcholine levels in the brain by inhibiting acetylcholinesterase (enzyme that breaks down acetylcholine).

†One agent is currently available that is not a cholinesterase inhibitor. Memantine acts by blocking the N-methyl-d-aspartate (NMDA) receptor and decreasing glutamate transmission.

not been studied.) They are effective in only a minority of patients, and people who are initially helped by the drugs eventually resume their decline. Donepezil has a major advantage over tacrine in that it does not cause liver damage. A newer agent, memantine, blocks the N-methyl-d-aspartate (NMDA) receptor, decreasing glutamate transmission. When used in combination with donepezil, it has been shown to help with cognitive decline, activities of daily living, behavior dyscontrol, and agitation in patients with moderate to severe Alzheimer's dementia (Table 27-9).

If psychotic symptoms develop, they can be treated with antipsychotics. The atypical agents risperidone and olanzapine have mild side effects and are generally well tolerated by elderly patients with dementia, but recent studies suggest an increased incidence of CVA in elderly patients with dementia who use these drugs. Follow-up studies are in progress to assess their safety. The atypical antipsychotics are not approved by the Food and Drug Administration for behavioral dyscontrol and should be used with caution in elderly patients.

Is There Anything Besides Medication That Can Help in Alzheimer's Disease?

The patient's caregivers will require extensive advice and education regarding the dementia. For the most part, most interventions are geared to supporting the family or caregivers of the patient. Assisting caregivers in decisions regarding nursing home placement, home care, financial matters, legal matters, and living arrangements are often the major goals of treatment.

Support groups for caretakers have been helpful in decreasing some of their distress.

KEY POINTS

◆ Delirium always includes an altered level of consciousness.

◆ Delirium may represent an underlying medical emergency.

◆ The important part of evaluating a dementia and delirium is looking for potentially treatable causes.

Case 27-1

A 63-year-old woman with no prior psychiatric history and a history of breast cancer treated with right breast lumpectomy 34 years earlier comes to a hospital emergency department with a recent history of multiple falls and complaints of dizziness and lower back pain. Clinical examination reveals a right-sided firm indurated breast mass. Chest radiography shows hilar adenopathy. The patient refuses a lumbar puncture and a head CT scan because she had a CT scan in 1967 that was negative and she believes the staff wants to repeat these tests simply "to display her organs on a TV screen." Her mental status examination reveals a restless, agitated, and guarded woman who looks older than her stated age. Her speech is rambling and at times incoherent. She has emotional lability and loosely organized paranoid delusions. She is disoriented to time and place and has difficulty sustaining attention throughout the interview.

    A. Can a psychiatric diagnosis be made?
    B. What is the most likely diagnosis?
    C. How should she be managed?

Case 27-2

An 85-year-old man comes to his internist's office because he is concerned about having dementia. He has noticed that he is more forgetful of people's names and cannot remember isolated facts. The man retired from his practice of general surgery 10 years ago. Since that time he has remained active in hospital and community affairs. He travels extensively with his wife, and he manages their large portfolio of investments. Physical examination is unremarkable except for reduced deep tendon reflexes and impaired vibration sensation in his legs.

    A. Does the man have a dementia?
    B. Will MRI and head CT scan help to establish the diagnosis?

Case Answers

27-1 A. *Learning objective:* **Understand the basis for a diagnosis of delirium.** It is usually necessary to rule out an underlying medical condition before making a psychiatric diagnosis. Two exceptions are the syndromes of delirium and dementia, which are presumed in most cases to result from drug-related or medical problems. Although the woman has psychotic symptoms, she also has an altered level of consciousness, which is the defining feature of delirium.

27-1 B. *Learning objective:* **Recognize the variety of conditions that can cause delirium.** The history, physical examination, and chest radiograph all strongly raise the possibility of disseminated breast cancer as the cause for the woman's delirium, but further investigations including neuroimaging studies are necessary to confirm the diagnosis. It is important not to foreclose prematurely on other possibilities such as a brain infection or withdrawal from central nervous system sedatives.

27-1 C. *Learning objective:* **Be familiar with basic treatment approaches in delirium.** It is urgent to continue the woman's evaluation. Haloperidol is effective in controlling agitation and reducing psychotic symptoms and can be given intramuscularly if necessary. It may help to restore some clarity of thinking and regain the woman's cooperation. Involving family members who will be able to help in making important decisions in her evaluation and treatment may be necessary.

27-2 A. *Learning objective:* **Recognize the difference between dementia and age-related cognitive decline.** There is no evidence that the man has dementia. He is experiencing memory lapses and forgetfulness that are typical of advancing age. A diagnosis of dementia requires the presence of cognitive problems in addition to memory impairment and some disability.

27-2 B. *Learning objective:* **Understand the appropriate use of neuroimaging studies in evaluating dementia.** Dementia is a clinical diagnosis. It is based on signs, symptoms, and clinical course. Imaging studies such as a CT scan and MRI may help to establish the cause of dementia. Some brain changes occur with normal aging: atrophy and dilated ventricles are seen on a CT scan, and white matter hyperintensities are seen on MRI. The degree of atrophy correlates poorly with the degree of cognitive impairment. In addition, electroencephalograms often show slowing of normal background alpha activity in nondemented old people.

28

Personality Disorders

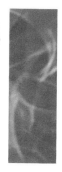

ZE'EV LEVIN

What Is Personality?

Personality can be thought of as a coherent organization of temperament, character, and psyche. Temperament refers to basic emotions and involves four major traits: harm avoidance, novelty seeking, reward dependence, and persistence. Character refers to the person's rational concepts of himself and his relationships. The psyche refers to the person's self-awareness.

What Are Personality Traits?

Personality *traits* are enduring patterns of thinking, feeling, and behaving over a wide range of a person's life.

What Are Personality Disorders?

Personality traits that are inflexible or maladaptive, that occur over long periods of time, that cause personal distress or social dysfunction, and that are present in people over the age of 18 constitute personality disorders.

Why Should I Know About These Disorders?

In the United States, at least 1 in every 5 to 10 people in the community has a personality disorder. About 50% of all psychiatric patients have personality disorders, which frequently coexist with Axis I disorders. Personality disorders predispose patients to other psychiatric disorders, such as substance abuse, suicide, mood disorders, impulse control disorders, eating disorders, and anxiety disorders, and increase the morbidity and mortality of these patients.

Are There Sex Differences in Personality Disorders?

There is a potential sex bias in diagnosing personality disorders. Certain disorders are diagnosed more in men, such as antisocial and schizoid, and others are diagnosed more frequently in women, such as borderline, histrionic, and dependent. Although real sex differences in prevalence may exist, we should guard against the social stereotypes about sex roles and behavior when making these diagnoses.

What Causes a Personality Disorder?

The causes of personality disorders are unknown, but we do have models that hypothesize about causality.

The *psychodynamic model* proposes that early trauma in the environment in which a person grows up, such as the loss of a parent, physical or mental abuse, or neglect (in combination with constitutional factors such as poor anxiety tolerance or high aggressiveness), results in a disordered personality. The individual shows a persistence of immature defense mechanisms and a poorly integrated sense of self as a person in the world.

The *spectrum disorder model*, which has received considerable research attention, proposes that certain personality disorders exist on a spectrum with the major clinical syndromes. Familial clustering of certain personality disorders with Axis I disorders suggests that they may be different clinical manifestations of a common underlying biologic predisposition. Examples include the mood disorder spectrum personality disorders such as borderline personality disorder, the schizophrenia spectrum personality disorders—schizoid, schizotypal, and paranoid personality disorder, and the anxiety spectrum personality disorders such as avoidant, compulsive, and dependent. Histrionic personality disorder has been thought of in the spectrum of somatoform and dissociative disorders.

The *psychobiologic model* is an integrative, multifactorial, and developmental etiologic model of personality and its disorders. This model proposes that genetics, learning, and neurophysiology interact to produce different cognitive styles, affect states, and behavior traits.

How Are the Personality Disorders Diagnosed?

Distinguishing between normal and abnormal personality is inherently relative and relies on arbitrary cutoff points on the continuum between two extremes of any behavior. It is also context dependent; the same behavior, manifested in different situations, can be considered as normal or maladaptive. Personality disorders also involve noninterpersonal traits, so we do not rely *only* on the social or situational context to establish these diagnoses. Both personal and social aspects account for the symptoms of personality disorders. You should consider these diagnoses when, through a series of diagnostic questions and knowledge of the descriptive characteristics of each disorder, you learn of your patient's history of chronic difficulties in relationships, work, and leisure activities. There is usually no clear onset of symptoms, the difficulties are experienced by the patient as "egosyntonic," and problems are usually externalized, experienced as a function of a difficult world as opposed to stemming from the patients themselves.

How Are Personality Disorders Classified?

According to DSM-IV-TR, the necessary criterion for distinguishing a personality disorder from abnormal personality traits is the evidence of long-term maladaptation and inflexibility, manifested as distress or impairment in social and occupational function, or both. DSM-IV-TR arranges personality disorders into three clusters, which share some clinical features. Studies support the construct validity of these clusters. Table 28-1 summarizes the three clusters.

Why Are Personality Disorders Coded on Axis II?

Personality disorders are Axis II disorders because they are typically life-long and reflect enduring, maladaptive patterns of an individual's internal experience and behavior. Axis I disorders are more typically the episodic eruption of symptoms against a background of more normal functioning. Personality disorders and mental retardation are the only two classes of mental disorders that are coded on Axis II. Axis I and II disorders can (and often do) coexist.

Can a Patient Have Both an Axis I Diagnosis and a Personality Disorder?

Yes. The disorders can and often do coexist. For example, patients who have borderline personality disorder are at significantly higher risk for developing mood disorders (dysthymia, major depression) as well as substance use disorders and anxiety disorders. Even in patients with the diagnosis of borderline personality disorder who do not have a comorbid mood disorder, there are likely to be significant emotional eruptions in response to life events—very often the vicissitudes of romantic relationships.

How Can I Tell if My Inpatient Has a Personality Disorder?

The diagnosis of a personality disorder is based on enduring, pervasive patterns of behavior, and neither the history of present illness nor the mental

Table 28-1

The Personality Disorders

Cluster A: "Odd" These people appear to have little interest in engaging with other people.
 Paranoid: Suspiciousness and hypervigilance but no delusions
 Schizoid: Social isolation because of lack of desire to socialize
 Schizotypal: Odd thinking and eccentric behaviors
Cluster B: "Dramatic" These people engage intensely with the people around them.
 Antisocial: Rejection and violation of laws and social norms
 Borderline: Wild swings between idealization and devaluation
 Histrionic: Attention seeking
 Narcissistic: Grandiosity and lack of empathy
Cluster C: "Anxious" These people long to connect with other people but are often unsuccessful.
 Avoidant: Social isolation related to fear of rejection
 Dependent: Excessive desire to be taken care of
 Obsessive-compulsive: Preoccupation with orderliness and control

Personality Disorders

status examination is likely to reveal the essential features of a personality disorder. Past history that includes the patient's childhood and adolescence, reported by the patient as well as by people who have been close to the patient for a long time, is often more helpful. During an acute inpatient admission, the full symptomatology of a personality disorder is often not revealed, and you may not be able to diagnose a personality disorder. It is also very difficult to get a good sense of patients' personality when they are in the midst of an exacerbation of a disorder that meets criteria for an Axis I diagnosis. For this reason, the diagnosis on Axis II is typically deferred during acute psychiatric hospitalizations.

Do I Need to Diagnose a Patient's Personality Disorder to Treat His Axis I Disorder on the Inpatient Service?

No. Axis I disorders such as schizophrenia, bipolar disorder, and major depressive disorder often have exacerbations that require acute care on an inpatient psychiatric unit and can be adequately treated with medications and psychotherapy even in the presence of an undiagnosed personality disorder. However, having an understanding of your patient's personality and being aware of the possibility of a particular personality disorder can greatly help you in your treatment plans. For example, if you suspect that your suicidal patient with major depressive disorder may also have schizoid personality features, you may choose to offer more individual and less group psychotherapy along with antidepressant medications.

Isn't There a Risk That Diagnosing Personality Disorders Simply Pathologizes Normal Varieties of Personality?

Yes, there is certainly such a risk. The DSM diagnostic system is *categorical* and classifies personality disorders as if they were discrete entities. According to DSM-IV-TR, a person either does or does not have a personality disorder. However, personality can also be thought of as consisting of a variety of traits (e.g., sense of humor, tolerance for risk, gregariousness), each of which can be evaluated on a scale from "a lot" to "none." Critics of the DSM-IV-TR categorical classification have argued in favor of such a *dimensional* approach that would allow a clinician to describe an individual's personality without having to label it pathologic or nonpathologic. Most individual personality styles should be considered part of the normal variety of human life, and the diagnosis of a personality disorder should be reserved for patients whose personalities clearly fall in the pathologic range because of the distress and disability they experience.

What Is a Hysterical Personality Disorder?

This diagnosis, sometimes used interchangeably with a histrionic personality disorder, does not exist in DSM-IV-TR. When someone is described as being "hysterical" in a clinical sense, it refers to a patient who has an intact sense of identity and the capacity for stable, emotionally rich relationships. The main defense mechanism used in these patients is repression. They are often emotionally labile, usually dramatic, and although they may appear superficial, their emotional experiences are authentic.

Is Obsessive-Compulsive Personality Disorder Related to Axis I Obsessive-Compulsive Disorder?

No. Although the two disorders have similar names and share some characteristics, there is evidence that the neurobiology underlying the two disorders is quite different. Unlike OCPD, which has no identifiable anatomic basis, OCD is sometimes linked to specific brain lesions (e.g., in the cingulate gyrus) that can be treated with psychosurgery. The clinical presentation is also distinct. Patients with OCD always have obsessions or compulsions, which they see as unwanted symptoms. People with OPCD have *no* obsessions or compulsions. They are perfectionists preoccupied with rules and order and are usually unconflicted about the way they are. It is useful to remember the triad of symptoms that is historically connected with patients with obsessive-compulsive personality disorder: orderliness, parsimoniousness, and obstinacy. (See Chapter 25 for a further discussion of OCD.)

TREATMENT

How Do I Treat Personality Disorders?

The treatment for personality disorders is usually long term. Most people with personality disorders perceive their lifestyles as normal and seldom seek or accept treatment. Typically, they seek help when their maladaptive behaviors result in marital, family, and work problems or for comorbid depression, anxiety, substance abuse, or eating disorders. Temperament traits are primarily treated with medications. Character, slow to change, is best managed with psychotherapy. Extreme temperament and immature character traits are best treated with combined psychotherapy and pharmacotherapy. Although you will not be able to treat your patient's personality disorder during an acute hospitalization for psychiatric or medical stabilization, an understanding of how a personality disorder can get in the way of treatment is helpful. For example, although you may not be able to treat narcissistic personality disorder during an admission for a major depressive episode, recognizing the patient's sense of entitlement and grandiosity as part of his personality disorder can help you set limits and control his destructive, maladaptive behavior on the unit. Treatment of personality disorders often combines psychotherapy and medication.

What Kind of Psychotherapy Is Most Effective for Personality Disorders?

Most personality disorders can be treated by different psychotherapies or by a combination of techniques from different psychotherapies. Dialectical behavioral therapy (DBT) and transference-focused psychotherapy (TFP) have been devised specifically for the treatment of borderline personality disorder. Table 28-2 describes the psychotherapy approaches to the three personality disorder clusters. Table 28-3 describes the goals and indications for some commonly prescribed psychotherapies. With all therapies, a main goal is to establish and maintain a stable therapeutic relationship and to provide reliable and consistent care. Behavior and feelings are often

Table 28-2
Psychotherapy Treatments for Personality Disorders

Cluster A: Patients rarely seek professional treatment. (Psychotherapy groups are often rejected.)
Supportive therapy
Cognitive-behavioral therapy (CBT)
Cluster B: Patients rarely respond fully to treatment.
  Dialectical behavioral therapy (DBT), especially for borderline personality disorder
  Transference-focused psychotherapy (TFP), especially for borderline personality disorder
  Cognitive-behavioral therapy
  Psychodynamic psychotherapy
  Group psychotherapy
Cluster C: Patients respond relatively well to treatment.
  Psychodynamic psychotherapy
  Cognitive-behavioral therapy
  Group psychotherapy

Table 28-3
Goals and Indications of Some Psychotherapies for Personality Disorders

Psychodynamic psychotherapy addresses the internal world of the patient's emotions and needs and regards symptoms as the external manifestation of internal motivations and conflicts.
Transference-focused psychotherapy is an adaptation of psychodynamic psychotherapy designed specifically for borderline patients. It is generally shorter and more focused on the transference.
Dialectical behavioral therapy also originated as a treatment for borderline personality disorder. It combines group therapy with individual therapy, both emphasizing behavioral approaches to symptomatic behavior.
Cognitive therapy helps patients correct distorted appraisal of environmental cues and underlying core beliefs that lead to maladaptive behavior.
Supportive psychotherapy works to strengthen behaviors and attitudes that are adaptive and minimize those that are maladaptive, often by surveying past experience to determine what worked and what didn't work.

the focus of therapy with the hope of establishing more flexibility and a greater repertoire of ways of interacting with other people and the world.

What Drugs Are Used in the Treatment of Personality Disorders?

There are no drugs that treat specific personality disorders. However, different symptoms, highly associated with specific personality disorders, can show improvement with medications. For example, mood stabilizers (such as valproate) and antipsychotics (such as clozapine) diminish the aggression and impulse dyscontrol found in borderline and antisocial personality disorders. Selective serotonin reuptake inhibitors (such as fluoxetine) treat the depression, anxiety, social phobia, and ruminative traits found in avoidant and obsessive-compulsive personality disorders.

Table 28-4 summarizes medications used for personality disorders. Most patients need a combination of psychotherapy and medication treatment.

How Do I Manage Manipulative Patients?

Some patients with borderline, narcissistic, or antisocial personality disorder are difficult and manipulative. At times, they may try to make you feel that you are the only person in the world who understands them and thus the only one who can save them. At other times, they may try to make you feel bad that you are unable to be of any help or even that you are directly responsible for their misery. Almost invariably, such attempts reflect the patient's psychopathology and internal struggles rather than your performance as a clinician. To be able to work effectively with these patients, it is necessary to develop professional distance from their provocations.

Table 28-5 summarizes some simple rules for observing proper boundaries with difficult patients.

What Do People Mean When They Say That a Patient with Borderline Personality Disorder Is "Splitting"?

Splitting was originally a psychoanalytic term used to describe unconscious and unobservable mental processes in which a patient—especially one with borderline personality disorder—cannot tolerate simultaneous good and bad thoughts and feelings about someone important. The good is *split* from

Personality Disorders

Table 28-4

Psychopharmacologic Treatments for Personality Disorders

Symptom	Medications
Dysregulated mood	
Depression	SSRIs, MAOIs, antipsychotics
Mood lability	Lithium, anticonvulsants, atypical antipsychotics
Emotional detachment	Atypical antipsychotics
Anxiety	SSRIs, MAOIs, benzodiazepines, GABAergic drugs, β-blockers, atypical antipsychotics
Dysregulated behavior	
Aggression/impulsivity	SSRIs, lithium, anticonvulsants, atypical antipsychotics, β-blockers, benzodiazepines

Medications are used adjunctively for particular symptoms and not for the treatment of a specific personality disorder.
GABA, gamma-aminobutyric acid; MAOI, monoamine oxidase inhibitor; SSRI, selective serotonin reuptake inhibitor.

Table 28-5

Boundaries to Observe with Patients

Do not become overinvolved with the patient.

Limit any physical contact with the patient to a handshake and to physical examinations, as indicated.

Do not share personal information with the patient, other than your name, your professional affiliation, your title, and your supervisor.

Outline clearly for the patient the consequences of his or her actions: "If you smoke on the unit, you will lose pass privileges."

Discuss difficult cases with your colleagues and supervisors. Do not feel embarrassed to ask for help when dealing with a difficult patient.

Avoid arguments and belabored explanations.

Resist the temptation to believe statements such as "Nobody understands me the way you do."

Do not give patients gifts.

the bad, with the result that the other person is seen as idealized (all good) or totally devalued (all bad). The term splitting is used these days on inpatient services to mean that one staff member is being pitted against another.

Multidisciplinary team members who treat borderline patients should be in very close communication with each other, talk about the patients' misdirected efforts, and plan coordinated care. It is destructive to staff functioning, and it is never helpful to patients, for the treatment team to start sharing some of the patient's beliefs that certain staff members are helping the patient and others are hurting her.

How Do I Treat My Patient Who Has Antisocial Personality Disorder?

Although most personality disorders respond best to supportive approaches, patients with antisocial personality disorder often need to be confronted and told in very clear terms what they are doing wrong—for example, "What you told me yesterday turned out to be a lie." Confronting antisocial patients may be helpful in curtailing their behavior, but neither supportive nor confrontational approaches have been shown to be helpful in changing the personality disorder itself. Mood stabilizers such as valproate and lithium have controlled impulsivity in some antisocial patients. Family psychotherapy can be helpful in reducing domestic violence. Approximately 60% of patients with antisocial personality disorder also have a substance use disorder and require addiction treatment.

KEY POINTS

◆ Personality disorders are typically lifelong and require long-term treatment.

◆ Personality disorders are difficult to diagnose during an acute psychiatric hospitalization.

◆ Setting clear behavioral limits and observing boundaries are essential in treating patients with personality disorders.

◆ Most patients with a personality disorder need a combination of psychotherapy and medication treatment.

Case 28-1

A 30-year-old man is admitted to the psychiatric inpatient service after extensive superficial bilateral cutting of his forearms. Initially, the nursing staff describes him as "normal," engaging, and even charming. However, within a few hours of his admission to the ward, he seems to have created havoc around him. People describe him as needy, nasty, and unpredictable. His nurse reports, "Yesterday he said I was the best nurse in the world and today he asked the head nurse to fire me." You have ruled out psychotic disorders, drug intoxication and withdrawal, and delirium. You have reason to believe from old hospital charts and discussion with collaterals that the patient has a personality disorder.

A. What is the likely personality disorder?
B. How do you treat the patient?
C. What do you tell the nurse?

Case 28-2

A 60-year-old employed woman with history of hypertension and diabetes comes to your primary care medical practice for the first time complaining of dizziness. When you suggest routine blood work, she refuses, stating, "I am not a guinea pig." You explain that the studies are solely for clinical management, but the patient is not convinced. The patient's daughter reports that her mother has made very few friends in her life because she is always suspicious of people. You maintain a supportive, nonconfrontational attitude and arrange for a follow-up appointment within a few days. When she returns, she voices her reservations but reluctantly agrees to the laboratory examinations.

A. Is the patient delusional?
B. Is the patient delirious?
C. How do you treat this patient?

Personality Disorders

Case 28-3

A 28-year-old medical resident with no past medical or psychiatric history comes to your gynecology clinic for routine examination and testing. Before seeing her, you realize that she switched the order of the charts in the nursing station so that she could be seen without waiting. Your administrative assistant points out to you that during a previous visit, the patient had reported that she was unemployed to avoid a $5.00 co-payment. When you bring these matters to the patient's attention, she says, "It's no big deal. It's not like I make much money as a resident."

A. What other information do you need to establish a personality disorder diagnosis?
B. Are there treatments for antisocial personality disorder?

Case Answers

28-1 A.   *Learning objective:* **Recognize the essential symptoms of the three personality disorder clusters.** The patient probably suffers from a cluster B personality disorder. In the absence of an acute Axis I or medical condition, the patient appears to be erratic, dramatic, and demanding. Although differentiating among the different cluster B personality disorders on the basis of the information presented in this case is very difficult if not impossible, the patient seems to experience the world as "black or white," all good or all bad, a characteristic of borderline personality disorder. Although borderline personality disorder is more commonly diagnosed in women, men are also affected and often misdiagnosed. The patient is unlikely to suffer from a cluster A personality disorder because he initially seemed well related; it is also unlikely that he struggles with a cluster C personality disorder as he is more dramatic and outwardly emotional than inwardly anxious and worried.

28-1 B.   *Learning objective:* **Know the treatment modalities for borderline personality disorder.** The hallmark of the treatment of borderline personality disorder is limit setting and clear understanding of these limits. Although several different psychotherapies have been tried for the treatment of borderline personality disorders, it appears that dialectic behavioral therapy may offer an advantage for severe cases.

28-1 C.   *Learning objective:* **Appreciate the importance of communication in a multidisciplinary treatment approach.** Discuss with the nurse the patient's psychopathology and his tendency to swing between idealization and devaluation, which is characteristic of a borderline personality disorder. (Psychiatric nurses on inpatient services will have a great deal to teach you about managing difficult patients.) Also, review with the other disciplines how to set consistent limits on the patient in order to reduce his destructive effects on the unit. Such discussions among different members of the treatment team are essential in reducing the demoralizing effect of the patient's accusations on the staff. They also help to refocus the team's efforts in treating the patient's illness.

28-2 A. *Learning objective:* **Distinguish paranoid thoughts from paranoid delusions.** She is probably not delusional. The patient displays paranoid thinking with marked suspiciousness and mistrust of people. However, with support from you and her daughter, it seems that she is able to be convinced and eventually agree with the plan. If she were delusional, she would have maintained her false belief despite any interventions. A paranoid idea becomes a paranoid delusion when the patient can no longer entertain any alternatives.

28-2 B. *Learning objective:* **Distinguish between a personality disorder and delirium.** She is probably not delirious. Medical problems can precipitate delirium, which can arise as paranoid thoughts or paranoid delusions. However, delirium usually has an acute onset and is always accompanied by an altered level of consciousness and often disturbances in orientation. The patient appears to suffer from chronic suspiciousness with some impairment in social relationships. You should consider paranoid personality disorder as a possible diagnosis, to be confirmed or ruled out on the basis of further information you will gather during the medical treatment of the patient.

28-2 C. *Learning objective:* **Recognize that building rapport is essential for patients with personality disorders.** You should treat the patient with respectful formality. An overly friendly or chummy approach will increase suspiciousness in a guarded patient. Establish rapport before pursuing diagnostic examinations or treatments that the patient finds suspicious. Trying to convince her that her idea is false by arguing or cajoling will not work. The paranoid ideas of patients with paranoid personality disorder often become self-fulfilling prophecies as physicians lose their patience, directly confront the false ideas, argue, and eventually become menacing in the eyes of the paranoid person.

28-3 A. *Learning objective:* **Recognize that the diagnosis of a personality disorder is based on pervasive patterns of behavior.** You need to establish that the patient's disregard for the rights of others extends well beyond your clinic before diagnosing antisocial personality disorder. Information from colleagues and family members may corroborate your suspicion that she deceives, lies to, and cons others for personal profit or pleasure on a regular basis; furthermore, she shows no remorse and rationalizes her behavior.

Personality Disorders

28-3 B. *Learning objective:* **Appreciate the limitations of psychiatric treatments.** There are no effective treatments for antisocial personality disorder. However, several symptoms associated with the disorder can be effectively managed with medications, individual psychotherapy, group or family psychotherapy, and substance abuse treatment, if applicable.

29

Eating Disorders

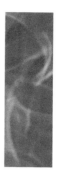

NATALIE GLUCK

What Is Anorexia Nervosa?

Anorexia nervosa is an eating disorder whose hallmark is a distorted perception of one's body and refusal to maintain a normal body weight. Anorexia nervosa has four cardinal features: preoccupation with or intense fear of gaining weight, a refusal to maintain at least 85% of expected weight, a distorted self-image of one's body size, and, in postmenarchial women, amenorrhea. There are two subtypes of anorexia nervosa. The *binge eating/purging type* is characterized by binge eating followed by a compensatory behavior, most frequently self-induced vomiting; patients with this type of the disorder sometimes use laxatives, diuretics, or enemas to rid themselves of the binge calories. The *restrictive type* is characterized by excessive dieting or fasting without any binge eating or purging behavior.

What Is Bulimia Nervosa?

Patients with bulimia nervosa have a similar preoccupation with body image but have regular menses and maintain normal or even above normal body weight. The hallmark of this disorder is episodic binge eating during which the patient feels a loss of self-control and may consume enormous quantities of food. Binge eating is followed by compensatory behaviors to avoid weight gain. Bulimia nervosa is classified as either *purging* type, in which the patient may use self-induced vomiting, laxatives, or diuretics to lose weight, and *nonpurging* type, in which patients attempt to control their weight with excessive diet and exercise.

How Common Are the Eating Disorders?

Eating disorders are more common in developed countries than in developing countries. In the United States, the lifetime prevalence of anorexia nervosa among women is 0.5% to 2%, and the lifetime prevalence of bulimia nervosa among women is 1% to 3%. Overall, the disorders are 10 times more common in females than in males, although the female-to-male ratio is lower in younger patients.

What Causes Anorexia Nervosa and Bulimia Nervosa?

The etiology of eating disorders is best understood through the biopsychosocial model of modern psychiatry. Some of the biologic, psychological, and sociologic underpinnings of eating disorders are summarized in Table 29-1.

When Do Eating Disorders First Appear?

Anorexia nervosa usually arises in early to middle adolescence, whereas bulimia nervosa first arises a little later during late adolescence to early adulthood. Young women with an extensive history of dieting are at higher risk for eating disorders. Traditionally, eating disorders are thought to be more prevalent in higher socioeconomic classes, but recent data suggest that middle-class and lower middle-class women may be equally affected.

Is Obesity an Eating Disorder?

Not necessarily. Although obese individuals suffer from higher than average rates of depression and anxiety, obesity is not considered to be a primary psychiatric disorder. However, between 25% and 50% of people with obesity have symptoms consistent with binge eating disorder, a subtype of eating disorder that is characterized by recurrent episodes of binge eating in the absence of inappropriate compensatory behaviors.

EVALUATION

How Do I Take a History from a Patient Who I Suspect Has an Eating Disorder?

Keep in mind that patients with anorexia nervosa do not appreciate their emaciated appearance. Their self-perception is usually distorted to the

Eating Disorders

Table 29-1
Factors Associated with Eating Disorders
Biologic factors
Female sex
Genetics: In anorexia nervosa, 55% concordance rate for monozygotic twins and 5% for dizygotic twins. In bulimia nervosa, the concordance rate is 35% for monozygotic twins and 30% for dizygotic twins.
Serotonin: High serotonin levels may result in a sense of fullness and decreased appetite.
Psychological factors
"Type A" personality, perfectionism and rigidity
Obsessional thinking
Impulsivity, negative emotionality and stress reactivity (bulimia)
Sociologic factors
Cultural preoccupation with thinness
Extremely thin role models (e.g., actors, dolls, cartoons)
Some professions that demand thinness (e.g., models, jockeys, gymnasts)

point that they insist that they are at a normal weight or even that they need to lose more weight. These patients rarely come to see the physician of their own volition and are often embarrassed or defensive, typically hiding their bodies in large clothes and providing vague histories. Talking with family and friends is often helpful in the assessment of eating disorders but of course requires the patient's permission. (You can talk with the parents of an adolescent without her permission, although it is essential to keep her as involved in the process of consultation as possible.) Adolescents are usually brought to medical attention at the insistence of their parents. Box 29-1 summarizes symptoms highly associated with anorexia nervosa and bulimia nervosa.

Do I Need to Look Out for Other Psychiatric Disorders?

Yes. Patients with anorexia and bulimia have high incidences of mood, anxiety, personality, and substance use disorders. Depression is present in approximately 65% of patients with anorexia, although whether it is a risk factor for or result of the eating disorder is still unclear. Anorexia is also associated with anxiety disorders in over 60% of cases and with obsessive-compulsive disorders in over 40% of cases. Patients with bulimia also demonstrate significant comorbidity with depressive and anxiety disorders, with a combined lifetime prevalence of 75%. Several studies have also shown that up to 30% of patients with bulimia suffer from a substance use disorder, most frequently involving alcohol or stimulants.

Are Patients with Anorexia Nervosa Psychotic?

Technically, no. Severe distortions of body perception, as seen in anorexia nervosa patients who believe they are fat, are usually described as "near delusional," although the intensity of the body distortion belief may render it indistinguishable from a frank delusion. These distortions, however, do not respond to antipsychotic medications.

BOX 29-1

SYMPTOMS OF ANOREXIA NERVOSA AND BULIMIA NERVOSA

Symptoms of Anorexia Nervosa

♦ Distorted perception of one's own body weight or shape
♦ Morbid fear of being or becoming fat
♦ Body weight less than 85% of normal
♦ Amenorrhea

Symptoms of Bulimia Nervosa

♦ Self-esteem based on body weight and shape
♦ Preoccupation with dieting but normal weight
♦ Binge eating with a sense of loss of self-control
♦ Inappropriate compensatory behaviors (e.g., self-induced vomiting, laxative abuse, excessive exercise)

Eating Disorders

What Kind of Personality Is at Risk for an Eating Disorder?

Patients who struggle with issues of rigidity and control may have both the restricting type of anorexia nervosa and obsessive-compulsive personality disorder. These patients are often consumed by attempts to be perfect and always in control in terms of work, school, and body fat. Recent research has implicated a particular personality cluster in patients with bulimia marked by a pattern of impulsivity and self-injurious behaviors such as cutting, traits most often associated with cluster B personality disorders.

What Are the Physical Findings?

For the diagnosis of anorexia nervosa, body weight below 85% of that expected for the patient's age, height, and gender is required. Body mass index (calculated by dividing weight in kilograms by height in meters squared) can help to establish the diagnosis of anorexia, with a BMI under 18 indicating a dangerously low weight. (See Box 29-2 for a list of BMI ranges.) Emaciation, bradycardia, hypotension, and hypothermia can be found on physical examination of patients with either binge eating/purging or restrictive-type anorexia nervosa. Some patients with anorexia also develop fine body hair called lanugo or show hair thinning. Figure 29-1 illustrates the extreme emaciation that is sometimes seen in advanced anorexia nervosa. Patients with anorexia nervosa of the binge eating/purging type or bulimia nervosa of the purging type who induce vomiting often have calluses on the back of their hands because their teeth rub against their skin when they induce vomiting. They also show dental enamel erosions from the lingual side resulting from the stomach acid hitting the upper teeth (Fig. 29-2). Large salivary glands often signify a recent history of repeated vomiting. Common physical findings are summarized in Table 29-2.

What Causes Amenorrhea?

Malnutrition and self-starvation result in hormonal changes including abnormalities in the circulating levels of follicle-stimulating hormone and luteinizing hormone, which in turn affect menses. However, amenorrhea in anorexia nervosa may also be mediated through a different mechanism as it sometimes *precedes* weight loss.

Eating Disorders

BOX 29-2

BODY MASS INDEX RANGES

- ◆ Underweight = <18.5
- ◆ Normal weight = 18.5–24.9
- ◆ Overweight = 25–29.9
- ◆ Obesity = BMI of 30 or greater

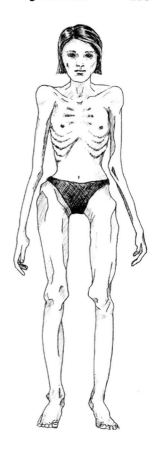

FIGURE 29-1 Extreme emaciation seen in advanced anorexia nervosa.

Are There Blood Tests That Help Make a Diagnosis of Anorexia Nervosa?

Yes. Although some patients with anorexia nervosa have no laboratory abnormalities, most patients exhibit laboratory findings consistent with the semistarvation state that is characteristic of anorexia. Table 29-3 lists common laboratory findings. In addition to electrolyte imbalances related to starvation, patients with anorexia nervosa may have endocrine abnormalities including low concentrations of luteinizing hormone, follicle-stimulating hormone, and estrogen. Low triiodothyronine can also be seen. Anorexics who induce vomiting may show low chloride and low potassium levels and an increase in serum bicarbonate related to metabolic alkalosis. Vomiting stomach hydrochloric acid renders the body alkalotic. On the other hand, patients who abuse laxatives may induce a metabolic acidosis.

However, none of these laboratory findings are pathognomonic for the presence of an eating disorder.

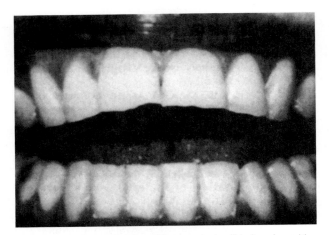

FIGURE 29-2 Dental erosion caused by repeated self-induced vomiting, with the characteristic finding of intact lower teeth and eroded upper teeth. (From Stege P, Visco-Dangler L, Rye L. Anorexia nervosa: Review including oral and dental manifestations. J Am Dent Assoc 1982;104:648–652. Reprinted with permission of American Dental Association.)

Table 29-2

Common Physical Signs Associated with Anorexia Nervosa and Bulimia Nervosa

Cachexia (extreme physical wasting)
Dry skin; lanugo (fine downy hair) on the back, forearms, and side of the face
Swelling of parotid and submandibular glands ("chipmunk cheeks")
Erosion of inner surface of front teeth
Cold hands and feet; hypothermia
Bradycardia; orthostatic hypotension; cardiac arrhythmias
Weak proximal muscles (elicited as difficulty rising from a squatting position)

Table 29-3

Laboratory Abnormalities Related to Starvation

Hematology	Low white blood cell count
	Low hematocrit
Chemistry	High blood urea nitrogen because of dehydration
	High cholesterol (hypercholesterolemia)
	High liver function tests (AST, ALT, alkaline phosphatase)
	Low phosphorus, magnesium, zinc, amylase levels
	Low estrogen levels in women
	Low testosterone levels in men

Self-induced vomiting can create a hypokalemic alkalosis.
ALT, alanine transaminase; AST, aspartate transaminase.

Eating Disorders

Are There Medical Conditions or Drug-Related States That Look Like Anorexia Nervosa?

Patients with gastrointestinal diseases such as malabsorption syndrome, endocrine diseases such as hyperthyroidism, cancer, and acquired immunodeficiency syndrome (AIDS) may present with significant weight loss, but patients with such diseases do not have a morbid fear of fatness and do not want to lose more weight. Patients who abuse stimulants such as methylphenidate, cocaine, ecstasy, or crystal methamphetamine may experience serious weight loss mimicking that in anorexia nervosa. Heavy marijuana use can result in significantly increased appetite followed by binge eating and purging in an attempt to compensate.

How Do I Rule Out Medical and Drug-Related Conditions?

Start with a thorough history and physical examination to evaluate weight loss, and follow up with laboratory testing and radiographic studies, as indicated. A history of unprotected sex or sharing intravenous needles requires testing for human immunodeficiency virus (HIV) infection. Cancer evaluation depends on the organs affected, and again a complete physical examination, including a breast examination, is essential. Although an elevated erythrocyte sedimentation rate may be a first clue of serious infection or cancer, it is also often elevated in patients with anorexia nervosa and thus is not as useful in the differential diagnosis. Most illicit substances are present in urine samples for only 48 to 72 hours after the most recent use. Therefore, urine toxicology examinations are usually not conclusive regarding substance abuse.

TREATMENT

What Are the Goals of Treatment?

First things first. Restoration of healthy weight and metabolic balance is the first goal of treatment. The second goal is to establish healthy eating routines and habits. The third goal is to change the distorted ideas the patient has about body shape, weight, fat, success, control, self-worth, and so forth. In other words, the goals of treatment are prioritized as (1) medical, (2) behavioral, and (3) cognitive. Because eating disorders often occur with depression, anxiety disorders, substance abuse, and personality disorders, ongoing assessment and specific treatments for such disorders should also be provided.

What Clinical Settings Are Appropriate for the Treatment of Eating Disorders?

It depends on the severity of illness. Inpatient treatment is almost always indicated if the patient has dangerously low weight or associated medical complications, such as an electrolyte imbalance, or both. Hospitalization may also be warranted if there is a risk of suicide, severe interpersonal problems at home, or failure of less intensive methods of treatment. Appropriate clinical settings are summarized in Table 29-4.

Eating Disorders

Table 29-4

Clinical Settings for the Treatment of Eating Disorders

Presentation	Treatment

Patient below 75% of expected weight for height, or history of rapid weight loss in an older patient, or electrolyte instability	Inpatient hospitalization
	  Medical stabilization
	  Medical model
	  General hospital

Patient requires acute weight restoration but is medically stable	Eating disorders program
	  Milieu based
	  Psychological model
	  Psychiatric unit or residence

Patient is stable but still symptomatic	Outpatient program
	  Individual and/or group therapy
	  Psychological model
	  Office or clinic

How Do I Talk to My Patient with an Eating Disorder?

Appreciate the disorder as a life-threatening illness over which the individual has lost control. Approach the patient with a nonjudgmental, nonpunitive attitude and avoid arguing, persuading, and cajoling.

What Kind of Psychotherapy Should I Use?

Individual cognitive-behavioral therapy (CBT) is the most commonly used psychotherapy. CBT is a structured therapy that uses an active approach, such as assigning homework exercises and encouraging journal keeping, to modify maladaptive thoughts and behaviors. CBT teaches patients to be aware of their negative thought patterns and to challenge their overvaluation of shape and weight, their eating habits, and self-image. Patients are encouraged to keep daily journals to monitor their food intake, their binging and purging, and the feelings and emotions aroused by their eating behaviors. In patients who are out of the acute phase of an eating disorder, an insight-oriented or psychodynamic therapy can also be useful. This kind of treatment may focus on identifying the underlying conflicts that lead to self-punishing behaviors and on helping the patient to recognize and assert her autonomy in healthier ways.

Are Any Medications Helpful in the Treatment of Eating Disorders?

Yes and no. In the acute phase, antidepressants are generally ineffective for weight restoration. Appetite-stimulating medications such as tetrahydrocannabinol (THC) or olanzapine are also ineffective, as the problem in eating disorders is not simply a loss of appetite. After nutritional balance has been established, antidepressants may be useful adjunctive treatment, particularly with bulimia. The selective serotonin reuptake inhibitors

(SSRIs) are generally safe and help treat the depression, anxiety, obsessive thinking, and low self-esteem associated with eating disorders. Even in the absence of depression or anxiety, studies have demonstrated that SSRIs reduce binging and purging behaviors. The atypical antidepressant bupropion is contraindicated because it increases risk of seizures in patients with electrolyte disturbances.

Is There Anything Else I Can Do to Help?

Yes. Family therapy, couples therapy, and group psychotherapy all have been shown to help as adjunctive treatments. Nutritional counseling, self-help books, food diaries, 12-step programs, and support groups can also be invaluable components of a comprehensive treatment plan.

What Is the Prognosis for My Patient with an Eating Disorder?

In general, one third of patients recover fully with treatment, one third continue to have some symptoms but no longer meet diagnostic criteria for an eating disorder, and one third remain chronically ill. Anorexia nervosa is associated with the highest mortality of all psychiatric disorders, with up to 10% of patients eventually dying from complications of the disease, including suicide. The most frequent causes of death in anorexia are cardiac arrhythmias and complications secondary to starvation, such as infection and multiorgan failure. Bulimia is rarely fatal but can have serious medical complications including Mallory-Weiss tears of the esophagus or even complete esophageal rupture, a phenomenon known as Boerhaave's syndrome.

KEY POINTS

◆ Patients with anorexia nervosa are significantly underweight, whereas patients with bulimia nervosa maintain normal weight.

◆ Self-induced vomiting can be associated with either anorexia nervosa or bulimia nervosa.

◆ Patients with anorexia nervosa have not lost their appetite.

◆ Anorexia nervosa may be a medical emergency with significant mortality.

Case 29-1

A 22-year-old woman comes to your office and immediately says, "I have terrible attention-deficit disorder and the only thing that has ever helped me is Ritalin. Ritalin 60 mg a day." When you ask her if she would like to take off her large overcoat, she refuses and says, "What do you want me to undress for? You want to see my tits or something? I told you, I just need Ritalin." The patient looks pale, emaciated, and depressed. The nurse provides you with the following information: blood pressure 95/60 mm Hg, heart rate 55 beats per minute, height 5 feet 8 inches, and weight unavailable (nurse's note: "patient refuses").

A. How do you respond?
B. What other information would you like?
C. What treatments do you suggest?

Case Answers

29-1 A. *Learning objective:* **Recognize that building a therapeutic alliance is an indispensable initial step in almost any treatment.** Although you suspect that the patient suffers from anorexia nervosa and she may not want to take her coat off because she is trying to conceal her weight loss, you should not insist on her taking off the coat right away. At this stage, you may also think that the patient is delusional or simply just cold intolerant and rude. Reassure the patient and explain that you would like to provide the best possible care for her, including a complete evaluation of her attention problems before prescribing medications. You should ask if you can talk with her parents.

29-1 B. *Learning objective:* **Know the key elements in the assessment of eating disorders.** The patient may not be able to provide a reliable history. If possible, involve the patient's family in the treatment, both for diagnostic and for therapeutic purposes. Ask the parents about weight loss, dieting, physical symptoms, attention problems, depression, and drugs. After obtaining a full history from the parents and developing basic rapport with the patient, perform a physical examination. You should then obtain an electrocardiogram, order a urine toxicology examination, and obtain laboratory tests, including complete blood cell count, electrolytes, HIV antibody test, liver function tests, and thyroid function tests to complete the assessment.

29-1 C. *Learning objective:* **Know the different treatment options for anorexia nervosa.** The patient may need to be hospitalized for medical stabilization and weight restoration. If you conclude that the patient suffers from anorexia nervosa, cognitive-behavioral psychotherapy will help this patient with her eating disorder. Following weight restoration, the patient should be evaluated for depression and offered an antidepressant if needed. Fluoxetine would be a good first-line choice as it has been shown to benefit patients with depression and eating disorders.

Eating Disorders

30

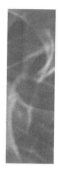

Sleep Disorders

MYRL R. S. MANLEY

Why Are Sleep Disorders Classified as Psychiatric Conditions?

Good question. Probably no other group of disorders points up the limitations of specialty classification as much as sleep disorders, which can involve emotional, neurologic, genetic, behavioral, cardiac, endocrine, and pulmonary factors. Most people with sleep complaints do not come to psychiatrists, and most sleep disorders are treated by physicians who are not psychiatrists. Nevertheless, psychiatrists must understand sleep disorders (and they are classified as Axis I disorders in DSM-IV-TR) for at least a couple of reasons. First, a large number of psychiatric disorders such as mania, depression, and anxiety can include sleep disturbances, and it is essential to be able to distinguish primary from secondary sleep problems. Second, many sleep disorders cause associated emotional and behavioral problems that may require psychiatric treatment.

How Do I Ask My Patient About Sleep Problems?

There is usually no difficulty in getting patients to acknowledge and discuss sleep problems because they can be so distressing. There may, in fact, be the risk that sleep complaints mask more serious symptoms. Keep in mind that insomnia is a symptom, not a diagnosis, and that it must be explored in the same way as any physical symptom. When did it start? How has it progressed? What makes it worse? What makes it better? Are there associated symptoms? Has it happened before? Most people tend to be inaccurate reporters of their own sleep. The patient who says "I didn't sleep a wink last night" may be reporting the level of subjective distress more than historical accuracy. General statements such as "I haven't been sleeping well at all" or "I slept really well last night" are notoriously unreliable and difficult to use diagnostically. Consequently, it is necessary to be quite specific when reviewing sleep complaints. Questions you may need to ask include, "What time did you go to bed? When did you fall asleep? Did you wake during the night? How often? How long did it take you to fall back asleep? How many hours of sleep have you had in the last 24 hours? How many hours do you *normally* sleep in 24 hours?"

What Tests Are Available to Diagnose Sleep Disorders?

Specific laboratory studies help diagnose a medical condition causing a secondary sleep disturbance. Polysomnographic sleep laboratory studies and the multiple sleep latency test are of considerable use in diagnosing some specific disorders. These tests are discussed more fully in Chapter 19.

What Treatments Are Available for Sleep Disorders?

The treatment for a secondary sleep disorder is of course directed to the underlying cause, but symptomatic relief may also be an appropriate adjunct. For example, a manic patient might be given lithium to control the mood disturbance but also a short course of the hypnotic zolpidem or a sedating atypical antipsychotic such as quetiapine or olanzapine to help with sleep right away. Symptomatic treatment, and the treatment of primary disorders, can be psychotherapeutic (usually cognitive-behavioral), somatic, or both. These are discussed more fully in the next sections.

PRIMARY INSOMNIA

ETIOLOGY

What Causes Primary Insomnia?

As the name makes clear, it is not caused by a psychiatric or medical condition or by drugs. Patients simply cannot sleep well. They can't fall asleep, they can't stay asleep, and sleep is not refreshing. Some primary insomnia is a behaviorally learned state. After a random bad night of sleep, for example, some people start to worry about sleeping well the next night, and the anticipatory anxiety starts to interfere with good sleep. The fear of not sleeping becomes self-fulfilling. Some primary insomnia is idiopathic and is probably the result of dysregulation of sleep/wake brain mechanisms. And some primary insomnia probably results from sleep state misperceptions in which the degree of subjective distress does not correlate with objective measures. These possible causes are not absolute or distinctive; there is often considerable overlap for individual patients.

EVALUATION

How Do I Evaluate Someone for Primary Insomnia?

In addition to getting a good sleep history, you will need to rule out secondary causes. Consequently, a good, thorough medical and psychiatric evaluation is necessary. Some clinicians ask their patients to keep a sleep log, writing down when they go to bed, when they rise and how often, and for how long they wake during the night. Sleep logs may increase the accuracy of information, but they also carry the risk, by so intensely focusing the patient's attention on sleep, of unintentionally making sleep worse.

Sleep Disorders

Are Laboratory Studies Useful?

Mostly to rule out secondary causes. If there is persistent uncertainty about the accuracy of a patient's self-report, sleep laboratory studies give an objective measure of sleep onset, duration, and characteristics.

Can Primary Insomnia Be Treated without Drugs?

Very often it can. With behavioral therapy using principles of sleep hygiene outlined in Box 19-1 and using techniques such as daytime sleep restriction and stimulus control, 70% to 80% of people benefit and 30% become good sleepers. Cognitive therapy may help in decreasing the emotional distress associated with chronic insomnia. Cognitive-behavioral therapy is probably an underused treatment for insomnia because of a shortage of trained practitioners and the ready availability of medications.

What Medications Can Be Used to Treat Primary Insomnia?

Benzodiazepines and the closely related drugs zaleplon (Sonata) and zolpidem (Ambien) are safe and effective but are recommended only for short-term use. The nonbenzodiazepine hypnotics eszopiclone (Lunesta) and ramelteon (Rozerem) can be used for longer periods. Barbiturates and chloral hydrate are very effective in decreasing sleep latency, but the quick development of tolerance to these drugs, the serious adverse medical reactions (respiratory depression with barbiturates, gastrointestinal irritation with chloral hydrate), and the feeling of drug hangover the day after they have been used make them appropriate only for patients who have not been helped by other measures and then only for very short periods—one or two nights.

Aren't Benzodiazepines Addictive?

Tolerance to the benzodiazepines (requiring ever-increasing doses) develops slowly and is not usually a significant problem, even with long-term use. Patients who have taken benzodiazepines for many nights may experience rebound insomnia and anxiety when the drug is stopped. This can be quite uncomfortable for some patients and can be minimized by a slow taper off the drug. As with all medications, the risk of treatment must be weighed against the risk of nontreatment. There is reason to believe that the dangers of benzodiazepines have been overstated. In one call-in sample of patients who had been taking benzodiazepines, only 10% reported withdrawal symptoms on discontinuation—the same proportion who experienced withdrawal after stopping over-the-counter remedies. A more recent controlled study found that rebound insomnia after 4 weeks of treatment was greater for people taking a placebo than for those taking a benzodiazepine.

Can Cognitive-Behavioral Therapy and Medication Be Combined?

Controlled data show that therapy without medication has the best long-term outcome. In clinical practice, however, medication is commonly used because it offers much quicker relief and because it disrupts the vicious cycle of preoccupation with sleep leading to increasingly poor sleep.

PRIMARY HYPERSOMNIA

ETIOLOGY

What Causes Primary Hypersomnia?

It isn't clear. There are probably multiple causes. Some cases are believed to be a forme fruste of narcolepsy.

EVALUATION

How Do I Evaluate a Patient for Hypersomnia?

You will need to rule out psychiatric, medical, and drug causes of excessive somnolence (Table 30-1). Both narcolepsy and sleep apnea commonly present with heavy daytime sleepiness and may require sleep laboratory studies for a definitive diagnosis.

How Much Sleep Is Too Much?

The amount of sleep considered normal varies widely from person to person. Assessing whether a person sleeps too much or too little can be done

---

Table 30-1

Some Causes of Hypersomnia

Psychiatric
    Breathing-related sleep disorders
    Narcolepsy
    Atypical depression
    Schizophrenia (especially prodrome and residual phases)
    Bipolar disorder, depressed phase
    Adjustment disorders
Medical conditions
    Influenza
    Hypothyroidism
    Hyperglycemia
    Trypanosomiasis
Drugs
    Central nervous system sedative intoxication
    Central nervous system stimulant withdrawal
    Antipsychotics (especially clozapine, quetiapine, olanzapine, and low-potency typicals)
    Antidepressants (tricyclic antidepressants, selective serotonin reuptake inhibitors,
        trazodone, mirtazapine)
    Antihistamines
    Anticholinergics

Sleep Disorders

only in regard to what is normal for that individual. In addition, sleep needs change as a person gets older. Children and adolescents tend to sleep much more than adults (12 to 15 hours compared with 7 to 8 hours). To qualify as a disorder, the hypersomnia must be severe enough to cause distress or impairment.

TREATMENT

Can Primary Hypersomnia Be Treated?

The treatment is similar to the treatment for narcolepsy: behavioral and pharmaceutical. Behavioral techniques involve establishing regular and consistent sleeping hours and the prescription of short naps throughout the day. Central nervous system stimulants such as methylphenidate are effective in increasing daytime alertness. Modafinil (Provigil) appears to promote alertness without generalized central nervous system stimulation. It is approved for the treatment of daytime sleepiness associated with narcolepsy, obstructive sleep apnea, and shift work changes (a circadian rhythm disturbance). Modafinil is widely used to treat primary hypersomnia.

NARCOLEPSY

ETIOLOGY

How Is Narcolepsy Different from Primary Hypersomnia?

They may be different points on the spectrum of a common disorder, but the clinical picture is distinct. Both are characterized by excessive daytime sleepiness and increased overall sleepiness, but narcolepsy always includes sudden, paroxysmal irresistible attacks of sleep that result in short, refreshing naps. In addition, ancillary symptoms are seen in about two thirds of patients with narcolepsy: cataplexy, hypnagogics, hypnopompics, and sleep paralysis.

What Causes Narcolepsy?

Narcolepsy is a neurologic disorder of sleep regulation with a strong genetic component. It is not caused by underlying psychiatric problems, although many people with narcolepsy experience emotional difficulties in attempting to deal with the disorder. The prevalence among first-degree relatives is 50 to 100 times the prevalence in the general population (which is quite low: 0.02% to 0.16% for adults, with equal occurrence among males and females). Cataplexy, hypnagogics, hypnopompics, and sleep paralysis are believed to result from the intrusion of rapid eye movement (REM) sleep into the transition between sleep and wakefulness and sometimes are referred to as "REM intrusion phenomena" (Box 30-1). The suspicion of a genetic basis has been strengthened by the recent identification of a single gene abnormality in dogs with narcolepsy. The abnormal gene results in impaired recognition of the transmitter hypocretin-2 in the hypothalamus.

BOX 30-1

REM INTRUSION PHENOMENA

Cataplexy: sudden loss of all muscle tone
Hypnagogic: hallucinatory-like perception as a person falls asleep
Hypnopompic: hallucinatory-like perception as a person wakes up
Sleep paralysis: momentary (few seconds) inability to move on waking up

How Is Narcolepsy Diagnosed?

There are two approaches. One makes the diagnosis only on the basis of clinical symptoms and course—the approach used in DSM-IV-TR—in which the sleep attacks must be accompanied by cataplexy or REM intrusion phenomena. The other approach uses the diagnostic markers provided by sleep laboratory polysomnographic studies or the multiple sleep latency test. Sleep laboratory studies show sleep-onset REM (as opposed to the usual 90 minutes between the onset of sleep and the first episode of REM sleep). In the multiple sleep latency test, an individual is instructed to take four to six naps during the day at 2-hour intervals. The time taken to fall asleep for each nap and the presence of REM sleep in two or more naps are used to help confirm a diagnosis of narcolepsy.

TREATMENT

How Is Narcolepsy Treated?

Some patients benefit by scheduling short naps throughout the day. Patients needing medication are most often given a psychostimulant such as methylphenidate, pemoline, or modafinil. Cataplexy and REM intrusion phenomena can be treated with antidepressants (tricyclics, monoamine oxidase inhibitors, and selective serotonin reuptake inhibitors), usually at one fourth to one half the dose used to treat depression.

BREATHING-RELATED SLEEP DISORDERS

ETIOLOGY

What Are Breathing-Related Sleep Disorders?

In breathing-related sleep disorders—also called sleep apnea—the person stops breathing (or breathes poorly) while asleep. The periods of apnea last for about 20 to 40 seconds and result in multiple wakenings through the night. People who have sleep apnea are often aware only of the heavy sleepiness they feel throughout the day and not the difficulty they have with sleep and breathing.

Sleep Disorders

What Causes Sleep Apnea?

The two most common causes of sleep apnea are *obstructive* and *central*. (A third cause is central alveolar hypoventilation.) In obstructive sleep apnea, mechanical obstruction such as fatty tissue collapses the larynx and impedes air flow. Central sleep apnea is caused by a failure of brain stem respiratory control. With obstructive sleep apnea, there is inspiratory effort but no air flow. In central sleep apnea, there is no inspiratory effort.

EVALUATION

How Do I Assess for Sleep Apnea?

Polysomnographic sleep laboratory studies are diagnostically definitive (Fig. 30-1), but your level of suspicion may be high even before referral

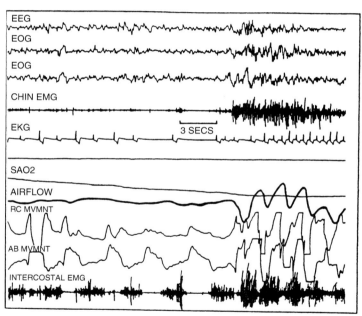

FIGURE 30-1 Sleep polysomnographic recording of sleep apnea. There is inspiratory effort (rib cage movement [RC MVMNT] and abdominal movement [AB MVMNT]) but no air flow. There are electrocardiographic changes as blood oxygen saturation (SAO2) falls and rebound tachycardia when the subject is aroused. EEG, electroencephalogram; EKG, electrocardiogram; EMG, electromyogram; EOG, electro-oculogram. (From Moore CA, Williams RL, Hirshkowitz M. Sleep disorders. In Sadock BJ, Sadock VA [eds]. Comprehensive Textbook of Psychiatry, 7th ed. Philadelphia, Lippincott Williams & Wilkins, 2000. p. 1688)

Sleep Disorders

to a sleep laboratory. Obstructive sleep apnea is the most common cause of excessive daytime sleepiness in middle-aged men, especially if overweight. The individual is unlikely to report poor sleep, but bed partners often describe horrific snoring, snorting, grunting, gasping, and restless sleep on the part of the patient—sometimes to such a degree that the partner sleeps in a different room. The heavy snoring is caused as the inspiratory air flow pushes past the obstruction. It is not usually a complaint made by the patient himself, although occasional sleepers snore so heavily that they wake themselves up. Symptoms associated with sleep apnea are headache, trouble concentrating, and mood disturbances.

Is the Physical Examination Helpful?

In addition to obesity, patients with breathing-related sleep disorders often have mild systemic hypertension with an elevated diastolic pressure. Individuals with chronically low oxygen saturation are predisposed to develop pulmonary hypertension, which can lead to right-sided heart failure, hepatic congestion, and ankle edema.

What Laboratory Abnormalities Are Seen in Patients with Breathing-Related Sleep Disorders?

In addition to the data from polysomnographic studies, patients may have arterial hypoxemia or hypercarbia on waking. (Arterial blood gases when fully awake are most often normal.) Cardiac arrhythmias during sleep are common. Elevated hematocrit or hemoglobin values can result from repeated nocturnal hypoxemia.

TREATMENT

How Are Breathing-Related Sleep Disorders Treated?

Some people benefit from noninvasive behavioral interventions such as losing weight or learning to sleep on their side rather than on their back. Continuous positive airway pressure (CPAP) is the mainstay of treatment (Fig. 30-2). The individual wears a mask or nasal prongs attached to a compressor that delivers air during sleep at pressures sufficient to maintain adequate ventilation. CPAP is most effective for obstructive sleep apnea but is used with benefit for some people with central sleep apnea as well. In some individuals with obstructive sleep apnea, surgical reconstruction of the soft palate, or the creation of an elective tracheostomy that is closed during the day and opened at night, can bring significant relief when more conservative measures have failed.

Are Sleeping Pills Helpful?

No. Sedative-hypnotics, including alcohol, exacerbate breathing-related sleep disorders. They prolong the apneic episodes, increase the risk of cardiac arrhythmias, and may in extreme cases be fatal.

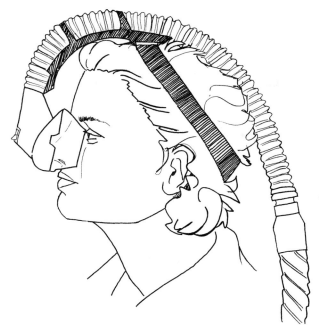

FIGURE 30-2 A woman wearing a continuous positive airway pressure (CPAP) device used to treat obstructive sleep apnea.

PARASOMNIAS

ETIOLOGY

What Are Parasomnias?

The prefix *para* means "alongside." For example, a paralegal works alongside a lawyer. Parasomnias are abnormalities that occur alongside—in the context of—otherwise normal sleep. The sleep itself is not disturbed, and patients do not complain of insomnia, fatigue, or somnolence. A list of common parasomnias is given in Table 30-2.

What Causes Parasomnias?

Parasomnias are part of the normal neurodevelopmental process in children. They do not indicate psychopathology, and they usually do not require treatment. Parasomnias in adults are more likely to be associated with psychiatric disorders. For example, recurrent nightmares are believed to be more common in adults with post-traumatic stress disorder or other anxiety disorders than in the general population. However, most of the

Sleep Disorders

Table 30-2
Some Common Parasomnias

Associated with stage II sleep
  Bruxism (teeth grinding)
Associated with stage IV sleep
  Somnambulism (sleepwalking)
  Somniloquy (sleep talking)
  Nocturnal enuresis (bed-wetting)
  Night terrors

literature on adult parasomnias is anecdotal and lacking in controlled, longitudinal studies.

How Common Are Parasomnias?

Very common in children. Between 10% and 50% of children between the ages of 3 and 5 years have nightmares bad enough to disturb their parents, and as many as 50% of adults report having an occasional nightmare. Sleepwalking episodes are reported to occur in 10% to 30% of children and 1% to 7% of adults. The prevalence of sleep terrors is believed to be between 1% and 6% of children but less than 1% of adults.

EVALUATION

How Do I Assess for Parasomnias?

A good history and description of the event (from parents for children, bed partners for adults) is usually sufficient to establish the diagnosis. Sleep laboratory studies are rarely indicated. It is especially useful to note the presence or absence of vivid dreams, which help distinguish nightmares and REM sleep behavior disorder (where they are present) from night terrors (where they are absent).

TREATMENT

How Do I Treat Parasomnias?

You may not need to. When they occur in children, they are often outgrown by adolescence. When they are persistent or cause a great deal of distress, a variety of treatment approaches are available. Sleepwalkers should be protected from harm, for example, by locking bedroom windows and removing objects of potential harm. Behavioral interventions such as relaxation exercises and systematic desensitization have been shown to reduce nightmares, and hypnosis may decrease sleepwalking and night terrors. In addition, nighttime benzodiazepine or antidepressant medications are reported to help some people with nightmares, sleepwalking, and night terrors. Serious damage to teeth caused by nighttime grinding (bruxism) can be reduced when a rubber guard is fitted over the teeth at night. An important aspect of treatment is to reassure parents

Sleep Disorders

that parasomnias in children are developmentally normal and that they do not signal current or future psychopathology.

KEY POINTS

◆ Insomnia is a symptom not a diagnosis. Not all insomnia requires medication.

◆ Sleep laboratory studies may be helpful in establishing a diagnosis of narcolepsy and breathing-related sleep disorders.

◆ Parasomnias are normal in children and usually do not require treatment.

Case 30-1

A 25-year-old medical student comes to the student health service with a request for something to help him sleep. He describes difficulty sleeping the night before important examinations and is worried about a pathology final in 10 days. He normally has no difficulty sleeping and usually gets 7 to 8 hours of uninterrupted, restorative sleep. However, on the night before his last two examinations, it took nearly 2 hours for him to fall asleep, and then he slept only fitfully. He is certain that his performance the next day was adversely affected by his lack of sleep. He has no significant medical or psychiatric history and he reports no allergies.

    A. Should he be medicated?

    B. Are any other interventions appropriate?

Case 30-2

A 60-year-old retired man comes to his primary care physician with a complaint of being sleepy all the time. He describes no difficulty falling asleep, and he usually sleeps for about 7 hours. He does not use an alarm clock, and he typically wakes with a dull, bifrontal headache, feeling groggy and disoriented. He has extreme difficulty staying awake during the day and takes naps whenever he is able. His daytime somnolence has seriously interfered with his family life and recreational pursuits. "I might as well be dead," he says. "I have no life, feeling tired all the time." He uses no drugs or medications and drinks no alcohol. Physical examination reveals a moderately obese middle-aged man with a blood pressure of 150/100 mm Hg. His red blood cell count is elevated. No other abnormalities are discovered.

    A. What is the most likely diagnosis?

    B. Are further investigations warranted?

    C. Considering the most likely diagnosis, what is the best treatment?

Case Answers

30-1 A. *Learning objective:* **Understand the appropriate use of hypnotic medication.** The history is one of purely situational insomnia. There is nothing to suggest insomnia secondary to a psychiatric disorder or an underlying medical condition. Either zolpidem or zaleplon is appropriate. They will help him fall asleep quickly and will minimize nighttime wakening. Use will be short term—very likely for just one night. Both have a relatively short half-life (zaleplon's is longer). Neither is likely to interfere with memory or concentration the next day, and abuse and habituation are not serious risks.

30-1 B. *Learning objective:* **Be familiar with nonpharmacologic approaches to treating insomnia.** Improving sleep hygiene is usually the first step in treating chronic insomnia. Some of the principles such as using the bedroom only for sex and sleep are unlikely to be of immediate benefit. Nevertheless, it is useful to review common habits that can interfere with sleep. It is possible, for example, that he drinks lots of coffee the night before an examination in order to study later. Similarly, he may be in the habit of drinking alcohol at night as a (mistaken) way to promote sleep.

30-2 A. *Learning objective:* **Know the major sleep disorder diagnoses.** Because the man wakes spontaneously after 7 hours, a primary or secondary hypersomnia is less likely than poor nighttime sleep. The most common cause of excessive daytime somnolence in middle-aged men is obstructive sleep apnea. His headache, high blood pressure, polycythemia, and obesity are all consistent with this diagnosis.

30-2 B. *Learning objective:* **Know the medical differential of major sleep disorders.** It doesn't seem likely that his sleepiness is due to drug or medication use. It is important, however, to rule out an underlying medical or psychiatric cause. No suspicious abnormalities showed up in his medical work-up, but the thoroughness of his examination is not described. More history, the mental status examination, physical examination, and laboratory studies should rule out the common medical and psychiatric causes of daytime somnolence: hypothyroidism, Addison's disease, hyperglycemia, hypercalcemia, an occult malignancy, and major depression. Information from a bed partner may also be useful (heavy snoring, restless sleep), but sleep laboratory studies would confirm a diagnosis of obstructive sleep apnea.

30-2 C. Losing weight and learning to sleep on his side may give some benefit, but a treatment more likely to be immediately helpful is continuous positive airway pressure. It is safe and noninvasive and effective the first night.

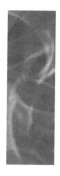

31

Sexual Dysfunctions

MICHELLE ROTTENSTEIN

What Causes Sexual Dysfunctions?

The causes may be physiologic or psychological. Physiologic causes are multiple and include medical conditions such as diabetes and the effects of drugs such as alcohol or antihypertensive medication. Psychological causes involve both an immediate cause—a thought or feeling that interferes with sexual pleasure—and remote causes arising from early experiences, parental attitudes, and interpersonal relationships. Table 31-1 provides a description of the individual sexual dysfunctions.

How Common Are Sexual Dysfunctions?

Good data do not exist. As a group they appear to be very common, although individual disorders (e.g., dyspareunia in men) may be rare. They are seen in every medical specialty. As you might expect, good sexual history-taking increases the likelihood of recognizing and treating dysfunctions.

What Medical Conditions or Drug-Related States Are Most Likely to Cause Sexual Dysfunctions?

Just about any illness can interfere with sexual desire and performance. Among the common medical causes are diabetes mellitus and cardiovascular or neurovascular diseases. Common drugs are alcohol, antihypertensives, cocaine, opioids, and many psychiatric medications including antipsychotics and antidepressants (see Table 20-2).

How Do I Talk with My Patient about Sex?

In the same way you would discuss any other medical issue: frankly, openly, empathetically, and nonjudgmentally. If a particular sexual topic makes you embarrassed, try to understand why. An embarrassed

Table 31-1

Sexual Dysfunctions

Each of the following may be lifelong or acquired, situational or generalized, and due to psychological or combined psychological and organic factors.

Hypoactive Sexual Desire Disorder
Occurs in both men and women. Involves decrease in libido (desire and interest in sex). May be lifelong but more commonly acquired. Associated with stress and interpersonal problems such as intimacy and commitment.

Sexual Aversion Disorder
Aversion to and avoidance of sexual genital contact with a partner (more rarely, an aversion to one's own genitals). May manifest as lack of desire, anxiety, or disgust.

Female Sexual Arousal Disorder
Inability to achieve adequate lubrication. Minimal if any subjective experience of arousal. Often accompanied by disorders of desire and orgasm.

Male Erectile Disorder
Inability to attain an erection, loss of erection before penetration, or loss of erection after penetration but before orgasm. Often associated with anxiety and worries about sexual performance.

Female Orgasmic Disorder
A delay or absence of orgasm after a normal excitement phase. Must take into account the wide variety in women's capacity for orgasm (e.g., not all women are able to reach orgasm with penetration alone). More commonly lifelong than acquired and more common in younger women than older (the capacity for orgasm increases with age for women). Orgasmic dysfunction in an otherwise healthy woman is generally due to psychological causes.

Male Orgasmic Disorder
Delay or absence of orgasm after a normal excitement phase. Most commonly involves inability to reach orgasm with intercourse but no problem with masturbation or oral stimulation.

Premature Ejaculation
Ejaculation with only minimal stimulation. Ejaculation occurs before the man wants it. Generally less a problem with masturbation. Most commonly due to psychological factors. The most treatable of sexual dysfunctions.

Dyspareunia
Genital pain with intercourse. Far more common with women than men, in whom it is almost always due to a medical or urologic condition such as phimosis.

Vaginismus
Involuntary contraction of the perineal muscles surrounding the outer third of the vagina so that penetration is difficult or impossible. May be associated with sexual abuse or trauma.

Sexual dysfunction due to a general medical condition

Substance-induced sexual dysfunction

Table 31-2

Outline for Sexual History-Taking

I. Current activity
   A. Currently sexually active or not
   B. Recent changes in sexual activity
   C. Preferred partner or partners
   D. Preferred activities
   E. Safe sex practices
   F. Any problems to discuss
II. Past activity
   A. When became sexually active
   B. Changes in sexual activity over the years
   C. Any prior difficulties
III. Developmental
   A. Childhood sexual exploration
   B. Any history of physical or sexual abuse
   C. Onset of puberty and menarche
   D. Adolescent sexual experiences

interviewer inevitably leads to an embarrassed patient and a consequent distortion of the information being gathered.

Do I Need to Ask All of My Patients about Sex?

It's a good idea. Many patients do not volunteer information about sexual symptoms unless specifically asked. Good sex screening questions are "Are you sexually active? Have you noticed any change in sexual functioning? Are there any issues about sex you would like to discuss?" For patients who mention a problem, a more detailed history is necessary.

What Words Should I Use in Discussing Sex with My Patients?

Good question. You will want to avoid street terms that sound obscene or make you uncomfortable as well as scientific or technical terms that are obscure and likely to be misunderstood. A good guideline is to follow your patient's lead and use common lay terms. For example, if a male patient talks about "coming too soon," it is perfectly acceptable to use that phrase instead of "premature ejaculation." Don't let lay terms obscure accuracy and precision, however; if a woman describes pain in her "privates," you must determine whether she means labia, vagina, urethra, or something else.

If My Patient Does Have a Sexual Symptom, What Else Should I Ask?

As with all other areas of psychiatry and medicine, your knowledge of the complex of symptoms and signs that constitutes specific diagnoses guides your questioning. Your goal is to obtain sufficient information to establish a credible diagnosis. That will allow you to make a good prediction about the likely response to treatment and the future course of the disorder. An outline for sexual history-taking is given in Table 31-2.

Do All My Patients with Sexual Dysfunctions Need a Medical Work-up?

A physical examination should be performed and consideration given to screening for common medical causes of dysfunctions such as diabetes. However, the indication for medical work-up varies depending on the nature of the sexual dysfunction. For instance, referral for gynecologic evaluation is often indicated for dyspareunia. Patients with generalized erectile dysfunction warrant urologic evaluation; patients with premature ejaculation do not because it rarely has an organic cause. Disorders that are clearly situational (e.g., erectile dysfunction with one partner but not with all) are unlikely to need extensive medical evaluation. Table 31-3 lists some common sexual dysfunctions for which a medical work-up is usually indicated.

TREATMENT

How Are Sexual Dysfunctions Treated?

When organic causes of dysfunction are excluded, treatment usually consists of a psychodynamically informed cognitive-behavioral approach addressing both the immediate behavioral and the long-term psychological causes.

Can I Treat My Patient's Sexual Dysfunction?

You may well be able to treat medical or drug-induced dysfunctions by treating the underlying medical condition or by changing your patient's medication. You will probably not be able to treat other sexual dysfunctions, and for those you will need to make a referral to a qualified sex therapist. Sex therapists are clinicians from a variety of disciplines—psychiatry, psychology, social work, nursing—who have had special training in sex therapy techniques.

What Happens in Sex Therapy?

Treatment of the immediate cause focuses on the thoughts, feelings, and behaviors that occur right before the symptom and that interfere with sexual feelings. Specific exercises are then prescribed as "homework,"

Table 31-3
Common Sexual Dysfunctions in Which a Medical Work-up Is Indicated (Especially When the Dysfunction Is Acquired and Generalized)
Hypoactive sexual desire Female sexual arousal disorder Male erectile disorder Dyspareunia

to be carried out at home by the patient and partner to correct previously maladaptive behavior.

What Kinds of Specific Exercises Are Prescribed?

A wide range of various techniques has been perfected for specific disorders, but a common starting point is for the therapist to proscribe sexual intercourse temporarily. This reduces the anticipatory anxiety that underlies many dysfunctions and allows the patient and partner to focus more on the exercises.

Treatment of *vaginismus* involves the woman's inserting a series of vaginal dilators, starting very small and progressing to larger sizes as she feels comfortable. The gradual dilation desensitizes the conditioned response of spasms.

Premature ejaculation is treated using the "stop-start" technique, whereby the patient's partner is instructed to stimulate him manually, while he focuses on the erotic sensations until he is near the point of orgasm. The patient then tells his partner to stop. Before the erection is lost, the patient asks his partner to resume stimulation, which again is stopped just before orgasm. This is repeated several times until the stimulation is allowed to proceed to orgasm.

Treatment of *anorgasmia* generally proceeds from exercises involving masturbation and the use of a vibrator and, once orgasm is achieved in these circumstances, to sexual intercourse.

Are Homosexuals Treated in the Same Ways?

Yes. Lesbians and gay men are vulnerable to the same sexual dysfunctions as heterosexual men and women. The same treatment approaches are effective for both.

Is Sex Therapy Better for a Couple or for an Individual Patient?

Ideally, the patient's partner should be involved in treatment and attend the sex therapy sessions because this significantly improves prognosis. If the patient does not have a partner, consideration could be given to using a sexual surrogate. However, sexual therapy can be effectively given for a single individual without a partner or whose partner is unwilling to attend the treatment sessions.

Are Sexual Surrogates Prostitutes?

No, although some prostitutes advertise themselves as "surrogates." Qualified sex surrogates receive special training and work closely with the treating sex therapist. Most prostitutes want to work as quickly as possible and avoid an emotional relationship. Surrogates understand the importance of working as slowly as necessary and are attuned to emotional issues.

Are Medications Used in Treating Sexual Dysfunctions?

They may be useful, especially when an organic disorder is identified. In addition, psychotropic medications are often indicated when the sexual dysfunction is secondary to a psychiatric disorder. For example, low libido associated with major depression is corrected by treating the underlying depression.

Sildenafil (Viagra) and tadalafil (Cialis) both increase blood flow to the genitals in the presence of sexual stimulation. (They do not cause erections when a man is not sexually stimulated.) Both are used in the treatment of men with erectile dysfunction. The potential for erections lasts up to 6 hours with sildenafil and up to 36 hours with tadalafil. There is some indication that they may also be useful in women with problems of arousal or anorgasmia, especially when these are related to medical issues such as menopause.

Yohimbine, an alkaloid derived from the bark of the African yohimbe tree, is a presynaptic α_2-antagonist that also has actions at acetylcholine, dopamine, and vasointestinal peptide receptors. It increases sympathetic activity and therefore epinephrine and norepinephrine release. It appears to increase penile blood flow and is sometimes used in the treatment of erectile dysfunction. There is no evidence that it is useful in the treatment of sexual dysfunctions in women.

Alprostadil, prostaglandin E_1, is also used for erectile dysfunction. It is a potent vasodilator that is injected into the corpora cavernosa or used intraurethrally before sexual activity, resulting in an erection.

Are Surgical Treatments Used?

In some cases of erectile dysfunction caused by neurologic or vascular disease, a semirigid malleable rod (which provides a constant erection) or an inflatable prosthesis (which can be inflated or deflated on demand) may be surgically inserted in a man's penis. Occasionally, microvascular surgery may be performed in cases in which erectile dysfunction is due to abnormal blood flow secondary to trauma.

KEY POINTS

◆ Each of the sexual dysfunctions is specific to a particular stage of the sexual response cycle.

◆ Sexual dysfunctions that are purely situational are more likely to be due to psychological factors than to underlying medical illness or drug-related effects.

◆ Cognitive-behavioral therapy is the main treatment modality for sexual dysfunctions.

Case 31-1

A 26-year-old single man presents with the complaint that he is unable to maintain an erection whenever he attempts to have sexual intercourse. He states that he has had this symptom since adolescence and that it has occurred every time he has attempted intercourse. He has never been able to maintain an erection long enough to achieve vaginal penetration. He states that he is very embarrassed by his inability to perform and that he has recently begun avoiding situations in which he might become sexually involved with a woman. His only relationship was at age 17, and it lasted 3 months. He states that he broke off the relationship soon after his first attempt to have sexual intercourse with his girlfriend. He reports that his sexual fantasies are about women only. There is no history of homosexual activity and no history of sexual abuse. There is no psychiatric or medical history of significance, and he denies substance abuse. He reports normal morning erections and that he has no difficulty maintaining an erection when he is masturbating. He reports intense anxiety during sexual situations, with the thought that he will not be able to perform adequately.

A. Is the man's erectile dysfunction likely to be of physiologic or psychological etiology?
B. Is the erectile dysfunction primary or secondary?
C. What is the immediate cause of the symptom?
D. How could his disorder be treated?

Case Answers

31-1 A. *Learning objective:* **Recognize that a sexual disorder that is purely situational is likely to have a psychological etiology.** The man reports that his difficulties occur only when he is attempting to have sex with a partner and that he has normal physiologic morning erections and no difficulty in maintaining his erections when he is masturbating.

31-1 B. *Learning objective:* **Know the difference between primary and secondary sexual dysfunctions.** The man reports having had no period of normal functioning, as he has never been able to achieve penetration. His disorder is therefore primary.

31-1 C. *Learning objective:* **Be able to identify the immediate causes of a sexual dysfunction.** The man reports both a feeling (anxiety) and a thought (that he will be unable to perform) that are distracting him from sexual feelings and thoughts and that are interfering with his ability to become involved with the sexual act.

31-1 D. *Learning objective:* **Be aware that addressing the immediate causes of the dysfunction can treat sexual disorders that have a psychological component.** In this case, the focus would be on enabling the patient to identify and therefore change the interfering feelings and thoughts and encouraging the patient's involvement in sexual fantasy during sexual activity.

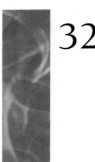

32

Adjustment Disorders

SERENA YUAN VOLPP

What Is an Adjustment Disorder?

It is the development of emotional or behavioral symptoms in response to a specific identifiable stressful event. The symptoms are severe enough to cause trouble in social interactions or with work or to cause subjective distress.

What Kinds of Situations Cause Adjustment Disorders?

They are often common situations such as a change in employment, a sudden financial loss, the breakup of a romantic relationship, or the death of a family member. Stressors can also be less common catastrophic events such as natural disasters. Even happy events such as the birth of a child, a significant promotion at work, or winning a lottery require adaptation and can lead to adjustment disorders for some people.

How Common Are Adjustment Disorders?

Prevalence estimates depend widely on the population being studied. They range from 2.3% of adult patients at a walk-in clinic to 10% to 20% of patients seen in general hospital psychiatric consultations to up to 65% of children presenting with a psychiatric disturbance.

What Causes an Adjustment Disorder?

Adjustment disorders are considered stress related: symptoms arise from a maladaptive response to stress. Normally, a person's response to a stressful event such as a divorce resolves soon after the event is over. If the stressor persists—if, for example, divorce proceedings go on for years—the person achieves a new level of adaptation to the stress. Some people have trouble with this. How well an individual person deals with stress is probably influenced by a number of factors, including her prior experience (has she ever overcome this type of stress before?), her social support system, as well as psychological strengths such as reality testing ability, frustration tolerance, and mood regulation. A minor stressor superimposed on a chronic major stressor can have a significant additive effect. Although an adjustment disorder is one of the few diagnoses in DSM-IV-TR that is definitively linked to psychosocial stress, there are many unanswered questions about why some people develop pathologic reactions to stress and some do not.

At What Age Do People Get Adjustment Disorders?

From young to old. Children requiring psychiatric services often receive a diagnosis of an adjustment disorder.

EVALUATION

Why Should I Give a Psychiatric Diagnosis to Someone Who Is Merely Responding to Stress?

People are given this diagnosis when their reaction to the stress is maladaptive and is interfering with their ability to function well. Diagnosis guides treatment. People's normal reactions to stress resolve over time. In adjustment disorder they do not go away and psychotherapy or medication may be helpful.

What Do I Need to Look for to Make a Diagnosis of an Adjustment Disorder?

There is no checklist of symptoms for adjustment disorder. Symptoms can be emotional or behavioral or both. They occur within 3 months of a stressful event, and they do not last longer than 6 months after the event has ended. If a person meets DSM-IV-TR criteria for another Axis I disorder such as a major depressive episode or post-traumatic stress disorder, that diagnosis takes precedence and the diagnosis of an adjustment disorder no longer applies. Nevertheless, adjustment disorders can include serious symptoms such as suicidal thoughts and actions. Because there is no operationalized symptom checklist, interrater reliability of the diagnosis is poor. The development of symptoms must occur within 3 months of an identified stressor.

What Are the Different Subtypes of Adjustment Disorders?

Subtypes are defined by the predominant symptoms—in particular depressed mood, anxiety, and behavioral disturbances. Disturbance of conduct means behavior that violates social norms or the rights of others, such as fighting, truancy, vandalism, and reckless driving. If the disturbance lasts less than 6 months, it is deemed acute; if it has lasted for 6 months or longer, it is deemed chronic. Table 32-1 lists subtypes of adjustment disorders with brief examples.

What Is the Difference between an Adjustment Disorder and Bereavement?

Bereavement—sadness and intense grief after the loss of a loved one—is normal. According to the DSM-IV-TR, normal bereavement reactions last up to 2 months, but there are many people in the field who say this period

Table 32-1

Clinical Examples of Subtypes

Adjustment disorder with depressed mood: An 80-year-old woman moved out of her family home into a small apartment in a retirement complex 1 month ago. Since then she rarely sees friends, does not go to her clubs, and has frequent crying spells throughout the week.

Adjustment disorder with anxiety: Two weeks ago a 65-year-old man found out that he was cheated out of a major investment and that he has lost half of his life savings. He has been having trouble falling asleep, is waking up early, feels jittery during the day, cannot concentrate at work, and is constantly worried about how he will support himself after retirement.

Adjustment disorder with mixed anxiety and depressed mood: A 37-year-old woman discovered a month ago that her husband was having an affair. When confronted, he moved out and is requesting a divorce. She has been having trouble sleeping and is feeling anxious, irritable, angry, and worthless; at times she feels suicidal.

Adjustment disorder with disturbance of conduct: A 17-year-old boy was informed 2 months ago that his grades are insufficient for graduation from high school. Over the past month, he has started engaging in physical fights with peers and has been stealing cars and taking them on joyrides.

Adjustment disorder with mixed disturbance of emotions and conduct: A 15-year-old girl was diagnosed with diabetes mellitus 3 weeks ago. She has been feeling sad, irritable, and angry. She started skipping school and admits to having shoplifted some items from the local drug store.

of time should be extended. A person may be diagnosed with an adjustment disorder or another Axis I disorder (such as a major depressive episode or brief psychotic episode) if the grief lasts longer than 2 months or if it is accompanied by marked functional impairment, morbid preoccupation with worthlessness, suicidal ideation, psychotic symptoms, or psychomotor retardation. Keep in mind that a diagnosis of "adjustment disorder" is appropriate only for people who do not meet criteria for another condition.

What Do I Need to Rule out When Making a Diagnosis of Adjustment Disorder?

Distinguishing between a chronic adjustment disorder and an anxiety disorder not otherwise specified (NOS) or depression NOS can be difficult; these syndromes do not need to be associated with a stressor, however. If the stressor is a rare, catastrophic event such as a natural disaster or violent crime, look for symptoms of acute stress disorder or post-traumatic stress disorder; adjustment disorder is more commonly associated with everyday events such as parental separation, academic failure, change of employment, financial losses, or ending of relationships. Before labeling someone with adjustment disorder, make sure that they do not meet criteria for major depressive disorder or other Axis I condition; an inaccurate diagnosis may result in inaccurate treatment.

TREATMENT

Do Adjustment Disorders Get Better without Treatment?

There are few data addressing this question. The prognosis for adults with adjustment disorder is better than that for children or adolescents. In one longitudinal study, 71% of adults at 5-year follow-up were completely well versus 44% of adolescents. Adolescents were more likely than adults to have developed major mental illness such as schizophrenia, bipolar disorder, major depressive disorder, antisocial personality disorder, and substance abuse. In the adolescent group, presence of behavioral symptoms was the best predictor for major pathology at follow-up.

What Works Better for Adjustment Disorders—Medication or Psychotherapy?

Psychotherapy is generally considered the mainstay of treatment for adjustment disorders. There are no published trials comparing psychotherapy and medication for adjustment disorders. In some patients, particularly in those with chronic adjustment disorders or those who are not responding well to psychotherapy, antidepressant or anxiolytic medication may be helpful.

What Type of Psychotherapy Should I Prescribe for a Patient Who Has an Adjustment Disorder?

Supportive psychotherapy is the psychotherapy of choice. In supportive psychotherapy, you help the patient reduce the level of stress and, if that is not possible, help the patient in his adaptation. This includes helping him verbalize his feelings about the stressor (expressing himself in words, not destructive actions), enhancing his coping skills (e.g., teaching him techniques for anger management and relaxation), and helping the patient maximize his support system.

Should I Refer My Patient with an Adjustment Disorder for Group Therapy?

Group therapy, in addition to individual therapy, may be particularly helpful for patients going through similar stressors such as adjusting to a new diagnosis of cancer or getting used to retirement.

KEY POINTS

◆ For a diagnosis of adjustment disorder to be made, there needs to be an identifiable stressor or precipitant.

◆ Adjustment disorders can arise in a variety of ways: with depressive symptoms, anxiety, and/or behavior problems.

◆ A diagnosis of adjustment disorder is not made for people who meet criteria for other Axis I disorders.

◆ A person with an adjustment disorder often responds to supportive psychotherapy and may not need pharmacologic treatment.

Case 32-1

A 45-year-old woman is referred to a psychiatric outpatient clinic by her primary care physician because of anxiety that is interfering with her ability to concentrate at work and to sleep at night. One month ago her father suffered a stroke, and he is now partially paralyzed on one side of his body. The woman has been spending most evenings after work and all of her weekends with her father. Her partner complains that she is never around; they have been getting into frequent verbal arguments.

A. What is your diagnosis?
B. How would you treat the woman?

Case Answers

32-1 A. *Learning objective:* **Understand the definition of adjustment disorder.** You diagnose Ms. A with adjustment disorder with anxiety (acute). The symptoms precipitated by her father's stroke are impairing her ability to function and interfering in her personal relationship. There is not enough information presented to justify another Axis I diagnosis. Her symptoms have occurred within 3 months of the stressful event.

32-1 B. *Learning objective:* **Be familiar with treatments for adjustment disorder.** Weekly supportive psychotherapy is the treatment of choice. The goals of therapy will be to help the woman verbalize her feelings about her father's sudden deterioration. She should be able to express fear about her father's mortality, fear about her own mortality, and anger about the sudden reversal in their roles. Therapy may help appease any feelings of guilt about not being with her father full-time and emphasize the importance of not neglecting herself or her relationship with her partner. You may also decide to prescribe an antidepressant or an anxiolytic, depending on the severity of her symptoms and the response to therapy alone.

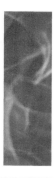

33

Dissociative Disorders

SERENA YUAN VOLPP

What Is Dissociation?

Normal consciousness is the integration of several mental functions including perception of one's surroundings, past memories, and sense of identity. Dissociation describes a breakdown of this integration. It occurs on a spectrum and at the mild end can include everyday experiences such as daydreaming or "getting lost" in a movie. Dissociation is the hallmark of the dissociative disorders, but it can also be a symptom of other disorders such as panic disorder and posttraumatic stress disorder (PTSD). DSM-IV-TR includes four dissociative disorders and a residual category for people who do not meet criteria for one of the four main disorders. These are summarized in Table 33-1. Chronic dissociation may be a coping mechanism that serves to ward off a situation or an experience that is too traumatic to be integrated into consciousness. The five core symptoms of dissociation are amnesia, depersonalization, derealization (a sense that oneself or the world is unreal), identity confusion, and identity alteration.

Who Gets Dissociative Disorders?

As just implied, dissociative disorders are thought to affect individuals who have experienced severe trauma, particularly in childhood. Dissociation may initially occur as a defense during trauma. Children who dissociate during a traumatic experience may start automatically using dissociation in other situations when they feel anxious or threatened and may then continue to use dissociation chronically, even after the traumatic experiences are over.

Do Dissociative Disorders Affect Either Men or Women More Frequently?

Women are diagnosed more frequently with dissociative disorders than men. Dissociative identity disorder in particular may be about five times more common in women than in men. There is current debate, however,

329

Table 33-1

The Dissociative Disorders

Dissociative Identity Disorder
(Formerly, "multiple personality disorder"). An individual has two or more separate and distinct personalities that influence behavior.

Dissociative Amnesia
Memory loss—usually of important personal information—not caused by medical illness or drugs.

Dissociative Fugue
A person travels away from home, loses memory of his past, and is confused about his identity or assumes a new identity.

Depersonalization Disorder
A persistent, distressing sense of not being real, of seeing oneself from the outside as if watching a movie.

over whether dissociative disorders are truly more common in women or whether they are only diagnosed more often.

Why Are Dissociative Disorders Often Misdiagnosed?

People with these disorders can be completely unaware of the dissociation and may spend years in treatment without an accurate diagnosis. Many of the symptoms that lead a person with dissociative disorder to seek treatment, such as mood swings, anxiety, and uncontrollable rituals, are common to other psychiatric diagnoses.

DISSOCIATIVE IDENTITY DISORDER

ETIOLOGY

What Causes Dissociative Identity Disorder?

Multiple models, physiologic and behavioral, have been proposed to help explain dissociative identity disorder (DID), formerly called multiple personality disorder. None are proved. However, DID is often associated with severe trauma in childhood, and the disorder is now conceptualized as a complex developmental trauma disorder.

How Common Is Dissociative Identity Disorder?

There are no good data. In the past, the validity of the diagnosis itself was challenged. Most clinicians and researchers now believe the diagnosis describes a clinical reality. Common estimates of lifetime prevalence range from 1% to 3%. Over the past several years, DID has been diagnosed more frequently, but it is not clear whether this reflects increased awareness of the disorder or overdiagnosis among suggestible individuals.

EVALUATION

At What Age Does Dissociative Identity Disorder First Appear?

DID can be diagnosed in childhood. It usually appears in adolescence or in the 20s. Note, however, that individuals often go many years before diagnosis.

How Many Personalities Can a Person with DID Have?

"Alter" is another word for identity or personality state. Individuals with DID have at least two separate and distinct alters, which may manifest with different speech, mannerisms, thoughts, memories, gender identity, and sometimes with different physical properties such as right- or left-handedness and allergies. Individuals with DID have been known to have as many as 100 alters, but the average is around 10.

Why Do People with DID Seek Help?

People with DID seek help for varied reasons. Some may not even be aware that they have the condition but may be worried about lapses in time or episodes of amnesia. People with DID almost as a rule have comorbid psychiatric issues for which they may be seeking help, including PTSD, depression, self-injurious behavior, mood swings, eating disorders, sleep disorders, substance use disorders, borderline personality disorder, and auditory or visual hallucinations.

Are People with DID Psychotic?

This is an interesting question. The auditory hallucinations that people with DID sometimes experience, including voices arguing with each other, are generally described as originating from within the person and being heard inside the head; these are more accurately called pseudohallucinations. People with DID often have other symptoms that might be considered psychotic if a careful history is not taken, including thought withdrawal and insertion, and influences playing on the body. Again, in general, these are experienced as internal, not external, in origin. About half of individuals with DID are misdiagnosed as having schizophrenia at some point during their contact with psychiatrists. Children with DID are especially likely to be misdiagnosed as having schizophrenia. Typically, these psychotic-like symptoms do not improve with antipsychotic medication.

TREATMENT

How Is DID Treated?

Psychotherapy, hypnosis, and pharmacotherapy are all used for DID. Psychotherapy must first be directed at safety, as patients with DID often engage in potentially dangerous behaviors and may have difficulty controlling aggression and violence. Clinicians who provide psychotherapy for patients with DID must be comfortable with a wide range of techniques. Pharmacotherapy generally targets treatment-responsive symptoms (e.g., mood symptoms) rather than dissociation itself. The quasipsychotic symptoms generally do not respond well to antipsychotic medication. Family therapy, art therapy, and movement therapy are helpful adjunctive treatments.

How Do I Form an Alliance with a Patient Who Has DID?

In many patients, it is necessary to form an alliance with all the patient's alter states. All of the alters need to be held accountable for the patient's behavior. Maintaining firm boundaries with the patient is critical, and actively structuring sessions is important in limiting regression. Given that most patients with DID have experienced severe trauma, it is common for the therapist to be experienced as potentially abusive or uncaring. Clinicians working with DID patients are likely to feel overwhelmed and unskilled.

Is It Important to Talk about Traumatic Memories with a Patient Who Has DID?

After an alliance is well established and when drug or alcohol use and other injurious behaviors are under control, processing traumatic memories can be therapeutic. A goal for any patient with DID is to consolidate and integrate the different personality states.

◼ DISSOCIATIVE AMNESIA

ETIOLOGY

Is Dissociative Amnesia Caused by Head Trauma?

No. In fact, DSM-IV-TR criteria for dissociative amnesia specifically state that the disturbance is not due to physiologic effects of a substance or to a medical or neurologic condition such as head trauma. A history of emotional trauma, however, does seem to be associated with dissociative amnesia. Trauma can include but is not limited to childhood abuse, incest, rape, combat experience, being a witness to violence, kidnapping, or other threats of death or physical violence. Dissociative amnesia is probably the most common of all the dissociative disorders.

EVALUATION

What Are the Different Subtypes of Dissociative Amnesia?

There are five types of dissociative amnesia: (1) *localized amnesia*, or failing to recall events during a specific period of time; (2) *selective amnesia*, or ability to recall some but not all of the events during a specific period of time; (3) *generalized amnesia*, or failure to recall one's entire life; (4) *continuous amnesia*, or inability to recall events after a specific time up to and including the present; and (5) *systematized amnesia*, or inability to recall information related to certain categories (e.g., memories related to one's family). The first two types are more common than the last three types.

What Do I Need to Rule out When Someone Presents with Memory Loss?

You first need to rule out any organic etiology, such as head trauma, drugs, or alcohol. Dissociative amnesia can be difficult to diagnose because patients may not come in complaining about the amnesia but rather with anxiety, depression, difficulty concentrating, or confusion. The amnesia cannot be directly observed by the clinician (except in cases of generalized amnesia). Vagueness and inconsistency as well as difficulty with narrating past events may suggest amnesia. However, dissociative amnesia is not inefficient retrieval of memory related to cognitive or language dysfunction. It generally involves autobiographical memory and does not involve implicit memory such as knowing how to type or ride a bicycle. Chapter 27 includes a more detailed discussion of amnesia with medical or drug-related causes.

TREATMENT

Do Patients with Dissociative Amnesia Ever Recover Their Memory?

Most people with dissociative amnesia do recover. Removing the individual from a stressful or threatening situation and exposing her to cues from the past can help restore memory. The more acute and more recent the onset, the more likely the amnesia is to resolve quickly. Hypnosis can also be helpful; during hypnosis patients may be asked to reexperience a time before the onset of the amnesia and then be reoriented to events that occurred during the amnestic period. If traumatic memories are regained, the patient will need support from a therapist to help process the integration of these memories into conscious awareness. Retrieval and recollection should be done carefully and at a controlled pace. Group therapy can be helpful. There are no double-blind controlled trials of medication treatment for dissociative amnesia.

DISSOCIATIVE FUGUE

ETIOLOGY

How Is Dissociative Fugue Different from Dissociative Amnesia?

Individuals with dissociative amnesia cannot recall important personal information. In a dissociative fugue (formerly called psychogenic fugue) state, an individual may also have trouble recalling the past but in addition suddenly and unexpectedly travels away from home or workplace. He does not exhibit any obvious pathologic signs or cognitive deficits to those around him. People in a dissociative fugue are often discovered in a new community by family members who have been looking for them.

Dissociative Disorders

This is frequently preceded by a traumatic experience such as a natural disaster, military combat, or loss of a loved one.

EVALUATION

How Long Does Dissociative Fugue Usually Last?

Usually days to weeks, although a dissociative fugue can last less than an hour or as long as a year.

Do People in a Dissociative Fugue Lose Their Identity?

Individuals in a fugue state have confusion about their identity. It used to be thought that individuals would commonly assume a new identity, but this is now thought to be rare. When a new identity is assumed, the new and old identities do not alternate, as in DID.

What Kind of Work-up Do I Need to Get for Someone in a Fugue State?

Fugues can be psychological or medical in origin. It is thus critical for any patient in a fugue state to have a thorough physical examination including a detailed neurologic examination. Baseline blood chemistries, drug screening, blood alcohol, electrocardiogram (ECG), and electroencephalogram (EEG) should be obtained. The most common medical cause of a fugue is temporal lobe epilepsy. Other possible causes include brain tumor, head trauma, migraine, cerebrovascular accident, hypertensive neuropathy, hypoglycemia, uremia, and dementia.

TREATMENT

What Do I Do if Someone Is in the Middle of a Fugue State?

Spontaneous remission (without treatment) can occur. Short-acting sedatives such as sodium amobarbital are sometimes used to "break" the fugue state. Medications can be avoided through the use of hypnosis. As with dissociative amnesia, hypnosis can be used to help the patient remember personal information that has been forgotten. Both methods should be used with care; sudden recovery of past memories may precipitate depression or anxiety.

How Do I Help Someone Who Has Recovered from a Fugue State?

When the fugue state has resolved, the patient will need your help to understand what she has just experienced. In addition, the patient will need your assistance in learning coping mechanisms other than dissociation. Over half of those who experience dissociative fugues have more than one episode. Patients who uses dissociation often have difficulty gauging their own reactions to stress; you can help them learn to recognize and express their feelings.

DEPERSONALIZATION DISORDER

ETIOLOGY

What Causes Depersonalization?

The term describes a sense of unreality that many people experience as subjectively distressing. It is experienced in a wide and diverse number of conditions and commonly follows stress or trauma. It is possible that the sense of detachment from extreme situations serves an adaptive purpose. However, the neurobiologic mechanisms are not well understood. It is believed that over half of adults have experienced at least one brief period of depersonalization. The prevalence of the disorder—in which symptoms persist—is unknown.

EVALUATION

How Do People with Depersonalization Disorder Describe Their Symptoms?

Individuals with depersonalization disorder may describe feeling as if they are outside their own bodies—that they are observing themselves as if they were in a dream or in a movie. They may state that they do not recognize themselves in the mirror, or they may feel as if their body parts are detached or unreal. Patients may not spontaneously report symptoms of depersonalization for fear of being seen as crazy. Unlike someone with psychotic symptoms, however, they are aware of a distortion in their perceptual experiences

Are Laboratory Tests Needed to Make the Diagnosis of Depersonalization Disorder?

Laboratory tests and a medical examination are essential to rule out a substance-related or general medical condition. Depersonalization disorder also often co-occurs with other psychiatric disorders such as PTSD or other anxiety disorders. In fact, symptoms of depersonalization may be experienced by up to 80% of psychiatric patients. If the symptoms of depersonalization occur only in the context of another disorder, a separate diagnosis of depersonalization disorder is not given.

TREATMENT

What Kind of Psychotherapy Should I Prescribe for a Patient with Depersonalization Disorder?

Depersonalization may not need any psychotherapy at all; it sometimes remits without any formal treatment. If symptoms are persistent and bothersome to the patient, several different types of therapy may help. Cognitive approaches to help reduce anxieties (particularly in patients with trauma histories) include techniques such as grounding, reorienting, creative visualization, and distraction. Self-hypnosis during which patients learn to induce transient depersonalization symptoms helps some people to better control or modify them when they occur spontaneously.

Do Medications Help Patients with Depersonalization Disorder?

There have been no double-blind trials of medication for depersonalization. Case reports have noted improvement of symptoms with antidepressant and antianxiety medications such as selective serotonin reuptake inhibitors and benzodiazepines.

KEY POINTS

◆ Dissociative symptoms are often precipitated by traumatic or life-threatening events.

◆ For all of the dissociative disorders, it is critical to rule out any organic etiologies, particularly any neurologic diseases such as temporal lobe epilepsy, brain tumors, cerebrovascular accidents, or head trauma.

◆ The five core symptoms of dissociation are amnesia, depersonalization, derealization, identify confusion, and identity alteration.

Case 33-1

A 28-year-old woman is admitted to an inpatient psychiatric service after a suicide attempt. When she is asked during the admission interview about any history of trauma, she glazes over and states that she does not remember her life before the age of 10. Upon further questioning, she becomes childlike and states in a young girl's voice, "I promise I won't tell anyone—I promise, I promise—please don't hurt me." A few seconds later, she suddenly appears older again and flirts with the interviewer.

A. What is your diagnosis?
B. How would you treat her?

Case 33-2

A 50-year-old man never returns from his lunch break at work. His wife alerts the police. Two weeks later, he is brought to the emergency room in a neighboring state by police who found him wandering on the street in the cold, unable to state his name or address. His driver's license is found in his wallet and his wife is notified.

A. What laboratory tests do you need to order?
B. How can you help this man?

Case 33-3

A 43-year-old woman is referred by an outside therapist to a clinic for a consultation because of a lack of full recovery from her depression. She states that her sleep and appetite have been restored to her baseline, but she continues to feel detached and numb, almost as if she is watching herself "in a dream."

   A. What further questions can you ask about depersonalization?
   B. Does this patient have depersonalization disorder?

Case Answers

33-1 A. *Learning objective:* **Recognize the high comorbidities with dissociative identity disorder.** This patient probably has dissociative identity disorder; that is, she has two or more distinct identities that take control of her behavior. This is probably not the diagnosis that precipitated her admission to the hospital, however. She must be screened for comorbid symptoms including depression, self-mutilation, risk-taking behaviors, and substance abuse.

33-1 B. *Learning objective:* **Be familiar with treatment for dissociative identity disorder.** Individual and milieu therapy on the inpatient unit should be focused on safety and maintaining firm boundaries with the patient. Pharmacotherapy should target comorbid symptoms, for example, by treating depressive symptoms with an antidepressant. She will need long-term psychotherapy after discharge. When core symptoms are stabilized, processing of traumatic memories may be helpful in consolidating the patient's identity.

33-2 A. *Learning objective:* **Be familiar with the medical differential for the dissociative disorders.** This man may be in a dissociative fugue. However, there are multiple medical conditions that can cause a fugue state and the other dissociative disorders. The most common is epilepsy, especially temporal lobe epilepsy; the patient needs an EEG. You also should order a head computed tomography study to rule out a brain tumor, head trauma, or a stroke. He should receive an ECG, blood chemistries, a drug screening, and a blood alcohol level measurement; in addition to drugs, alcohol, and some medications, other conditions that can cause fugue include hypoglycemia, uremia, dementia, and hypertensive neuropathy.

33-2 B. *Learning objective:* **Be familiar with the treatment for dissociative fugue.** The fugue may remit spontaneously—most last from a few days to a few weeks. If the fugue does not remit, hypnosis may be helpful. Psychotherapy needs to be supportive; dissociative fugue is often precipitated by a traumatic event and a patient recovering from a fugue state may become depressed or suicidal.

33-3 A.   *Learning objective:* **Understand how patients with depersonalization describe themselves.** Depersonalization is a feeling of detachment from the self. Patients describe this as feeling unreal, light, or dead; feeling as if they are floating and watching themselves or observing a movie of themselves; feeling as if their body parts are disconnected. They may look different to themselves every time they look in the mirror. Note that they maintain reality testing (i.e., they recognize what is real) but may say that things don't *seem* real.

33-3 B.   *Learning objective:* **Be familiar with the diagnostic criteria for depersonalization disorder.** Depersonalization occurs on a spectrum. If this woman's depersonalization is persistent or recurrent and causes her clinically significant distress or impairment in functioning, she may very well have depersonalization disorder. You need to be sure that the depersonalization does not occur solely during the course of another mental disorder and that it is not due to a substance or a medical condition.

Dissociative Disorders

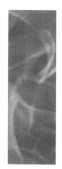

34

Somatoform and Factitious Disorders

MYRL R. S. MANLEY

 SOMATOFORM DISORDERS

What Are Somatoform Disorders?

Somatization is a general term for describing the tendency to express emotional problems through physical symptoms. Somatoform disorders are conditions in which that tendency is carried to such an extreme that the symptoms have begun to cause significant stress or impairment in social and work functioning. DSM-IV-TR describes five separate somatoform disorders, which are listed in Table 34-1. The boundaries between them are not discrete, and many patients fail to meet full diagnostic criteria for a specific disorder or meet different criteria at different times. Although the distinct categorical diagnoses are a useful way to organize your thinking about somatizing, their limitations in the care of individual patients must be kept in mind.

Are There Important Differences among the Somatoform Disorders?

Yes. Body dysmorphic disorder is the only one that does not arise with physical signs and symptoms but rather with a preoccupation with a perceived body defect and an exaggerated sense of its impact. It is probably only superficially related to the other diagnoses in this category. Pain disorder differs from the others in calling for specific pharmacotherapy and other physical interventions. Somatization disorder, conversion disorder, and hypochondriasis are conceptually distinct but the most fluid in clinical practice.

Why Is Pain Disorder Considered a Psychiatric Condition?

The classification of pain disorder as one of the somatoform disorders is a holdover from a time when pain was thought to be either real and physical or psychogenic. Pain specialists now recognize that all pain is both physical and psychological; psychological factors play an important part in

339

Table 34-1

The Somatoform Disorders

Somatization disorder: Multiple and varied symptoms occurring for a long time for which no medical basis can be found

Conversion disorder: A single, prominent symptom or sign, usually involving voluntary muscles or the sensory system

Hypochondriasis: Unrealistic worry of having a serious illness

Body dysmorphic disorder: Preoccupation with an imagined body defect, serious enough to be disruptive

Pain disorder: Chronic severe pain with no discernible physiologic basis or clearly in excess of known pathology

modifying peripheral pain signals, either amplifying or diminishing them. The relative importance of psychological factors and peripheral stimuli in the final perception of pain varies considerably from individual to individual. There are people for whom the psychological component is the more important. They experience pain in the absence of any identifiable medical disease or greatly in excess of what can be explained medically. The psychiatric diagnosis of pain disorder is intended to describe these people.

ETIOLOGY

What Causes Somatoform Disorders?

There is much speculation and little consensus about the causes of somatization and somatoform disorders or the psychological mechanism by which emotions are transformed into physical symptoms. Some patients appear to have a real underlying medical illness whose symptoms are exaggerated. Others appear to have no medical illness whatsoever; the physical symptoms derive wholly from psychological factors. In all cases the production of physical symptoms is *unconscious*. Patients are not trying to fool the physician. They are not trying to get insurance benefits or work exemptions, and they are unaware of the emotional distress that is postulated to underlie the symptoms. Their physical complaints are true reports of subjective experience. There is high comorbidity with other psychiatric disorders, particularly depression, anxiety, and personality disorders. Some cases of body dysmorphic disorder appear to be variants of obsessive-compulsive disorder.

How Common Are Somatoform Disorders?

The prevalence of somatoform disorders in the general population is unclear. Estimates vary widely and, for somatization disorder, may be as high as 2% of women in the general population. Women are diagnosed with somatization and conversion disorders five times as often as men. Sex ratios for the other somatoform disorders appear to be more equal. What is certain is that these conditions are much more common in clinical settings than in the general population. All physicians, regardless of specialty, are likely to deal with patients with one or another of the somatoform diagnoses. It was estimated that 4% to 6% of patients coming to one medical clinic qualified for a diagnosis of hypochondriasis.

What Is the Usual Clinical Course for Somatoform Disorders?

For the most part, these disorders are chronic. The symptoms often wax and wane in intensity, sometimes in response to stress. There are some exceptions. One is conversion disorder, in which the conversion symptom is likely to emerge abruptly and then resolve after a few days. It is estimated that 75% of people with conversion symptoms that have resolved have no recurrence. Hypochondriacal concerns are common after major illness or injury. For example, people who have had a heart attack and have fully recovered are often preoccupied with cardiac symptoms in the months following the attack. When such symptoms do not become chronic, they are regarded as the normal, adaptive hypervigilance following a life-threatening situation and are not considered a psychiatric disorder. A final exception to the generalization that somatoform disorders are chronic is body dysmorphic disorder occurring in childhood or adolescence. Preoccupation with perceived body defects is common in young people (skin condition, genital and breast size, height) and often resolves as the individual grows older and socially matures.

EVALUATION

What Findings in the History and Mental Status Examination Help in Diagnosing Somatoform Disorders?

The somatoform disorders are diagnoses of exclusion. Your history, physical examination, and mental status examination will look for evidence of a true medical condition or an underlying psychiatric disorder that could be presenting with physical symptoms. Some of these are listed in Table 34-2. Because of the high incidence of psychiatric comorbidity, you will also need to assess carefully for other psychiatric disorders, even if they are not directly contributing to physical symptoms.

There are no specific findings that in themselves are diagnostic of somatoform disorders, but they may be suggested by a history of chronic, vague, shifting medical complaints that have not responded well to treatment and whose etiology is unclear. *La belle indifférence* has sometimes been described as a characteristic of somatoform disorders, especially conversion disorder. The term describes a bland unconcern about even serious disability such as blindness or paralysis. It is unquestionably present in some patients but not reliably enough to use as a diagnostic marker. In addition, there are patients who work hard to put up a courageous front and who, to the casual observer, appear to be unconcerned. To describe such patients as having la belle indifférence is unhelpful. Body dysmorphic disorder, a diagnosis based on the patient's thinking rather than on physical complaints, is somewhat more straightforward and easier to diagnose on the basis of the psychiatric evaluation alone. Because it

Table 34-2

Some Psychiatric Disorders That Can Present with Physical Symptoms

Depression	Fatigue, anorexia, weight loss, insomnia, decreased libido, multiple aches and pains
Panic disorder	Shortness of breath, palpitations, chest pain, paresthesias during the attack
Generalized anxiety disorder	Gastrointestinal symptoms (cramps, nausea, diarrhea), palpitations, headaches, shortness of breath, diaphoresis
Schizophrenia and other psychotic disorders	Somatic delusions—sometimes bizarre: a person's heart has been removed; sometimes nonbizarre: a patient reports (falsely) copious bleeding from the rectum. Some patients ask to have healthy teeth pulled because of a belief that a transmitter or microphone is embedded in the tooth.

describes an exaggerated response to perceived physical imperfection, there is no underlying disease to rule in or out.

What Aspects of the Physical Examination Help in Making a Diagnosis of a Somatoform Disorder?

The concept of somatoform disorders is based on the premise that physical complaints are caused by emotional distress rather than by tissue pathology. The *absence* of physical signs is consistent with the diagnosis of a somatoform disorder; any positive physical finding leads away from it. Physical findings that are nonphysiologic or nonanatomic, although not proving a somatoform disorder, raise the suspicion. For example, a patient with a limb paralysis may have normal muscle tone and intact deep tendon reflexes.

Do Somatoform Disorders Occur with Other Psychiatric Disorders?

Comorbidity is common. Especially frequent are major depression and dysthymia, anxiety disorders, and personality disorders. If another psychiatric condition is present, you must make sure that it is not the cause of the patient's physical symptoms. For example, profound fatigue could result from major depression.

Are There Laboratory Investigations for Diagnosing Somatoform Disorders?

As with the physical examination and the history, laboratory investigations are used to rule out real medical disease. There are no findings that are specific for somatoform disorders. The *absence* of findings is consistent with the diagnosis. Depending on the particular complaints, specialized studies such as electromyography or nerve conduction studies may be necessary.

Do a Normal Physical Examination and Negative Laboratory Studies Mean That My Patient Has a Somatoform Disorder?

Not at all. Some medical conditions are purely clinical diagnoses. Grand mal seizures, for example, are diagnosed on the basis of the clinical syndrome of tonic-clonic convulsions, not on electroencephalographic findings. A negative electroencephalogram does not rule out true seizures. Moreover, it is not correct to think that our medical knowledge is complete or that available technology is adequate to detect all diseases that ever have been or ever will be known. Good medical follow-up of some patients who have somatoform features will ultimately show them to have had a real but previously undetected medical illness.

Is It Ever Appropriate to Withhold Further Investigations in Somatoform Disorders?

Yes. Whether to pursue aggressive and invasive studies will be based on the patient's overall history, past findings, and the present indications for such studies. One of the long-term complications of somatoform disorders is the morbidity associated with repeated and uninformative invasive procedures such as exploratory laparotomies. You will need to make a considered medical judgment about the relative risks and likely rewards of further studies. Keep in mind that if you forgo aggressive testing, it need not be for all time. If your patient develops new symptoms or physical findings, new testing may be appropriate.

If I Give My Patient a Placebo and He Gets Better, Does That Mean the Complaint Was Somatoform?

A placebo response is poorly understood, and the very existence of placebo response has recently been called into question. Some researchers have suggested that endorphins may be released in placebo responders, but the exact neurophysiologic mechanisms are not understood. A positive response to placebo has no diagnostic use and cannot be used to rule out a true medical or psychiatric condition.

What Is an "Amytal Interview"?

Amytal (amobarbital) is a barbiturate that has sometimes been used to diagnose and treat conversion disorder. Other sedative-hypnotics such as lorazepam are also occasionally used.

Patients are given an intravenous dose of the drug to the level of mild sedation and then interviewed about their lives and symptoms. While some patients are under the influence of barbiturate intoxication, it is believed that they will give up their conversion symptoms.

Does an Amytal Interview Work?

Most of the literature on Amytal interviewing (also called narcoanalysis) is anecdotal. If a patient does lose a particular symptom such as blindness or paralysis while intoxicated with amobarbital, it is convincing evidence that the disability was not caused by physical pathology. The reverse is not true. It is not known how many people with conversion symptoms do not get better with amobarbital. Amytal interviewing works best for symptoms of recent onset and less well for chronic symptoms. It is impractical for long-term therapy.

TREATMENT

What Happens if Somatoform Disorders Are Untreated?

The somatoform disorders are associated with morbidity and even mortality. Treatment is difficult but should be attempted. Patients are at risk for multiple repeated invasive diagnostic procedures. They may develop secondary complications from investigations themselves, such as abdominal adhesions from exploratory surgery. Patients with body dysmorphic disorder may submit to a series of cosmetic procedures and still feel dissatisfied with their appearance. Patients with pain disorder are at increased risk for suicide. After a period of time, people with somatoform disorders may find that their medical complaints are no longer taken seriously by their physicians, and they face the added risk of real medical diseases going undetected. Apart from medical complications, many people with somatoform disorders lead unhappy, frustrated lives. The somatic preoccupation limits productivity, well-being, and pleasure. It is often off-putting to friends and family and can lead to serious disruptions of important relationships (Table 34-3).

Should Patients with Somatoform Disorders Be Referred to a Psychiatrist?

Psychiatric referral can be extremely difficult. Almost by definition, the diagnosis of a somatoform disorder means that the person has a psychological investment in believing symptoms to be physical rather than emotional. Many patients react to the request for psychiatric consultation as if it were dismissive and as though their complaints were not being taken seriously, with the result that physical symptoms intensify. They may leave a physician who raises psychiatric concerns and find another whose focus is purely medical. Even among the patients who do agree to see a psychiatrist, resistance to self-reflection and emotional exploration can

Table 34-3
Complications of Somatoform Disorders
Impaired work and social relationships
Unnecessary investigations and procedures with secondary complications
Substance abuse and dependence
Disregard or dismissal by medical personnel
Suicide

be so intense that meaningful therapy is not possible. The best treatment is coordinated between a primary care physician and a psychiatrist.

How Should I Ask My Patient with a Somatoform Disorder to See a Psychiatrist?

The best referrals reassure patients that their complaints are still being taken seriously. Primary care physicians should emphasize the *effect* of symptoms rather than their cause. They can observe that the patient is truly suffering, that the physical symptoms are stressful, and that stress can make the symptoms even worse. They can recommend pragmatism, noting that it is worth considering any approach that has the possibility of helping the patient feel better. The primary care physician should make it clear that he or she is not getting rid of the patient but rather that a psychiatrist is being brought in as a part of the treatment team.

What Psychotherapy Approach Is Best for Treating Somatoform Disorders?

There is no single approach that works well for all patients. Because the disorders are postulated to arise from unresolved emotional conflicts, you might think that a psychoanalytic approach that aims to resolve those conflicts would be best. In practice, however, many patients with somatoform disorders are too resistant to psychological exploration to benefit much from psychodynamic exploration. Cognitive-behavioral therapy has been successful with some patients, particularly those with hypochondriasis. Hypochondriacal patients misread and amplify normal body sensations, mistaking them for signs of serious illness. Mild gastrointestinal distress may be interpreted as evidence of colon cancer. Cognitive-behavioral therapy attempts to correct these distortions. Psychotherapy can also be effective in decreasing associated anxiety and depression, even in noninsightful patients. That relief may be enough to reduce the intensity of physical symptoms.

Should I Tell My Patient with a Somatoform Disorder to Stop Seeing Her Internist?

No. On the contrary; the best approach for people with somatoform symptoms—especially somatization disorder and hypochondriasis—is a routine of frequent office visits that are scheduled in advance and not prompted by new symptoms or intensification of old symptoms. This approach provides the reassurance of ongoing medical care and at the same time helps to break the cycle that rewards new symptoms with more attention. Many experienced primary care physicians ask somatoform patients to come in for brief visits once a month or every 6 weeks. At the same time, they try to avoid unnecessary procedures and investigations, using their growing personal knowledge of the patient as a commonsense guide. For the patient with a somatoform disorder, an attentive, monthly physical examination is more reassuring, less costly, and more therapeutic than specialized technological investigations of ever-increasing sophistication.

Factitious Disorders

Should Medication Be Part of the Treatment of Somatoform Disorders?

The judicious use of medication can help control associated anxiety and depression, but you must be cautious. Substance abuse is a frequent complication of these disorders—through either self-medication or misuse of prescription drugs. Patients become addicted to benzodiazepines and abuse painkillers. When the original somatoform symptoms are complicated by an overlay of benzodiazepine or opioid dependence, evaluation and treatment become even more difficult. All medication must be monitored closely. Body dysmorphic disorder resembles obsessive-compulsive disorder and may respond to antiobsessive medications such as selective serotonin reuptake inhibitors (SSRIs). Some principles of treating somatoform disorders are presented in Box 34-1.

How Do I Manage a Patient with Pain Disorder?

Treatment of acute pain differs from treatment of chronic pain. The goal in treating acute pain is to eliminate it with analgesics, including opioids. The goal for chronic pain is to control the pain and to minimize its disruptive impact in a person's life. You should avoid the extended use of opioid analgesics in treating chronic pain because of the risks of tolerance and dependence. Supportive psychotherapy and cognitive-behavioral therapy are helpful for certain patients. Some antidepressants such as tricyclics and SSRIs have analgesic properties and are a beneficial option in managing chronic pain. Alternative approaches include acupuncture, biofeedback, and hypnosis. Surgical intervention is sometimes necessary. The evaluation and treatment of pain has become a medical specialty in its own right. Many medical centers across the country have established multidisciplinary pain clinics providing a coordinated approach, commonly including psychiatry, neurology, internal medicine, and anesthesiology.

How Do Antidepressants Reduce Pain?

The mechanism is unknown. Analgesic effect is observed for both serotonergic and noradrenergic drugs and is independent of the antidepressant

Factitious Disorders

BOX 34-1

PRINCIPLES OF TREATING SOMATOFORM DISORDERS

1. Reassure patients that their complaints are taken seriously.
2. Recommend a broad-based treatment approach that includes psychiatry but does not exclude medicine.
3. Frequent, scheduled evaluations are better than evaluations prompted by new or more serious symptoms.
4. Avoid unnecessary investigations and procedures.
5. Use medications judiciously to avoid creating dependence.
6. Remember that even hypochondriacal patients can get sick.

effect. Nondepressed patients obtain as much relief as depressed patients. The tricyclic antidepressants are the most effective, although some pain control has been reported with monoamine oxidase inhibitors and SSRIs. The analgesic effect of tricyclics, like the antidepressant effect, is delayed, usually taking several days to weeks.

What Kind of Pain Do the Tricyclics Treat?

They are first-line drugs for treating pain related to neuropathies such as postherpetic neuralgia or diabetic neuropathy. They are used in many other conditions as well and often make possible lower doses of narcotic analgesics when used in combination.

What Dose of Tricyclic Should I Use?

The analgesic effects of tricyclics are seen at lower doses than those used to treat depression. Amitriptyline is the most studied; a reasonable starting dose is 25 mg/day. The dose should be increased slowly, balancing symptom relief against side effects.

FACTITIOUS DISORDERS AND MALINGERING

ETIOLOGY

What Are Factitious Disorders?

The diagnosis of factitious disorder is used to describe someone who intentionally fakes signs or symptoms of an illness to assume the sick role and not because of any external tangible benefit such as insurance compensation or exemption from jury duty. Such a person may, for example, add blood to a urine sample to create the impression of hematuria or hold a thermometer next to a light bulb to make it look as though she has a fever. The deception can be more invasive and self-destructive. Patients have been known to inject themselves with fecal material to create septicemia or to take oral hypoglycemics or anticoagulants to create factitious physical signs. The diagnosis of factitious disorder is also used for people who fake psychiatric illness. They may claim to be experiencing auditory hallucinations or may actually take psychotropic medication to cause psychiatric signs and symptoms.

Why Would Anyone Want to Assume the Sick Role?

A number of psychological explanations have been proposed: that the factitious patient unconsciously wants to defeat or devalue the caring physician, that early abuse or neglect may lead some people to associate love and caring with submissiveness and pain, or that factitious signs and symptoms are reinforced by the medical attention they receive. Each of these explanations is speculative and may play a greater or lesser role for the individual patient. Some reported cases of factitious disorder have been in people with serious personality disorders, especially borderline and antisocial personality disorders. There is no evidence of a genetic vulnerability, and no credible neurobiologic explanation has been proposed.

How Common Are Factitious Disorders?

The prevalence remains as elusive as the etiology. The diagnosis is difficult to make, and factitious disorder patients are seldom cooperative or reliable historians. It is possible that the suggested prevalence rates for chronic factitious disorder are overstated because a single patient may see multiple physicians, each of whom reports the case. Factitious disorder is believed to be more common in men than in women.

EVALUATION

How Is a Diagnosis of Factitious Disorder Made?

The thrust of your evaluation is twofold: to rule out real medical disease and psychiatric disorders and to establish that signs and symptoms are consciously being fabricated. (You will also need to rule out the presence of external incentives for faking illness.) A good history, attentive physical examination, and observant mental status examination are necessary first steps to rule out a real medical condition.

How Can I Tell if My Patient's Signs and Symptoms Are Being Faked?

Unless your patient is directly observed inflicting self-injury or otherwise creating physical signs, it may be impossible to know with complete certainty and the diagnosis may remain presumptive. There are some attributes that should raise the suspicion of a factitious illness, however. These are summarized in Box 34-2.

Is Munchausen's Syndrome the Same Thing as Factitious Disorder?

Munchausen's syndrome (not described separately in DSM-IV-TR) is a particular kind of chronic factitious disorder. Patients go from hospital

Factitious Disorders

BOX 34-2

FACTORS ASSOCIATED WITH FACTITIOUS DISORDERS

1. Patients present the history in an elaborate, engaging manner but are vague or inconsistent about details.
2. Patients seem to know a great deal about medicine and hospital routines.
3. Patients do not have visitors.
4. New complaints emerge when original symptoms have been treated.
5. Patients do not complain of pain or ask for analgesics.

to hospital, emergency department to emergency department, and even city to city presenting with fabricated signs and symptoms and submitting to an endless series of medical investigations and treatments. The syndrome can so dominate a person's life that the person is left without family, friends, or employment.

What Is Munchausen's Syndrome by Proxy?

Called "factitious disorder by proxy" in DSM-IV-TR, it is used for a person who makes somebody else sick to assume the role of concerned caregiver or, indirectly, the sick role. Sadly, Munchausen's by proxy often involves seriously disturbed parents who make their young children sick and then rush them to medical attention. Deaths of infants and young children have resulted.

How Does Factitious Disorder Differ from Malingering?

Malingering is not a psychiatric diagnosis in DSM-IV-TR. In both factitious disorder and malingering, the person knowingly and intentionally fakes illness (unlike the situation in somatoform disorders, in which symptom creation is unconscious), but the motivation is different. In factitious disorder, it is for internal, psychological reasons that the patient may not understand or be aware of. In malingering, it is for clearly defined external gain. People who pretend to be sick to get out of jury duty, receive worker's compensation, or win a lawsuit are all malingering.

How Can a Psychiatrist Know When a Patient Is Malingering?

It may be impossible with practiced liars. Unlike diagnosis in physical medicine, psychiatry relies almost wholly on self-report. There are no verifiable physical signs or laboratory tests to corroborate what the patient tells you. Your suspicion may be aroused when the degree of disability is disproportionate to the actual findings or when the evaluation is immediately followed by a request—for example, for legal documentation or for narcotic pain medication.

TREATMENT

How Can People with Fake Symptoms Be Treated?

The goal of treatment in factitious disorder is damage control—to disrupt the cycle of symptom creation and medical intervention and to prevent complications and unnecessary procedures. The person suspected of a factitious illness should be confronted, ideally by a group of people involved in the patient's care, such as internist, nurse, and psychiatrist. To the extent humanly possible, the confrontation should be nonaccusatory and nonhostile and presented as an offer to help by shifting the focus from inappropriate medical treatment to psychiatric treatment. Most patients, however, become indignant, vehemently deny faking illness, and abruptly leave the hospital against medical advice. There will be some patients whose factitious behavior is potentially so self-injurious—for example, swallowing razor blades—that involuntary transfer to a locked psychiatric unit is justified.

KEY POINTS

◆ Somatoform symptoms are not consciously created. Patients are reporting their true experience and are not making up symptoms to get attention.

◆ Signs and symptoms are consciously created in both factitious disorder and malingering. The purpose in factitious disorder is to assume the sick role. The purpose in malingering is to get some external, tangible reward.

◆ All pain involves peripheral stimulation and psychological modification.

Case 34-1

A 48-year-old accountant believes he has AIDS, despite the fact that he has been celibate for many years, has never used recreational drugs, and has never received blood transfusions. He describes a chronic cough, fatigue, and weakness lasting 3 years. When asked why he thinks he has AIDS, he answers, "What else could it be? I know it's serious." Physical examination, chest radiographs, chest and abdominal computed tomography (CT) scans, and extensive laboratory investigations including six HIV tests and multiple CD4 counts have failed to demonstrate any abnormality. When presented with negative test results, he is initially reassured but slowly begins to brood about the possibility of laboratory error and false-negative test results. His preoccupation with AIDS is interfering with work, and during the past year, his accounting practice has fallen off significantly.

A. Is the man suffering from a somatoform disorder?
B. What is the most likely diagnosis?
C. What treatment strategies might help this man?

Case 34-2

A 32-year-old woman comes to the physician with complaints of abdominal pain. The complaints are poorly localized but cause her considerable discomfort. She has a 10-year history of multiple changing symptomatic complaints, including headache, shortness of breath, paresthesias in her arms and legs, pelvic pain, weakness, and fatigue. Over the years, multiple physical examinations, laboratory studies, radiographs, and CT scans have failed to reveal any abnormalities. She has never had psychiatric treatment of any kind. On this occasion, her physical examination is unremarkable: complete blood cell count, electrolytes, blood urea nitrogen, creatinine, liver function tests, cholesterol, triglycerides, amylase, glucose, and sedimentation rate are within normal limits. The woman asks for an exploratory laparotomy and is willing to sign a waiver against any damage.

A. What is the most likely diagnosis?

B. What should her physician do?

Case 34-3

A 50-year-old man has been suffering from severe facial pain for 6 months. The pain is in the distribution of the left trigeminal nerve. He has been treated with nonsteroidal anti-inflammatory drugs, aspirin, acetaminophen and codeine, and narcotic analgesics but with modest benefit at most. The man has no prior medical or psychiatric history.

A. What treatment do you recommend?

Case Answers

34-1 A. *Learning objective:* **Understand the concept of a somatoform disorder.** It sounds like it. Although it is a diagnosis of exclusion, the information is consistent with a diagnosis of a somatoform disorder. He has complained for a long time of physical symptoms for which no physical or laboratory evidence of medical disease has been found. There is not enough information to diagnose a psychiatric disorder such as major depression. The fact that he is momentarily reassured by negative test results strongly indicates that his beliefs aren't delusional. His somatic concerns are serious enough to cause disruption of his business.

34-1 B. *Learning objective:* **Understand the major differences among somatoform disorders.** His symptoms and course are most consistent with a diagnosis of hypochondriasis. Although he complains of multiple vague symptoms over a long period of time, he is fixated on a specific, serious diagnosis, a feature more characteristic of hypochondriasis than somatization disorder. His complaints do not focus on pain (pain disorder) or a perceived body deformity (body dysmorphic disorder). The fear of disease is more prominent than a single dramatic symptom or sign, as would be true for conversion disorder.

34-1 C. *Learning objective:* **Be familiar with treatment strategies for somatoform disorders.** The man's fear of AIDS can't be dismissed, but regular, frequent medical visits that are scheduled in advance and not prompted by new worries or symptoms may be reassuring and decrease the need for additional unnecessary testing. Exploratory, supportive, or cognitive-behavioral therapy may help lessen the impact on his life of his medical concerns. There is a hint of social isolation in his history (years of celibacy) that may be a source of tension or unhappiness that could be further explored in psychotherapy. Medication may be useful for any associated symptoms of depression, anxiety, or insomnia.

34-2 A. *Learning objective:* **Recognize the major somatoform disorders.** Because of the difficulty in proving a negative—in this case, the absence of physical disease—a medical condition cannot be definitively ruled out. However, it is made much less likely by the absence of physical findings and by her long history of changing symptomatic complaints. The most likely diagnosis appears to be somatization disorder.

34-2 B. *Learning objective:* **Understand the basic principles of managing somatoform disorders.** Invasive procedures such as an exploratory laparotomy should be avoided without some objective indication. Her willingness to sign a waiver does not relieve the physician of the obligation to do what is in the patient's best interest. Because she has had no previous psychiatric treatment, a referral to a psychiatrist may feel dismissive and risks breaking the established relationship she has with her physician. A better approach would be to schedule frequent short follow-up visits. This approach offers reassurance that her complaints are being taken seriously, minimizes the risk that true physical pathology will be overlooked, and avoids the expense and potential morbidity of unnecessary procedures.

34-3 A. *Learning objective:* **Be familiar with strategies for managing pain.** Tricyclic antidepressants such as amitriptyline or imipramine are effective in controlling or reducing pain—especially neuropathic pain, which this appears to be. The tricyclic can be used alone or in combination with anti-inflammatory or analgesic agents. The addition of a tricyclic often makes lower doses of opioid analgesics possible.

Factitious Disorders

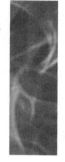

35

Disorders of Childhood and Adolescence

CARMEN M. ALONSO, GARY GOSSELIN, AND ERIC TEITEL

 OVERVIEW

How Common Are Psychiatric Disorders in Children and Adolescents?

Mild, transient emotional or behavioral problems are common. The diagnosis of a "disorder" is warranted when (in addition to fulfilling DSM-IV-TR diagnostic criteria) the severity of the condition leads to functional impairment and, less often, to a perceived need for mental health services. Using these guidelines, the prevalence of childhood and adolescent psychopathology is about 11%. The major disorders—and the ones to be discussed in detail—are listed in Table 35-1.

Is a Child Psychiatric Assessment the Same as an Adult Assessment?

Although child and adult psychiatric evaluations are organized in similar ways, there are significant differences in *how* the information is obtained. Most children referred for a psychiatric evaluation have behaved in ways intolerable to others, especially at school. Unlike adults, who have at the least accepted the possibility that their distress warrants a mental health evaluation, children, and sometimes their parents, may have little sense of why a psychiatric evaluation is recommended or what it entails. Children's problems generally affect their adaptation to multiple environments—school, friends, after-school activities, babysitters, and so forth. It is thus necessary to obtain information from all of these sources. (Parental consent is always a prerequisite to obtaining information about the child.)

How Do I Do a Psychiatric Assessment of a Child?

You will usually see a child's parents or primary caretakers alone for the initial intake. Allow them to discuss issues that might not be appropriate to discuss in front of their child. Set the stage for a collaborative working

353

Table 35-1

Disorders of Childhood and Adolescence

I. Disruptive behavior disorders
   A. Attention deficit/hyperactivity disorder
   B. Oppositional defiant disorder
   C. Conduct disorder
II. Mood disorders
III. Separation anxiety disorder
IV. Pervasive developmental disorders—autistic disorder
V. Mental retardation

relationship. In addition to parents' customary worries about a physician's finding something wrong with their child, they are contending with guilt over their possible failures related to their child's upbringing, fear that they will be blamed for the child's disorder, frustration with the child's behavior or referring agency (school), and anger or distrust of mental health professionals because of the stigma associated with mental illness. It is therefore necessary first to put the parents at ease by educating them about the process of the evaluation and their role in assisting the physician. It is instructive to ask parents whether the child knows they are seeing you and what the child has been told because this may reflect the parents' feelings about the child's difficulties and attitudes toward seeking mental health care.

Do I Evaluate Adolescents the Same Way?

Adolescents are typically interviewed before the parents in order to respect the adolescent's increasing autonomy and need for privacy. This allows the adolescent to explain her views on the issue rather than just responding to parental reports. You should clarify issues of confidentiality right at the start: you will not tell the parents anything the adolescent says without her permission except for issues of danger. Both parents and adolescent (or child) should participate in the feedback session at the termination of the evaluation to allow them to question the diagnosis and treatment recommendations.

How Do I Talk to Children?

A developmental perspective is essential. Infants and toddlers are best evaluated with the primary caretaker. Given that children's abilities to separate from their parents and interact with strangers develop slowly over time, the examiner must be sensitive to the child's and parents' readiness to tolerate the interview process. The younger the child, the more likely it is that you will have to engage him or her through play or art because the child will quickly lose interest in a solely verbal approach. Rather than asking about presenting problems, try to learn more about the child in general (e.g., school, friends, family, hobbies) before inquiring about potentially threatening or troubling issues.

Child psychiatrists generally approach children and families in a warm, active, and supportive fashion, not from a neutral, observing stance. The physician must convey a nonaccusatory, helpful attitude toward both parents and children, engaging everyone in a collaborative problem-solving endeavor. Rather than focusing exclusively on determining a diagnosis, the process aims to find assets and strengths that will be used to formulate treatment recommendations. Flexibility is key.

ATTENTION DEFICIT/HYPERACTIVITY DISORDER

ETIOLOGY

How Common Is Attention Deficit/Hyperactivity Disorder?

Attention deficit/hyperactivity disorder (ADHD) affects approximately 3% to 5% of school-aged children, with prevalence rates ranging from 4% to 12% in school and community-based studies. (Similar rates have been found worldwide.) ADHD is the most frequently encountered childhood-onset neurodevelopmental disorder in primary care settings. Elementary school-aged boys outnumber girls by 9:1 in clinical settings but only by 4:1 in community surveys.

What Causes ADHD?

The etiology of ADHD is unknown, although a combination of psychological, environmental, and biologic factors contributes. There is a genetic factor: concordance rates are 51% in monozygotic twins and 33% in dizygotic twins. Studies of brain structure and function have shown significant *group* differences between healthy controls and subjects with ADHD, but individual differences cannot yet be used for diagnostic purposes. Prefrontal cortex dysfunction modulated by norepinephrine and dopamine has been implicated. There is also evidence that serotonin may influence the hyperactive and impulsive components of ADHD.

Isn't Diagnosing ADHD Just an Attempt to Medicalize Normal, Active Children?

Probably not. The group differences just mentioned suggest a true medical condition, albeit one in which symptoms are increased or decreased by what goes on in the environment. More important, children who receive the diagnosis are at long-term risk for poor school performance and impaired interpersonal relationships. These risks are reduced with appropriate treatment.

EVALUATION

When Is ADHD First Diagnosed?

Although school concerns about a child's inattentiveness, distractibility, hyperactivity, and impulsiveness are the most common reason for referral, many parents report their child's having had these core ADHD symptoms from the time he was a toddler. Because a child's behavior changes in different settings, it is essential to obtain reports from multiple informants before diagnosing or ruling out ADHD on the basis of parents' report alone and a brief office visit.

Are There Medical Conditions That Look Like ADHD?

There are some known medical disorders (fragile X syndrome, fetal alcohol syndrome, a rare generalized resistance to thyroid hormone, G6PD deficiency, and phenylketonuria) that can present with ADHD symptoms. Given the low prevalence of these disorders in children with ADHD, laboratory screening is not warranted unless the physical examination and history suggest it. All children with ADHD should be evaluated for the presence of vocal and motor tics. Children who go on to develop Tourette's syndrome may manifest symptoms of ADHD months to years before the onset of tic activity.

What Drugs Cause ADHD Symptoms?

Medications do not cause ADHD. Medications with central nervous system activity can cause behavioral toxicity. Manifestations of behavioral toxicity include mood irritability, diminished frustration tolerance, impaired attention, and reduced impulse control. When evaluating a child or adolescent it is important to take a complete medication history, to check side effect profiles, and to clarify dose-response effects. Behavioral toxicity is transient and occurs as a clear dose-response effect when a medication trial is being initiated or a dose is being adjusted.

Are There Other Psychiatric Disorders That Look Like ADHD in Children?

Yes. Anxiety disorders and mood disorders—especially a manic or hypomanic episode—may include restlessness, hyperactivity, and impaired concentration. In mood disorders, these symptoms stand out against a background of normal child development and behavior. The presence of other symptoms such as hypersomnia or insomnia, dysphoria, and somatic symptoms may also help distinguish mood disorders from ADHD in children. Children with ADHD often have significant impairments in school function, and robust associations with ADHD and learning disorders have been noted (Table 35-2).

Are There Blood Tests or Imaging Studies That Help Make the Diagnosis of ADHD?

ADHD is a clinical diagnosis. There is no test for ADHD. However, standardized ADHD-specific parent and teacher behavior rating scales are useful in distinguishing normal variants of attention, impulsivity, and activity from ADHD and serve as a baseline from which to assess treatment response.

Childhood and
Adolescence

Table 35-2

Attention Deficit/Hyperactivity Disorder Comorbidity

Community Samples	Primary Care Settings
Oppositional defiant disorder (33%)	Oppositional defiant disorder (38%)
Anxiety disorder (38%)	Anxiety disorder (25%)
Conduct disorder (25%)	Conduct disorder (9%)
Depressive disorders (20%)	Depressive disorders (9%)
Learning disabilities (12%-22%)	

What Do I Look for in Evaluating ADHD?

The core symptoms of ADHD are problems with impulse control, sustained attention, distractibility, and motor restlessness or hyperactivity. These lead to difficulties in academic and peer interactions that usually lead to referral, although behavioral issues at home may have been present for years. Given the frequency of comorbid disorders, your evaluation must seek to rule them out. The types and frequencies of comorbid disorders are presented in Table 35-2.

TREATMENT

How Should I Treat My Patient with ADHD?

Stimulants (methylphenidate, dextroamphetamine) are the drugs of choice for the treatment of ADHD. Start with a low dose and keep increasing it while monitoring for side effects until there is no more room for improvement as assessed by parent and teacher rating scales completed before each visit. Common side effects are transient decrease in appetite and increase in time to fall asleep. Although there has been concern about the potential for abuse of stimulants, emerging evidence shows that pharmacotherapy of ADHD decreases the risk for substance abuse.

Does It Matter Which Stimulant I Use?

There are few distinctions among stimulants, but it is not unusual for a child to respond to one after not having responded to another. Compliance with taking stimulants two or three times a day and rebound effects (which could resemble worsening of original symptoms) seen as the last dose of the day wears off are the most significant clinical problems. Some long-acting preparations of methylphenidate (Concerta) and dextroamphetamine (Adderall XR) require once-a-day dosing and reduce problems of rebound, and many argue that these preparations should be considered first-line treatment.

Childhood and
Adolescence

Are Other Medications Used?

Yes, noradrenergic partial agonists (clonidine and guanfacine hydrochloride) might be used alone to treat ADHD if stimulants are ineffective. Sometimes they are used in combination with stimulants to augment a treatment response. The antidepressant bupropion (Wellbutrin) is sometimes used to treat ADHD symptoms but is not considered a first-line agent. The Food and Drug Administration (FDA) requires a black box warning about possible increased suicide risk when using antidepressants to treat children and adolescents. Anyone considering the use of antidepressants in a child or adolescent must balance the increased risk of suicidal thinking with the clinical need for the drug. Signs and symptoms of comorbid disorders should also be addressed in the treatment plan when treating any disorder (see Table 35-2).

Is Psychotherapy Helpful in Treating ADHD?

The Multimodal Treatment Study of Children with ADHD (MTA), a national multisite study involving the largest sample of rigorously diagnosed children with ADHD, concluded that for ADHD symptoms, careful titration of stimulants with monthly feedback from teachers before the child's clinic visit with his or her parent is superior to behavioral treatment and to routine community care that included medication. The combination of behavioral treatment with medication management did not yield significantly greater benefits than medication management alone for core ADHD symptoms but may have provided modest advantages for non-ADHD symptoms and for long-term outcome. Despite the lack of empirical evidence for the benefit of psychotherapy, the treatment of ADHD generally includes environmental modification (including parent training) to address behavioral symptoms and remediation to overcome deficits in academic and social skills.

Psychoeducation about ADHD for patients, parents, and teachers continues to be considered standard practice, although it has not been systematically evaluated. Support groups, such as Children and Adults with Attention Deficit Disorders (CHADD), are helpful in decreasing the stigma of the disorder and educating parents about resources for their children. Federal mandates require educational and testing accommodations for people diagnosed with ADHD.

What Happens When ADHD Is Not Treated?

Gross hyperactivity may decrease with age, but ADHD does not disappear with the onset of puberty. A large proportion (30% to 50%) of children with ADHD still meet criteria for the disorder as adults. A variety of social and emotional difficulties lead to problems in social relationships (increased marital disruption, impaired parenting skills), higher education (reduced academic achievement), and work (vocational instability).

Childhood and
Adolescence

OPPOSITIONAL DEFIANT DISORDER

ETIOLOGY

How Common Is Oppositional Defiant Disorder?

Most parents will agree that occasional oppositional behavior is ubiquitous in childhood and adolescence. However, the consistent pattern of noncompliance and defiance characteristic of oppositional defiant disorder (ODD) is less common: 2% to 16% of children, depending on the measures used and the population sampled. ODD is more prevalent in boys before puberty, but the rates are similar in both sexes after puberty.

What Causes ODD?

The etiology is unknown. Children (particularly boys) with difficult temperaments (withdrawal from novel situations, slow adaptation to change, anger, and irritability) are at higher risk for developing a behavior disorder. Whether this is due to the child's innate temperamental characteristics or the poorness of fit between the expectations and demands on the child by parents and others in the child's environment is not clear. ODD is thought to be more common in families in which at least one parent has a history of a mood disorder, ODD, conduct disorder, ADHD, antisocial personality disorder, or a substance-related disorder. The relative contributions of biologic predisposition and family environment remain to be elucidated.

EVALUATION

When and How Does ODD Appear?

Oppositional behavior usually begins in the home in the preschool years. Many parents report that their child never left the "terrible two's," a sense that the child's quest to establish autonomy is fought out on a daily basis over issues such as dressing, bathing, eating, and sleeping. Adolescence, with its impetus to establish an autonomous self, is similarly fraught with an increase in oppositional behaviors. ODD may be seen only in the home, with the child not manifesting symptoms at school. However, most cases invariably show conflicts with teachers and peers.

How Do I Diagnose ODD?

A diagnosis of ODD should be given only if the behaviors occur more frequently than is typically observed in children of a comparable age *and* lead to significant impairment in social, academic, or occupational functioning. Children with ODD manifest a pattern of negativistic, defiant, disobedient, and hostile behavior toward authority figures, usually beginning with their parents, lasting at least 6 months but generally present for years before coming to clinical attention. These children are argumentative, refuse to comply with or defy adult requests, and deliberately annoy people. They are also easily annoyed by others and can be resentful and vindictive. Their hostility does not include physical aggression toward people or animals, destruction of property, or a pattern of theft and deceit seen in individuals with conduct disorder.

Does ODD Occur with Other Psychiatric Disorders?

The most common comorbid diagnosis found in children with ODD is ADHD. Other disorders associated with ODD are learning disorders and communication disorders. These comorbid disorders increase the child's exposure to frustrations and the likelihood of a worse prognosis. ODD can be a developmental antecedent to conduct disorder.

Can Medical Conditions Mimic ODD?

Parents and teachers know that many children "melt down" when tired or sleep deprived. Similarly, hospitalized children may become irritable because of their fears of pain and separation. Such transient behavioral difficulties do not warrant a diagnosis. Children who are treated with steroids sometimes manifest a dysphoric (sad or irritable) mood that may be similar to the negativistic behavior and easy annoyance by others of ODD.

TREATMENT

Can ODD Be Treated?

Yes, but family involvement is crucial. Psychoeducation of parents, with the aim of reassessing expectations and demands and improving *goodness of fit* between parent and child, is indicated. Preschoolers benefit from their parents learning effective and consistent parenting skills with appropriate rewards for decreasing oppositional and increasing compliant behaviors. Children with more ingrained behavioral problems need specific behavioral management plans along with the previously mentioned strategies. Family therapy may be necessary in high-conflict situations that interfere with the family's ability to engage in these treatments. The child may require individual treatment if behavior problems have led to demoralization and low self-esteem. Social skills groups may also help children whose symptoms make it difficult for them to get along well with others. Similarly, educational remediation of associated learning or communication disorders is indicated as soon as their diagnosis is confirmed.

Are Medications Useful?

Not for ODD itself, but treatment of comorbid disorders such as ADHD can lead to improved treatment outcomes.

CONDUCT DISORDER

What Is Conduct Disorder?

A diagnosis of conduct disorder (CD), unlike ODD, describes children and adolescents who persistently violate the rights of others or social

Childhood and Adolescence

norms. Examples of CD behavior include assaulting others, torturing animals, setting fires, and running away from home.

ETIOLOGY

How Common Is Conduct Disorder?

CD is one of the most frequently diagnosed disorders in child and adolescent psychiatry, with a general population prevalence between 1.5% and 3.4%. Rates vary significantly by setting (urban more than rural), sex (male-to-female ratio 5:1), age (gap between boys and girls closes in adolescence), and diagnostic methods. Poverty and socioeconomic disadvantage are associated with CD.

What Causes Conduct Disorder?

CD is a heterogeneous disorder with multiple risk factors for its development and predictors of its course. Although CD aggregates in families, the relative contributions of genetic and environmental factors are unknown. About 60% of children with CD do not go on to develop antisocial personality disorder (for which evidence supporting heritability exists). Children and adolescents with CD may have preexisting brain disorders or expose themselves to situations in which they are at risk for sustaining brain injuries, which may in turn exacerbate their cognitive deficits and low frustration tolerance. They are more likely to become involved in alcohol and drug abuse that may further disinhibit them and increase their propensity for involvement in antisocial activity. Risk factors associated with CD are listed in Table 35-3.

How Does Conduct Disorder First Appear?

Evidence supports an age-based distinction between early or childhood onset (before age 10—about 15% of all cases) and late or adolescent onset

Table 35-3

Risk Factors Associated with Conduct Disorder

Constitutional Factors	Family Risk Factors	Environmental Risk Factors
Difficult temperament	Marital discord	Negative peer relationships
Cognitive, speech, and language deficits	Poor or ineffective parenting (giving in to child's coercive behavior in an inconsistent fashion)	Negative role models
Chronic illness and disability	Family substance abuse	
Attention deficit/ hyperactivity disorder	Family psychiatric illness	
Early aggressiveness	Child abuse and neglect	

(after age 10—about 85 % of all cases). The early childhood subtype has a greater frequency of neuropsychiatric disorders, ADHD, low IQ, aggression, and familial clustering of externalizing disorders. These children exhibit a greater number of antisocial activities in different areas such as fighting and school truancy, school suspensions and expulsions, early drug abuse, stealing, and out-of-home placements with multiple placement failures and more overt aggression. Most cases of CD occur after puberty and appear to be more significantly affected by peer influences. Adolescent-onset CD is often transient and does not have the pervasive, persistent problems found in the early-onset type. Early-onset CD is more likely to lead to adult antisocial personality disorder.

EVALUATION

How Do I Evaluate a Child for Conduct Disorder?

Assessment of children and adolescents with CD has to be multidimensional and include multiple informants, given that patients tend to minimize their problems. Patients with CD may anger their examiners by rejecting or attempting to con them. However, it is essential not to be put off and to persist in comprehensively evaluating the patient.

Some children with CD may experience sporadic psychotic symptoms while presenting a normal facade when not under stress, and you should assess the presence of paranoid thoughts and auditory hallucinations. It is also imperative to obtain a thorough trauma history given the risk of exposure to physical or sexual abuse.

TREATMENT

What Happens When Conduct Disorder Is Untreated?

Untreated CD generally gets worse through adolescence and early adulthood but then lessens in intensity. However, the negative impact of CD on interpersonal relationships and on the abilities to maintain a healthful lifestyle, to achieve academic success, to be financially self-supporting, and to parent children in a consistent and noncoercive manner may be lifelong.

Can Conduct Disorder Be Treated?

Current research indicates that the most effective interventions appear to be early preventive measures rather than initiating treatment when the disorder is well established. Training parents how to interact with their young children, how to model adaptive behaviors, and how to handle the tantrums and noncompliant behaviors of preschoolers in a consistent and noncoercive manner can prevent a cycle of frustration, aggression, and disruptive behaviors from taking hold. School-aged children also benefit from skills training for their parents but need their own training in problem-solving skills and anger management to improve academic performance and social interactions. Family therapy and the parents' individual treatment may be indicated, depending on the degree of dysfunction in each domain.

Childhood and Adolescence

Are Medications Used to Treat Conduct Disorder?

Psychopharmacology consists of treating comorbid conditions, particularly ADHD, depression, and substance abuse. However, if there are no comorbid conditions, target symptoms such as aggression, mood lability, and impulsivity may warrant treatment if they are severe and do not respond to psychosocial interventions. Low-dose atypical antipsychotic medications are currently considered first-line agents when treating aggression and mood lability in CD. "Start low and go slow" is the primary rule for dosing. Lithium carbonate, anticonvulsants, propranolol, and partial alpha agonists (clonidine, guanfacine) are sometimes used to target aggression and mood lability.

 MOOD DISORDERS

ETIOLOGY

Are Mood Disorders as Common in Children as in Adults?

Probably not. Depression is thought to affect between 0.4% to 2.5% of children and 0.4% to 8.3% of adolescents. Depressive disorders do not demonstrate any sex differences before puberty but do show female predominance (female-to-male 2:1) after puberty. Bipolar disorders affect boys and girls equally, but the prevalence of bipolar disorders in children is not clear. Dysthymic disorder is thought to be as prevalent as depression.

EVALUATION

Do Mood Disorders in Children Look the Same as Mood Disorders in Adults?

They may, but there are more likely to be atypical features. Depressed prepubertal children may present with separation anxiety, phobias, irritable mood, somatic complaints (headache, stomachache), and behavioral problems. Children with psychotic features are more likely to have auditory hallucinations than the delusions that are common in adults with psychotic depression. Vegetative signs of depression in young children include failure to make expected weight gains. In adolescents, however, an *increased* appetite, particularly for sweets and carbohydrates, is common. Adolescent sleep disturbances may include *sleep reversal* (up all night, sleeping all day) and hypersomnia. Irritability and mood reactivity are common markers for adolescent depression.

Are There Differences in Bipolar Disorder between Children and Adults?

Manic episodes in adolescents are more likely than episodes of depression to include psychotic features and may be associated with school truancy, antisocial behavior, school failure, or substance abuse. A significant minority of adolescents appear to have a history of long-standing behavior problems that precede the onset of a manic episode. Manic episodes typically begin suddenly, with a rapid escalation of symptoms over a few days. They last a few weeks to months and are briefer and end more abruptly than major depressive episodes. Bipolar children younger than 9 present with irritability and emotional lability. Older children are more likely to present with the euphoria, elation, paranoia, and grandiose delusions seen in adults. Hyperactivity, pressured speech, and distractibility may be found in both.

TREATMENT

How Are Mood Disorders Treated in Childhood?

Various forms of psychotherapy are used. There is some empirical evidence that cognitive-behavioral and interpersonal therapies may be the most effective with adolescent outpatients with mild to moderate depression.

Are the Same Medications Used to Treat Children and Adults with Mood Disorders?

Selective serotonin reuptake inhibitors (SSRIs) are considered first-line agents when medications are indicated in the treatment of child and adolescent depression. However, the FDA requires a black box warning about possible increased suicide risk when using antidepressants to treat children and adolescents. Anyone considering the use of antidepressants in a child or adolescent must balance the increased risk of suicidal thinking with the clinical need for the drug. Randomized controlled trials are needed to evaluate the efficacy and risk of SSRI use in children and adolescents. Studies are under way attempting to clarify the relationship between antidepressant effects and suicide. Mood stabilizers (lithium, valproate) are used in patients with bipolar disorders, but they have not been assessed in randomized controlled trials with adolescents.

SEPARATION ANXIETY DISORDER

ETIOLOGY

How Common Is Separation Anxiety Disorder?

The prevalence of separation anxiety disorder (SAD) is about 4% of children and adolescents, without gender differences.

What Causes Separation Anxiety Disorder?

Fears are relatively common in childhood. Infants toward the end of the first year of life fear strange people and novel objects. Fears of the dark, animals, and imaginary creatures are common in preschoolers and young school-aged children. Children's fears become more realistic with age. By adolescence, they fear bodily injury, physical danger, natural hazards, and loss of loved ones, and they develop concerns about school achievement

Childhood and Adolescence

and social relations. *Separation anxiety* (protest at the mother's departure, distress caused by her absence, and anxiety about her anticipated absence) is thought to be a universal phenomenon that is adaptive in protecting infants from the danger of being alone. Entry into daycare or nursery school commonly elicits such anxiety. *Separation anxiety disorder* is distinguished by anxiety that is *developmentally inappropriate* and *excessive* to the point of causing impairment in social and academic functioning. It is not unusual for SAD to arise first after a significant stress such as a death in the family or a move to a new neighborhood.

When Does Separation Anxiety Disorder First Show Up?

Usually in school-aged children. When it appears before the age of 6 (early onset), the intensity, pervasiveness, and duration of symptoms warrant the diagnosis. It is more common during the early years of school, with peaks when children go to a new school, and it is usually the child's inability to sustain school attendance (school phobia) that leads to the referral. Some children with SAD may be excellent, conscientious students who develop somatic complaints that keep them from attending school, particularly after weekends and holidays.

EVALUATION

How Can I Recognize Separation Anxiety Disorder?

Usually by the severe distress a child manifests when separated from loved ones. This ranges from silent preoccupation about loved ones instead of participating in class activities, inconsolable crying, clinging to loved ones, and refusing to stay without them to aggressive outbursts on attempts at separation. Children do not usually talk about their separation fears and worries (such as harm befalling loved ones or themselves) unless directly asked. Fear of separation caused by sleep leads to attempts to stay with parents at night, resistance to falling asleep by oneself, and repeated nightmares. Adolescents may deny their fears and deprecate their parents despite their homebound behavior. Younger children appear despondent when separated from their parents but are all right in the safety of their homes. Adolescents may exhibit a more pervasive depressed mood and may qualify for an additional diagnosis of mood disorder.

TREATMENT

How Is Separation Anxiety Disorder Treated?

Cognitive-behavioral therapy is the treatment of choice. If the child's anxiety is so distressing that it interferes with his ability to participate in therapy, medications may be used. SSRIs are the first-line agents, along with anxiolytics, such as clonazepam, if necessary. School phobia requires the cooperation of the school in working with the therapist to move the child slowly back into a classroom setting. Homebound schooling is contraindicated because it makes the disorder worse. In severe cases in which the parents are unable to get the child to leave the home, psychiatric hospitalization may be necessary to stabilize the child with medication. Family therapy may also be called for if the family's unresolved and conflicting messages about separation undermine the child's ability to separate.

PERVASIVE DEVELOPMENTAL DISORDERS

What Is Autism?

Autism is a neurobehavioral syndrome, with onset of symptoms within the first 3 years of life, caused by brain dysfunction resulting in deviant, not just delayed, development. It is classified as one of the *pervasive developmental disorders* (Box 35-1). These disorders share varying degrees of the following triad: qualitative impairments in *social interaction*, qualitative impairments in *communication*, and restricted, repetitive, and stereotyped *patterns of behavior*.

ETIOLOGY

How Common Is Autism?

Autistic disorders may be more common than was once thought, occurring in 1 to 1.3 per 1000 children. There is ongoing controversy over whether there is an actual increase of these disorders or simply better identification of milder cases. The ratio of boys to girls is 3 to 4:1, with boys predominating in milder cases.

What Causes Autism?

Although it is generally accepted that autism is a biologically based condition affecting the central nervous system, extensive research has not yet identified any specific anatomic or neurochemical abnormalities. Monozygotic twins have a concordance rate for autistic spectrum disorders of 90%, whereas siblings have a concordance rate of 7%. In both cases,

---

BOX 35-1

PERVASIVE DEVELOPMENTAL DISORDERS

Autistic disorder: The classic disorder described by Kanner in 1943
Asperger's syndrome: Intact language and cognitive functioning, so usually diagnosed in children older than 3 years
Rett's disorder: Rare disorder with an identified gene defect on the X chromosome affecting primarily girls with severe retardation and hand wringing
Childhood disintegrative disorder: Rare dementing disorder in children aged 2 to 10 years

Childhood and Adolescence

concordance for severity of the disorders is less, suggesting nongenetic influences. Fewer than 20% of cases of autism have a known etiology such as intrauterine infections (rubella, cytomegalovirus, and herpes simplex), intrauterine toxins such as thalidomide, and known genetic syndromes such as *fragile X*.

Do Vaccinations Cause Autism?

No. Although there are anecdotal reports of children developing behavioral changes, having bowel disturbances, and being first diagnosed with autism after measles-mumps-rubella (MMR) vaccinations, there are no data suggesting that MMR vaccinations lead to autism.

How Does Autism Appear?

There are no markers for the diagnosis of autism at birth. Most parents only gradually become aware of their child's disability as he fails to achieve social and language milestones. The full syndrome of signs and symptoms is usually apparent only by age 3. Typical clinical features are presented in Table 35-4.

EVALUATION

Are There Blood Tests or Imaging Studies That Help Make the Diagnosis of Autism?

There are no specific medical tests that can be used to establish the diagnosis of autism. Comprehensive health evaluation should look for signs of associated medical conditions or genetic syndromes that are seen more frequently in children with autism. This should include hearing and vision assessment; a neurologic evaluation, including a sleep electroencephalogram (up to one fourth of children with autism develop epilepsy by adolescence); a skin examination (for signs of tuberous sclerosis or neurofibromatosis); blood lead level; a urine test for phenylketonuria (PKU); and a search for medical conditions, genetic syndromes, or other developmental problems that are sometimes associated with autism. After the diagnosis has been confirmed and associated medical issues clarified, a full developmental assessment, including evaluation of cognitive, communication, behavior, social interaction, and adaptive skills and of motor and sensory abilities, is indicated to devise an appropriate plan.

What Clues in the History and Psychiatric Assessment Raise the Suspicion of Autism?

Parents' concerns that a child's development is delayed or deviant (lack of eye contact, does not reach out to be picked up, lack of reciprocal smile, lacks social imitation, does not wave "bye-bye," language delays, does not acknowledge or respond to other people, lack of pretend play) should always be taken seriously. Delayed speech and language regression or stagnation should alert you to ask about other autistic symptoms. Other clues that should be investigated include lack of initiation of social play,

Table 35-4

Typical Clinical Features of Autism

I. Qualitative impairments in social interaction—Lack of reciprocal social interaction: Deficits in social relatedness
   A. Early: Baby has poor eye contact, stiffens when held
   B. Middle years: Child does not initiate or sustain play
   C. Adolescence: Lacks social judgment, does not pick up on social cues, unable to recognize feelings in others
II. Qualitative impairments in communication
   A. Majority of children do not use language for functional communication at the time of diagnosis
   B. They do not use or imitate gestures (shaking head yes/no) for purposes of nonverbal communication
   C. If present, language is rote and repetitive with characteristic
      1. Echolalia: Repetition of the last few syllables of words heard
      2. Confusion of personal pronouns: Referring to self in second or third person
      3. Verbal perseveration: Repetition of the same phrase, topic, jingle (television ads)
      4. Abnormalities of prosody: Rate, rhythm, inflection, or volume of speech
III. Restricted, repetitive, and stereotyped patterns of behavior, interest, and activities
   A. Repetitive actions: Flap hands, bang head, rock, spin, pattern of finger movements
   B. Preoccupied with small number of activities/objects to the exclusion of novel stimuli (play with string, reading subway maps)
   C. Compulsive adherence to routines, becoming agitated or losing control over minor deviations
IV. Unusual responses to sensory stimuli
   A. Sensitive and distressed by certain sounds, sights, smells, tastes, and tactile stimuli while being oblivious to commonly perceived sensory stimuli
V. Cognitive characteristics
   A. Most are mentally retarded
   B. Those with normal and higher IQs may exhibit difficulties with abstract concepts
   C. Some children have "splinter skills" (aptitude for rote memory or calculations far exceeding their other abilities)
   D. Few have "savant skills" or "Rain Man–like" abilities to perform complex calculations

lack of pointing at an object to get another person to look at it, unusual repetitive hand and finger mannerisms, and unusual reactions to sensory stimuli.

TREATMENT

How Is Autism Treated?

Behavioral and educational interventions are the usual approach. Many programs use a systemic behavioral approach referred to as *applied behavioral analysis* (ABA). It is recommended that these programs include a minimum of 20 to 25 hours per week of individualized behavioral intervention using ABA techniques, independent of time spent with parents. Parent training is an integral part of intensive behavioral intervention programs. Family support through needed respite care and assistance with long-term planning for their child must also be included.

Are Medications Helpful in Autism?

Medications are used to treat comorbid disorders such as anxiety, mood, and tic disorders or to manage maladaptive behaviors such as aggression or self-injury. Hormone therapies, such as ACTH and secretin; immunologic therapies, such as intravenous immune globulin; antiyeast therapies; and vitamin and diet therapies lack the scientific evidence to recommend their use.

What Happens to Children with Autism?

The prognosis for autism is still poor for a majority of children when defined by social and vocational adjustment and ability to function independently. However, with intensive behavioral approaches begun at an early age, children with milder cases may improve to near-normal functioning. There is some suggestion that early and intensive intervention results in better long-term outcomes.

■ MENTAL RETARDATION

What Is Mental Retardation?

Mental retardation (MR), coded on Axis II, is defined as significantly *subaverage intellectual functioning* (IQ of 70 or below) with *onset before the age of 18 accompanied by impaired functioning.* (When the onset is after age 18, it is called *dementia.*) The degree of intellectual impairment further determines the type of retardation; this is outlined in Table 35-5.

EPIDEMIOLOGY
How Common Is Mental Retardation?

MR affects 1% of school-aged children, with boys outnumbering girls by 1.5:1. Known causes of retardation account for only 30% to 50% of all cases in the developed world.

What Causes Mental Retardation?

Mild MR has been primarily related to social and environmental conditions (psychosocial deprivation), whereas severe MR has been related to underlying biologic conditions (inborn errors of metabolism, chromosomal anomalies, brain injury, toxins such as lead, prenatal infections such as rubella, postnatal infections such as meningitis). Fragile X syndrome is the most common known *inherited* cause of developmental delay (Fig. 35-1). Rates of fragile X syndrome among individuals with MR range from 0.5% to 5.4% worldwide. Fetal alcohol syndrome and fetal alcohol

Childhood and
Adolescence

Table 35-5

Levels of Mental Retardation

	Percent of Population with MR	IQ Level	Adult Mental Age (yr)	Academic Potential	Communication Skills	Living Arrangements	Patterns and Intensity of Support Needs (AAMR)
Mild	85	50-55 to 70	8-9 to <12	Sixth-grade level skills	Almost all have communication skills	Live in community	Intermittent
Moderate	10	35-40 to 50-55	6 to <9	Second-grade level skills	Most have communication skills	Live in supervised community settings	Limited
Severe	3-4	20-25 to 35-40	3 to <6	Preacademic skills	Limited language skills	Live in supervised settings only	Extensive
Profound	1-2	<20 or 25	<3		Few language skills	Live in sheltered settings	Pervasive

AAMR, American Academy of Mental Retardation

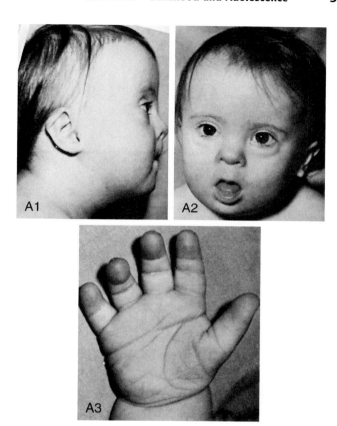

FIGURE 35-1 Fragile X syndrome. *A*, Young infant with a flat face, straight hair, protrusion of tongue, and single crease of inturned fifth finger. (From Smith DW. Recognizable Patterns of Human Malformation, 2nd ed. Philadelphia, WB Saunders, 1976.)

effects affect about 2 per 1000 children in United States, making them the most common cause of *preventable* retardation and developmental delays (Fig. 35-2).

When Is Mental Retardation Apparent?

The more severe types of MR are recognized in infancy and the preschool years because of the child's accompanying medical problems or severe delay in attaining normal developmental milestones, and they tend to require lifelong intervention and support. Milder forms may be revealed as lateness in meeting developmental (particularly language) milestones but may not be diagnosed until the child begins school and academic deficits become evident. Some children with mild MR are able to develop

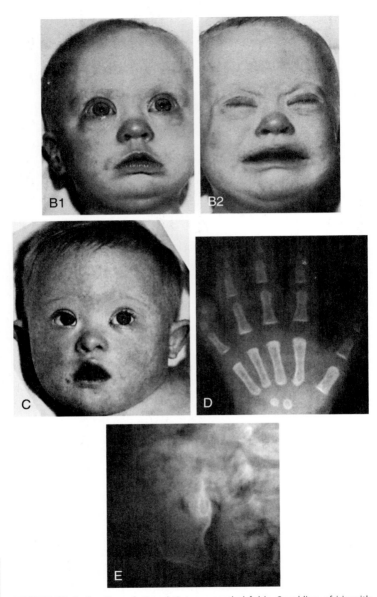

FIGURE 35-1 Continued. *B* and *C,* Inner canthal folds. Speckling of iris with lack of peripheral patterning. Small auricles are prominent at the right. "Pouting" expression is shown when crying. (From Smith DW. Compendium on shortness of stature. J Pediatr 1967;70:463-519.) *D,* Hypoplasia, midphalanx of fifth finger. *E,* Shallow acetabular angle with small iliac wings having the shape of elephant ears. (From Smith DW. Recognizable Patterns of Human Malformation, 2nd ed. Philadelphia, WB Saunders, 1976.)

vocational skills in nonacademic areas and improved adaptive functioning to the extent that they no longer meet the diagnostic criteria for MR as adults.

EVALUATION

How Is Mental Retardation Diagnosed?

The diagnosis of MR is based on the results of intelligence tests and adaptive functioning scales. Although there are no laboratory studies that are diagnostic of MR, further testing may be warranted to rule out accompanying general medical conditions.

Impairments in adaptive functioning are usually the presenting symptoms in individuals with MR and include areas such as self-care, communication, home living, social skills, health, and safety. Clinicians must be alert to the increased risk for physical and sexual abuse of mentally retarded children.

Are Down Syndrome and Mental Retardation the Same Thing?

Down syndrome is one known cause of MR. It occurs in approximately 1 in 1000 live births and is characterized by multiple physical malformations and varying degrees of MR. It is associated with extra genetic material from chromosome 21 (nonfamilial trisomy 21) in 95% of cases; the risk increases with maternal age.

When Is Down syndrome Diagnosed?

Usually at birth, based on associated facial dysmorphic features (epicanthal folds, depressed nasal bridge, Brushfield spots on iris), short stature, simian crease (single transverse palmar crease), congenital heart disease, and duodenal atresia (Fig. 35-3A and B). Children with Down syndrome are at increased risk for hearing and visual impairments, which can adversely affect their development. Down syndrome is associated with accelerated aging; most individuals demonstrate neuropathologic findings consistent with Alzheimer's disease by age 35, although they do not necessarily manifest clinical signs of dementia until ages 40 to 70.

TREATMENT

How Is Mental Retardation Treated?

The goal of treatment is nearly always to manage the cognitive disability rather than to reverse it. Early identification is essential to maximize benefit. In addition, families need to be trained in working with multiple systems (health, education, rehabilitation, and resources to assist them in maintaining their child at home or finding appropriate placement). Psychiatric referrals are usually secondary to behavioral problems or self-injurious behavior. Behavioral management strategies are usually the first type of treatment offered. Psychopharmacology is primarily indicated for treatment of comorbid disorders but has also been used to control aggressive or self-injurious behaviors.

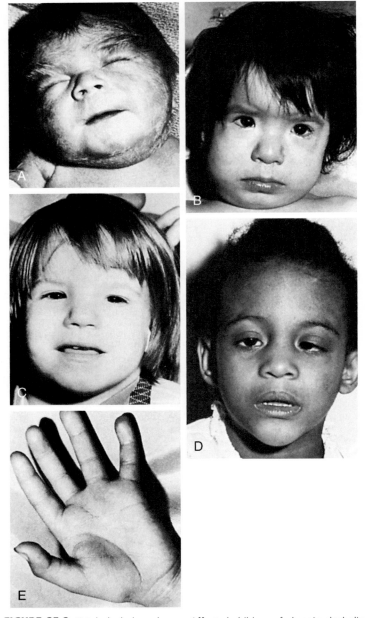

FIGURE 35-2 Fetal alcohol syndrome. Affected children of chronic alcoholic women at birth (*A*), 1 year (*B*), 2½ years (*C*), and 3¾ years (*D*). Note the short palpebral fissures in all children, strabismus (*B*) and (*D*), ptosis of the eyelid (*D*), and facial hirsutism in the newborn (*A*). *E*, The hand shows mildly altered upper palmar crease patterning. (*A* from Jones KL, Smith DW. Recognition of the fetal alcohol syndrome in early infancy. Lancet 1973;2:999-1001; *B* through *E* from Jones KL, Smith DW, Ulleland CN, Streissguth P. Pattern of malformation in off-spring of chronic alcoholic mothers. Lancet 1973;1:1267-1271.)

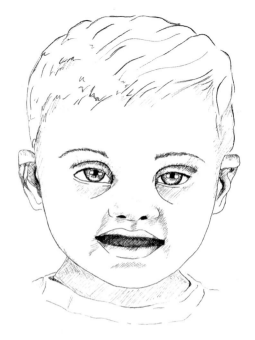

FIGURE 35-3A The typical facial features of Down syndrome.

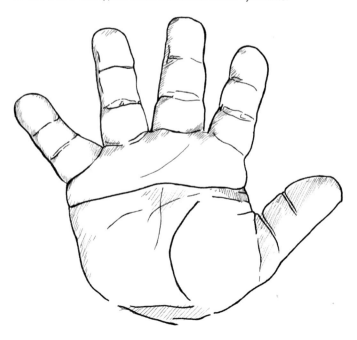

FIGURE 35-3B The transverse palmar crease seen in Down syndrome.

KEY POINTS

Attention Deficit/Hyperactivity Disorder

◆ Symptoms that increase the suspicion of ADHD:

Child appears driven by a motor on constant high gear (cannot sit through a meal or favorite television show)

Child is described as spacey, with peers complaining that he always misses the point

◆ Consider an underlying medical or drug condition as the cause of ADHD symptoms:

If there are physical signs

If you find abnormal laboratory results

If the onset was in a child older than 7 with no prior symptoms

◆ Stimulants are the treatment of choice for ADHD.

KEY POINTS

Oppositional Defiant Disorder

◆ Children with ODD are not just "going through a phase."

◆ Irritability and the reactive nature of oppositionality may become self-maintaining without intervention.

KEY POINTS

Conduct Disorder

◆ A persistent pattern of violating rules and the rights of others, along with the legal repercussions of such behavior, is characteristic of CD but not OD.

◆ Risk taking manifests as early and impulsive sexual behavior, cigarette smoking, and substance abuse.

◆ Suicidal thoughts and attempts are much more common in CD than in normal adolescents and sometimes surpass rates found in depression.

KEY POINTS

Mood Disorders

◆ The essential difference between childhood and adult-onset mood disorders is that in children the mood is more likely to be one of irritability or crankiness than of sadness.

◆ Childhood depressive disorders are generally comorbid with other psychiatric disorders.

KEY POINTS

Separation Anxiety Disorder

◆ Separation anxiety disorder frequently manifests as school phobia. Somatic complaints that prevent school attendance are a warning sign of school phobia.

◆ Separation anxiety disorder in adolescents is frequently accompanied by depression.

KEY POINTS

Pervasive Developmental Disorders

◆ Most cases of autistic disorder are of unknown etiology. The most common specific genetic disorder associated with autistic disorder is fragile X.

◆ Language regression is never insignificant in developing children.

KEY POINTS

Mental Retardation

◆ Mental retardation is defined by limitation in both intelligence and adaptive functioning beginning before age 18.

◆ The vast majority of people with mental retardation live in the community.

◆ Fragile X syndrome is the most common known inherited cause of mental retardation.

◆ Fetal alcohol syndrome is the most common known preventable cause of mental retardation.

Childhood and
Adolescence

Case 35-1

Jimmy is an 8-year-old second grader referred by his teacher because of problems at school. He is described as a wandering spirit, unable to remain in a given spot or activity without becoming interested in something else. He not only loses assignments but also loses his place while engaged in doing his work. Children resent his intrusive interruptions and the need for multiple repetitions of instructions if he is involved in a collaborative task. Jimmy has told his mother that no one likes him at school.

    A. What additional work-up would you want to do?

    B. What treatment, if any, would you recommend?

Case 35-2

Johnny is a 9-year-old boy brought in to the emergency department after losing control in his special education classroom. He bit and kicked his teacher when she held him back from stabbing a peer with a pair of scissors. Johnny is now calm, expresses no remorse, and justifies his actions: "He hit me first and she scratched me when she grabbed me. My mother told me you don't stay hit." His teacher reports that he is the class bully within a class of aggressive children. He is often late and truant, does no homework, and is not progressing academically, but his mother gets upset with the school because "They keep picking on him. He's got to be tough to survive in this neighborhood."

    A. What is the most likely diagnosis?

    B. What treatment, if any, would you recommend?

    C. What other interventions may help?

Case 35-3

Brian is a 2-year-old who is his parents' firstborn child. He was described as a placid baby who hardly cried. It was only toward the end of his first year of life that his mother began to notice his lack of babbling and emotional reactions but was told that boys speak later than girls. He walked on tiptoes and seemed to prefer flicking his fingers in front of his face to playing with toys. He ignored other children, pushing them aside as he might a toy to get to what he wanted. An evaluation was suggested when Brian's parents attempted to place him in daycare.

    A. What additional work-up would you want to do?

    B. What treatment, if any, would you recommend?

    C. What else can you offer his parents?

Childhood and Adolescence

Case Answers

35-1 A. *Learning objective:* **Be familiar with the ways in which ADHD is diagnosed.** Although Jimmy has the cardinal symptoms of inattention, impulsivity, and hyperactivity in the school setting, it is important to assess these symptoms across different domains and to quantify their severity using standardized scales to ensure that they are inconsistent with a child at this developmental level. Comorbid learning disorders need to be assessed before demoralization and poor self-esteem result from Jimmy's perception that he is treated as if he were lazy and not smart.

35-1 B. *Learning objective:* **Be familiar with basic treatment approaches to ADHD.** Psychostimulants will probably help Jimmy with many of his symptoms, but behavioral treatments may be necessary to teach him organizational, learning, and social skills.

35-2 A. *Learning objective:* **Be familiar with the major categories of child and adolescent psychiatric disorders.** The information provided—although incomplete—strongly suggests conduct disorder. Oppositional defiant disorder does not include physical aggression against others.

35-2 B. *Learning objective:* **Treat all comorbid disorders first.** Conduct-disordered children are difficult to treat because many of the adverse psychosocial circumstances surrounding them are not easily amenable to treatment. The best option is to treat underlying comorbidities, allowing the child the opportunity to participate appropriately in social and academic pursuits.

35-2 C. *Learning objective:* **Understand the need to address parent and other environment issues in treating children.** Conduct disorders are not an adaptation to impoverished, high-crime neighborhoods. Johnny's mother may be trying to protect him, but he is headed down a path of academic underachievement, illegal drug use, legal difficulties, physical injuries, poor work adjustment, and volatile interpersonal relationships. His aggression is likely to turn against himself as he ages because conduct disorder confers an increased risk of suicide attempts and completed suicides. The best way to protect him is to work with the school, after-school programs, therapists, and so forth in a multisystem fashion to teach him noncoercive ways of interacting with others.

35-3 A. *Learning objective:* **Understand the importance of developmental levels in assessing young children.** Lack of or delayed speech development warrants evaluation independent of the child's sex. Girls' tendency to speak earlier than boys generally no longer applies if the child is not speaking after 2 years of age. A child who has never babbled by age 1 or who has no words by 18 months warrants a hearing test at the minimum. Assessment of cognitive difficulties (mental retardation is a common cause of language delay) and a full language assessment are indicated.

35-3 B. *Learning objective:* **Know the basic treatment approaches to child disorders.** If the results of initial investigations confirm a diagnosis of autism, Brian should be enrolled in an intensive program using applied behavioral analysis as soon as possible. The child's ability to develop communicative language by age 5 is a significant prognostic factor.

35-3 C. *Learning objective:* **Be aware that treating a child often involves treating the whole family.** Caring for a child with autism places significant stress on a family. Adequate treatment demands the prevention of caretaker burnout through support and respite.

36

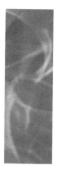

Medication-Induced Movement Disorders

ARTHUR SINKMAN

ETIOLOGY

What Movement Disorders Are Caused by Medication?

Psychotropic medications can cause several different types of movement disorders. These can be conveniently divided into early onset and delayed onset. The early-onset disorders include dystonia, akathisia, Parkinson's disease–like symptoms, and neuroleptic malignant syndrome. The delayed-onset disorders are tardive dyskinesia and tardive dystonia. See Table 36-1.

How Do the Early-Onset Side Effects Present?

The pseudo-Parkinson's side effects mimic the real condition of Parkinson's disease very closely. The classic symptoms of that condition are bradykinesia (slowness and difficulty initiating movements), rigidity, a pill-rolling resting tremor (three to five cycles per second), and postural instability including stooped posture and slow walking.

Dystonic reactions are muscle spasms that most commonly involve the head and neck but may affect any voluntary muscle. A dystonic spasm is painful and often disabling. It is often an acute problem and a medical emergency.

Akathisia is a subjective experience of restlessness that makes the patient feel compelled to pace or move. It is felt to be unpleasant. It is easily confused with anxiety and mistaken for a worsening of the patient's psychiatric illness. It is accompanied by restlessness and movement such as rocking from foot to foot while standing.

These side effects are referred to as extrapyramidal symptoms, often abbreviated as EPSs. (They lie outside the voluntary motor pathways that involve the pyramidal tracts at the back of the spinal cord.)

What about Neuroleptic Malignant Syndrome?

Neuroleptic malignant syndrome (NMS) is a serious and acute condition that can be life threatening. It is the most serious of the EPSs listed previously. It presents with severe rigidity. Other cardinal features include mental

381

Table 36-1

Main Medication-Induced Movement Disorders

Disorder	Characteristics	Treatment
Early Onset		
Parkinson's disease–like syndrome	Rigidity, pill-rolling tremor, slow movements	Anticholinergics
Dystonia	Muscle spasm, especially of head and neck	Anticholinergics
Akathisia	Subjective restlessness, inability to sit still	β-Blockers
Neuroleptic malignant syndrome	Rigidity, fever, confusion, vital sign changes	Stop neuroleptic, supportive measures, dantrolene, bromocriptine
Late Onset		
Tardive dyskinesia	Chewing, lip smacking, tongue thrusting, hands and feet moving	Early detection and stop medication, clozapine

confusion, fever, and unstable vital signs (pulse and blood pressure). NMS is caused by antipsychotic medication. It occurs shortly after a new medication has been started or after the dose of an existing medication has been increased. It is exceedingly unlikely to occur when a person has been taking stable doses of the same medication for a long time.

What Medications Are Involved?

For the group of EPSs, antipsychotic drugs are the prime offenders, but selective serotonin reuptake inhibitor (SSRI) and serotonin and norepinephrine reuptake inhibitor (SNRI) antidepressants can also cause some of these symptoms, particularly akathisia. Lithium frequently causes a tremor. The greatest risk is with high-potency typical antipsychotics such as haloperidol and fluphenazine. The atypical antipsychotics are much less likely to cause movement disorders but the risk is still present. Of the atypicals, risperidone has the highest risk for EPS (with aripiprazole posing a risk for akathisia). Similarly, the greatest risk for NMS is with high-potency typical drugs. NMS from low-potency typicals and from atypical antipsychotics is much less common but still possible.

How Common Are Antipsychotic-Induced EPSs?

Approximately 10% to 15% of patients treated with typical antipsychotics experience one of the acute EPSs. Fortunately, NMS is relatively rare.

What Do the Late-Onset Movement Disorders Look Like?

The late-onset or tardive dyskinetic movements are involuntary and rapid ticlike (choreiform) movements that usually involve the tongue, lips, face, and neck. That said, it must be noted that they frequently occur in other parts of the body, particularly the extremities, but also involving the muscles controlling breathing and body posture. The form of the movements is also quite variable with athetoid (slower writhing movements) and dystonic components occurring as well. Lip pursing, eye blinking, frowning, and tongue darting are common movements. Tardive dyskinesia (TD) is caused by long-term exposure to antipsychotic medication. As with other EPSs, it is less likely to occur with atypical antipsychotics.

Are the Acute EPSs and TD Caused by the Same Mechanism?

No. The acute EPSs are caused by the direct blockade of dopamine D2 receptors in the nigrostriatal system. (Antipsychotics are dopamine antagonists.) The cause of TD has not been definitely established but a likely mechanism is hypersensitivity of these dopamine receptors brought on by prolonged blockade. Because the cause of each is different, the treatment is also different.

How Common Is Tardive Dyskinesia?

It's common. With typical antipsychotics the annual risk for new-onset TD is about 5% each year during the first few years. The risk is cumulative; the longer the patient takes medication, the more likely it is to develop. The overall incidence is 15% to 25%, possibly higher. With atypicals it is much lower—about one fifth to one tenth the incidence seen with typical agents. Although TD usually occurs after several years of treatment, on occasion it can occur after just a few months, particularly in older patients.

What Are the Risk Factors for Developing Tardive Dyskinesia?

In addition to length of time on medication, age is an important risk factor. Old people taking antipsychotics are at much higher risk. There are other risk factors, summarized in Table 36-2.

Table 36-2

Risk Factors for the Development of Tardive Dyskinesia

Length of time on medication
Higher dose of medication
Greater cumulative dose
Advanced age
Female sex
Depression
Brain damage

EVALUATION

How Can I Tell if My Patient's Abnormal Movements Are Caused by Medication?

You can tell by the type of movement and their temporal relationship to the use of medication. If the movements look like one of the typical patterns and began soon after the medication was introduced, you can presume that they are medication related. This presumption is strengthened if the movements resolve when the medication is stopped.

How Can I Diagnose Neuroleptic Malignant Syndrome?

You should have a high index of suspicion for any patient taking antipsychotic medication who develops fever and rigidity. The temperature may be as high as 40 °C and is typically sustained (nonfluctuating.) The rigidity of NMS can be so extreme that it is difficult to flex or extend the patient's limbs passively. On mental status examination, the patient will show impairment ranging from lethargy and mild confusion to obtundation or coma. In addition, there is instability of the autonomic nervous system with changes in blood pressure and pulse, sweating, and pallor. Sustained muscle contraction causes damage to the muscle tissue and a significant elevation in creatinine phosphokinase (CPK) levels, often greater than 1000. Muscle breakdown products can get into the urine, causing myoglobinuria and eventual signs of impaired renal functioning. Leukocytosis can occur.

How Can I Detect Tardive Dyskinesia Early?

It is important to examine your patient regularly for the development of dyskinetic movements. It is a must to do so *before* you start prescribing an antipsychotic. This includes the atypical drugs even though they pose a lower danger of TD. The examination should be repeated at regular intervals. The Abnormal Involuntary Movement Scale (AIMS) is a structured guideline for observing and rating the severity of the movements. A copy of the scale is provided in Table 36-3. It is useful to practice doing the AIMS in order to be better able to identify TD movements. Movements are evaluated in seven different areas of the body: face, lips, jaw, tongue, trunk, upper extremities, and lower extremities. In addition, it is helpful to observe the patient's respiratory movements. TD movements in the feet and legs can be easily confused with the restlessness from akathisia.

Do I Really Still Need to Be Concerned about These Movement Disorders? Typical Antipsychotics Don't Seem to Be Used Very Much

Yes, you do. There are several reasons. First, typicals are still very much in use and their use has been increasing. Recent research has confirmed their effectiveness and equivalence to the newer atypical antipsychotics. In addition, the atypicals do cause EPSs, although much less often than the older antipsychotics. Finally, movement disorders can be caused by medications other than antipsychotics. Antidepressants can cause akathisia.

Table 36-3

Abnormal Involuntary Movement Scale (AIMS) Examination Procedure

Either before or after completing the examination procedure, observe the patient unobtrusively at rest (e.g., in the waiting room). The chair should be hard and firm without arms.

The patient should be rated on a scale of 0 (none), 1 (minimal), 2 (mild), 3 (moderate), or 4 (severe) according to the severity of symptoms.

Ask the patient whether there is anything in his or her mouth (e.g., candy), and if so to remove it.

Ask the patient about the current condition of his or her teeth. Ask whether the patient wears dentures. Do the teeth or dentures bother the patient?

Ask the patient whether he or she notices any movement in the mouth, face, hands, or feet. If yes, ask the patient to describe it and to what extent it bothers the patient or interferes with activities.

0 1 2 3 4	Have the patient sit in the chair with hands on knees, knees slightly apart, and feet flat on the floor. (Look at body for movements while in this position.)
0 1 2 3 4	Ask the patient to sit with the hands hanging unsupported—if the patient is wearing slacks, hands should be between the legs; if the patient is wearing a skirt, hands should be hanging over the knees. (Observe the hands and other body areas.)
0 1 2 3 4	Ask the patient to open the mouth. (Observe the tongue at rest within mouth.) Do this twice.
0 1 2 3 4	Ask the patient to protrude the tongue. (Observe abnormalities of tongue movement.) Do this twice.
0 1 2 3 4	Ask the patient to tap the thumb with each finger as rapidly as possible for 10 to 15 seconds; this should be performed first with the right hand, then with the left hand. (Observe facial and leg movements.)
0 1 2 3 4	Flex and extend the patient's left and right arms (one at a time).
0 1 2 3 4	Ask the patient to stand up. (Observe in profile. Observe all body areas again, hips included.)
0 1 2 3 4	*Ask the patient to extend both arms outstretched in front with palms down. (Observe trunk, legs, and mouth.)
0 1 2 3 4	*Have the patient walk a few paces, turn, and walk back to chair. (Observe hands and gait.) Do this twice.

*Activated movements.

TREATMENT

Are Treatments Available for the Medication-Induced Movement Disorders?

Yes. For the acute EPSs adequate treatment is available. It varies depending on the specific presentation. For Parkinson-like symptoms and dystonia, anticholinergic medication is effective. Acute treatment of dystonia often requires intramuscular injection. The oral route is too slow and also impractical because the muscle spasms may cause difficulty swallowing. Benztropine 2 mg or diphenhydramine 50 mg given intramuscularly usually suffices. Of course, discontinuing the offending medication is usually required. Not so with the Parkinson-like symptoms. The antipsychotic can be continued along with maintenance oral anticholinergics, such as benztropine 1 mg twice a day. Akathisia is best treated with β-adrenergic blocking agents such as propranolol 10 to 40 mg twice a day. For patients who cannot take such a medication, such as bronchial asthma sufferers, anticholinergics are used.

Should I Give My Patient an Anticholinergic Drug When I First Start an Antipsychotic?

Although starting an anticholinergic medication simultaneously with an antipsychotic minimizes the risk of EPS, it also exposes all patients to the anticholinergic effects of the additional drug, whereas only 10% to 15% will benefit from its positive effects. Therefore, it is general practice to withhold anticholinergics until there is a demonstrated need for them. The decision should also be based on your knowledge of the individual patient and the likelihood of his stopping medication or dropping out of treatment if EPSs do occur.

Are Treatments Available for Tardive Dyskinesia?

The only effective treatment is early detection and stopping the medication. There is a significant rate of improvement when the medication is stopped, but for some there is no improvement. Various treatment measures have been tried but without consistent or significant success. Clozapine has shown some promise. Choosing an atypical over a typical agent and prescribing the lowest possible dose are helpful preventive measures.

Do We Have a Duty to Warn the Patient Ahead of Time about This Possible Untreatable Side Effect?

It's complicated. Antipsychotics are used to treat people with severe illnesses that are often long term and chronic. In such patients, the danger of developing TD is real. Therefore, the patient should be informed of the risks and benefits of the treatment in order to give informed consent or to refuse treatment. In an acute setting in the emergency room or on a hospital unit, obtaining consent is neither practical nor reasonable as the patient is too ill and the treatment may be short term. Also, the patient is probably not in a mental state in which she could give informed consent. It becomes more of an issue when the patient is stable and being treated as an outpatient. However, even at those times obtaining informed consent can be a difficult issue as the patient may remain psychotic and impaired in his judgment. With typical antipsychotics this issue is more pressing than it is with atypicals, with which the frequency of TD is less.

What Should I Do if My Patient Begins to Show TD Movements?

You have several options. Stopping medication is preferable, but for many patients with recurrent psychotic disorders such as schizophrenia it is not feasible. It may be possible to lower the dose of the medication and still maintain good therapeutic control. Alternatively, you may want to switch medications to a drug less likely to cause TD, such as an atypical antipsychotic. Treatment with clozapine is an option. You will need to counsel your patient that if she stops or decreases the medication, the movements may become worse before they get better. Increasing the dose of the original medication may momentarily reduce the movements, but it is a bad choice because it perpetuates the underlying process and will make the TD worse in the long run.

What Can I Do if My Patient Develops Neuroleptic Malignant Syndrome?

You must immediately stop the antipsychotic medication, even if the symptoms of NMS are mild. It is often necessary to transfer the patient to a medical service or intensive care unit where he can receive the necessary medical care such as intravenous fluids, external cooling, and supportive maintenance of vital signs. Treatment includes a dopamine agonist, bromocriptine 2.5 mg by mouth three times a day, and a muscle relaxant, dantrolene 25 to 100 mg by mouth three times a day.

KEY POINTS

◆ The risk for acute EPS is greater with typical than with atypical antipsychotics.

◆ The abnormal movements of tardive dyskinesia can become irreversible; early detection is essential.

◆ EPSs are a common cause of noncompliance with antipsychotic medication; they are usually treatable.

Case 36-1

A 23-year-old unemployed man is brought to a local emergency department for evaluation. He was found pacing the halls at the residence where he has lived for the last 6 months. Three weeks earlier, he was brought in under similar circumstances. At that time he was evaluated and thought to have an acute exacerbation of his chronic psychotic disorder. He denied auditory or visual hallucinations, but he appeared to be agitated, pacing the hallways, even when being evaluated in the emergency department. His regular dose of haloperidol was increased from 15 to 25 mg every night. On examination he appears restless, constantly moving his legs up and down and refusing to sit still longer

Medication-Induced Movement

than a minute or two. His thoughts are logical and goal directed. There are no hallucinations or evidence of delusional thinking.

A. How can his current situation and response to the first intervention be explained?

B. What treatment plan is appropriate now?

Case Answers

36-1 A. *Learning objective:* **Recognize various presentations of medication-induced movement disorders.** The likelihood that an akathisia was not recognized when the patient first presented with symptoms becomes more obvious when the intervention of increasing his antipsychotic dose does not improve his condition.

36-1 B. *Learning objective:* **Be familiar with strategies for treating antipsychotic medication–induced movement disorders.** In this case, the possibility of adding a medication to treat the akathisia needs to be weighed against the strategy of changing the antipsychotic. The addition of propranolol is an effective treatment for akathisia in most patients. Alternatively, his dose of haloperidol could be decreased or another medication such as an atypical antipsychotic substituted.

37

Topics in Women's Mental Health

NATALIE GLUCK

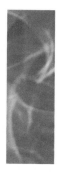

INTRODUCTION

Why Do Women Warrant Special Consideration in Psychiatry?

Several reasons. First, women as a group utilize health services, including mental health care, at much higher rates than men. Second, there are significant gender differences in the prevalence, phenomenology, and treatment response to various psychiatric disorders including depression, schizophrenia, anxiety, and eating disorders. Finally, the reproductive life cycle of a woman can be associated with a unique subset of psychiatric disorders, including premenstrual dysphoric disorder, pregnancy-induced mood disorders, postpartum disorders, and emotional changes related to menopause. The issue of treatment in pregnancy is of particular importance in psychiatry because of the complexities related to psychotropic medication use in pregnant women.

What Are the Gender Differences in Psychiatric Disorders?

There are significant differences between men and women in vulnerability, presentation, and treatment response in various disorders. For example, the lifetime prevalence of depression among women is double that of men. Further, women with depression tend to have a younger age of onset, are more likely to have a family history of mood disorders, and suffer from a more "atypical" type of depression characterized by hypersomnia and increased appetite. Although the rates of schizophrenia are equal among men and women, women tend to present at later ages, have fewer negative symptoms of schizophrenia than men, and are more responsive to treatment. Bipolar disorder is also equally diagnosed between the genders; however, women are more susceptible to rapid mood cycling. Finally, eating disorders afflict women at 10 times the rate of men.

389

What Biopsychosocial Factors Contribute to Psychiatric Disorders in Women?

Some of the biologic, psychological, and social factors that are unique to or predominately affect women are listed in Table 37-1.

PREMENSTRUAL DYSPHORIC DISORDER

ETIOLOGY

What Is Premenstrual Dysphoric Disorder?

Categorized as a "mood disorder not otherwise specified" and area for further research in the DSM-IV, premenstrual dysphoric disorder (PMDD) is a disturbance of mood associated with both emotional and physical symptoms that cause a marked impairment in school, occupational, or social functioning.

How Is PMDD Different from Premenstrual Syndrome?

Premenstrual syndrome, or PMS, is a mild syndrome experienced by up to 80% of women. It is usually associated with mostly physical symptoms and possibly some emotional changes as well. The key difference is that none of the symptoms of PMS are severe enough to interfere with a woman's functioning, as is the case with PMDD. Only about 5% to 15% of women endorse symptoms that meet criteria for PMDD.

What Is the Etiology of This Disorder?

The etiology of PMDD is not entirely understood. Research in this area has demonstrated that fluctuations in gonadal hormones, including

---

Table 37-1

Psychiatric Illnesses in Women: Clinically Significant Factors

Biologic Factors
Autoimmune diseases: increased prevalence among women; many have psychiatric
    manifestations (e.g., lupus, fibromyalgia, thyroid disease)
Sexually transmitted diseases that affect sexual functioning
Premenstrual dysphoric disorder and other menstrual cycle irregularities
Pregnancy (normal hormonal changes of pregnancy, postpartum disorders)

Psychological Factors
Increased lifetime risk of depression, anxiety, and eating disorders

Sociologic Factors
Increased vulnerability to domestic and sexual violence
Financial hardship: women tend to make lower wages and often head single-parent
    homes
Childrearing pressures, balancing dual roles of motherhood with career

luteinizing hormone, follicle-stimulating hormone, estrogen, and progesterone, all have psychoactive effects that can increase vulnerability to emotional disturbances. Estrogen in particular has been shown to affect neurotransmitters involved in the regulation of mood, behavior, and cognition. There is increasing evidence of a genetic component to PMDD, which suggests that certain women may be predisposed to the disorder, perhaps because of a hypersensitivity to hormonal changes in the brain.

EVALUATION

What Clues in the History Confirm the Diagnosis of PMDD?

To establish the diagnosis of PMDD, symptoms must be present during the late luteal phase (within the 7 days prior to menses) and remit 1 to 2 days after the onset of menstruation. Patients are asked to record symptoms prospectively over two menstrual cycles to confirm a cyclic pattern consistent with PMDD. A minimum of five symptoms must be present to meet criteria for the disorder. The common symptoms of PMDD are listed in Table 37-2.

Are There Physical Examination or Laboratory Findings Associated with PMDD?

There are no specific laboratory or examination findings that are needed to confirm the diagnosis of PMDD. However, obtaining a medical history and routine laboratory tests is important for ruling out other disorders such as thyroid abnormalities, endometriosis, or fibrocystic breast disease.

TREATMENT

How Do You Treat PMDD?

Mild PMDD can usually be managed with nonpharmacologic interventions such as psychoeducation and supportive psychotherapy. Oral contraceptive

Table 37-2
Premenstrual Dysphoric Disorder Common Symptoms
Depressed mood, feelings of hopelessness or self-deprecating thoughts
Decreased interest in unusual activities
Anxiety, feeling "keyed up" or on edge
Marked irritability or affective instability
Interpersonal conflicts
Lethargy/fatigue
Concentration difficulties
Changes in appetite or specific food cravings
Marked hypersomnia or insomnia
Subjective sense of feeling overwhelmed or out of control
Physical symptoms, e.g., bloating, breast tenderness, joint and muscle pains

pills can also be helpful, particularly if the patient suffers from predominately physical symptoms of PMDD. For more moderate to severe symptoms, the treatment of choice for PMDD is a selective serotonin reuptake inhibitor (SSRI), which is taken continuously throughout the menstrual cycle. Additional agents can be used to target specific symptoms of PMDD, such as alprazolam for anxiety or spironolactone for bloating and weight gain.

DISORDERS OF PREGNANCY

ETIOLOGY

What Are the Psychiatric Effects of Pregnancy?

Pregnancy was once thought to be relatively protective against psychiatric disorders such as depression or anxiety. However, the current understanding of psychiatric illness in pregnancy is that women do experience symptoms during pregnancy and that patients with premorbid illness tend to have worse outcomes if left untreated. Recent studies have demonstrated that pregnant women who suffer from untreated depression or anxiety have an increased rate of perinatal complications such as preeclampsia, preterm delivery, and low birth weight. Further, women with psychiatric symptoms in pregnancy are at a significant risk of suffering from postpartum disorders such as depression or psychosis, discussed in the following.

EVALUATION

How Do I Evaluate a Woman for Psychiatric Disorders in Pregnancy?

First, when treating any woman of reproductive age it is important to be aware of her potential to become pregnant. Any evaluation of such a patient should include questions regarding sexual activity, use of contraception, and future plans of conceiving. Important factors to consider for pregnancy consultation and planning include the patient's past psychiatric history; current use of medication; any drug, nicotine, or alcohol use; past reproductive history; and any history of postpartum depression or psychosis.

TREATMENT

How Do I Approach Treatment in Pregnancy?

Treatment decisions are optimally made before a patient becomes pregnant and should include nonpharmacologic alternatives, such as supportive psychotherapy, as well as medications. In determining which medication to use, you must weigh its potential benefits against the risk of teratogenicity or perinatal effects on the fetus, or both. It is equally important to explain the risks associated with not treating, as psychiatric symptoms in pregnancy increase the likelihood of noncompliance with prenatal care, of perinatal complications, and of a postpartum exacerbation of the underlying disorder.

What Medications Can Be Used during Pregnancy?

The use of psychotropic medication in pregnancy is complicated and still a subject of much research and debate among clinicians. Some psychotropic medications, such as lithium and valproic acid, are associated with a known risk of congenital defects, whereas for some of the newer medications such as olanzapine and aripiprazole there are limited data regarding use in pregnancy. One class of medication that has been extensively studied over the past two decades is the SSRIs. Although there is no evidence of teratogenicity with the SSRIs, there is a slight risk of perinatal "withdrawal" effects on the baby, which are usually transient and rarely, if ever, serious. Table 37-3 lists the potential teratogenic and perinatal complications of commonly used psychiatric medications.

What about Electroconvulsive Therapy?

Electroconvulsive therapy (ECT) is the "gold standard" for the treatment of depression in pregnancy. In practice it is used less frequently, partly because of the misconceptions about its safety and efficacy. However, there are no known adverse effects of ECT on either the fetus or the mother, and it is considered to be the safest option among all biologic interventions.

POSTPARTUM DISORDERS

ETIOLOGY

Are the "Maternity Blues" and Postpartum Depression the Same Thing?

No. Maternity or postpartum blues are the mildest of all postpartum syndromes and differ from postpartum depression in severity and time course. Postpartum blues are common, transient, and rarely require medical treatment. Postpartum depression is a psychiatric illness characterized by symptoms consistent with a severe major depression and almost always requires pharmacologic treatment.

How Common Are These Disorders?

Up to 85% of women experience the postpartum blues, but only 10% of women experience postpartum depression.

What Causes Postpartum Depression?

It is unclear why some women develop postpartum depression, but certain risk factors significantly increase a patient's risk for this disorder. These include a history of depression or a previous postpartum depression,

Table 37-3

Psychotropic Medications in Pregnancy: Effects of In Utero Exposure of Commonly Used Medications

Medication	Teratogenicity	Perinatal Effects
Lithium	Slightly increased risk of cardiac malformation, most commonly Ebstein's anomaly	Hypotonia, feeding difficulties, cyanosis, hypoglycemia, neonatal goiter, and diabetes insipidus have been reported
Valproic acid	Significant risk of neural tube defects with first-trimester exposure. Also risk of developmental delay, craniofacial defects, cardiovascular and urinary abnormalities, and fingernail hypoplasia	Hypoglycemia and hepatic dysfunction have been reported
Carbamazepine	Similar to valproic acid in risk of neural tube defects and other nonspecific congenital abnormalities	Hypoglycemia, hepatic dysfunction, and bleeding disorders have been reported
Typical antispychotics, high potency	No known congenital abnormalities	Transient perinatal symptoms of motor restlessness, tremor, hypotonia, hyperreflexia, irritability, and poor feeding
Low-potency antipsychotics	May increase risk of nonspecific congenital anomalies	Transient perinatal symptoms of motor restlessness, tremor, hypotonia, hyperreflexia, irritability, and poor feeding
Atypical antipsychotics	No data available	No data available
Selective serotonin reuptake inhibitors	No evidence of congenital abnormalities	Slight risk of perinatal complications, all of which are transient. These include jitteriness, tachypnea, respiratory distress, poor tone, lower Apgar scores
Bupropion	Preliminary data suggest an increased risk of spontaneous abortion	No data available
Benzodiazepines	Small risk of oral cleft defects	Transient perinatal toxicity that includes lethargy, hypothermia, and hypotonia may occur with regular use

depressive symptoms during pregnancy, marital discord, and poor social supports.

What Causes Postpartum Psychosis?

Postpartum psychosis can occur as a complication of postpartum depression or mania or can be a postpartum exacerbation of a chronic psychotic disorder. Risk factors include a history of bipolar disorder, a history of recurrent major depression, and any previous postpartum psychotic episodes. Women without any prior psychiatric history can experience a postpartum psychosis as well, although this is less frequent and may represent an unmasking of an underlying psychotic or mood disorder.

How Common Is Postpartum Psychosis?

Postpartum psychosis occurs 1 to 2 times per 1000 births.

EVALUATION

What Are the Major Symptoms of Postpartum Blues and Postpartum Depression?

Both postpartum blues and depression can be characterized by tearfulness, mood lability, irritability, and anxiety. However, postpartum depression tends to be marked by a persistently depressed mood, often associated with guilt, anxiety, fear of harm to the baby, or obsessional thoughts. Less frequently the depression is associated with psychotic symptoms, suicidality, or thoughts of infanticide.

What Is the Time Course for Postpartum Blues and for Postpartum Depression?

The blues usually appear within 2 to 4 days after birth and have fully remitted within the first 2 weeks after delivery. Postpartum depression tends to have a later onset of 2 to 4 weeks following delivery and persists for at least 2 weeks.

Are There Other Psychiatric Disorders with Postpartum Onset to Look out For?

Yes, less commonly women can present with a postpartum onset of an anxiety disorder such as obsessive-compulsive disorder (OCD) or panic disorder. Patients with bipolar disorder are at risk for developing a postpartum mania with psychotic features as well as postpartum depression.

TREATMENT

How Do I Approach a Patient with Postpartum Depressive Symptoms?

First, understand that the perinatal period is one marked by dramatic hormonal shifts that may contribute to excessive tearfulness or stress. That

Table 37-4

Postpartum Depression and Psychosis: Treatment Options

Disorder	Treatment Options
Postpartum blues	Psychoeducation
	Supportive therapy (individual, group)
Postpartum depression	Psychotherapy (individual, group)
	Social supports (e.g., family involvement, extra child care)
	Pharmacotherapy (SSRIs, atypical antidepressants)
	Consider hospitalization for suicidality, obsessional thoughts about harming the infant, or lack of social supports
	ECT for severe or refractory symptoms
Postpartum psychosis	Hospitalization warranted in most cases
	Antidepressants
	Antipsychotics
	Mood stabilizers for manic symptoms or if there is a history of bipolarity
	Anxiolytics
	ECT

ECT, electroconvulsive therapy; SSRI, selective serotonin reuptake inhibitor.

said, symptoms that do not recede after 2 to 4 days may signal a major depression. Postpartum depression is often worrisome as it can have the major impact of negative parenting behaviors and neglect of the child as well as self-neglect of the patient. A warm, nonjudgmental approach may help to encourage the patient to be forthcoming about her mood and feelings, particularly if they include negative thoughts toward her baby. Assessing for any psychotic symptoms is also important as they occur in up to 10% of patients with postpartum depression.

What Are the Treatment Options for Patients with Postpartum Depression and Psychosis?

The choice of treatment depends upon the severity of illness and the particular symptoms with which the patient is presenting. For example, a postpartum depression with severe melancholic or psychotic features may warrant hospitalization or ECT, or both. Treatment options are outlined in Table 37-4.

PSYCHIATRIC ISSUES IN MENOPAUSE

ETIOLOGY

When Do Menopause and Perimenopause Occur?

Menopause is the point in a woman's life at which ovulation has ceased and she permanently stops menstruating. Natural menopause usually occurs between the ages of 44 and 55. Perimenopause is the time of transition between regular ovulatory menstrual cycles and complete cessation of ovarian function. This typically occurs 5 to 7 years before menopause.

What Are the Major Physical Changes Associated with Menopause?

During perimenopause a woman's menstrual cycle becomes increasingly irregular, which is usually the first sign of decline in ovarian function and fertility. This process can be associated with physical changes including vasomotor symptoms (hot and cold flashes), sleep disturbance secondary to the vasomotor effects, dizziness, lightheadedness, decreased sexual functioning (urogenital atrophy, dyspareunia), and fatigue.

What Effect Does Menopause Have on Mood?

Despite the common perception of menopause as a time of emotional turbulence, long-term studies have not shown that menopause increases a woman's risk for depression. There is, however, an increased vulnerability to depression during perimenopause, the transitional period marked by major hormonal and physical changes. Certain physical symptoms, such as hot or cold flashes and sleep disturbance, are specifically linked to worsening mood symptoms. Other risk factors for depression in perimenopause include a prior history of depression, history of PMS or PMDD, and poor physical health. The major risk factors for depression in menopause and perimenopause are summarized in Table 37-5.

EVALUATION

How Do I Approach a Middle-Aged Woman with Depression?

When a woman presents with depression in middle age, it is important to review her psychiatric history to establish whether this is a first episode or part of a chronic mood disorder such as recurrent major

Table 37-5
Risk Factors for Depression in Menopause
History of depression, including postpartum depression and premenstrual dysphoric disorder
Sleep disturbances
Presence of hot flashes
Death of, divorce from, or separation from a partner
Chronic medical problems
Lower level of education
Unemployment
Financial hardship

depression or bipolar disorder. Any evaluation of a woman in this age group, particularly if this is a new-onset depression, should include an assessment of menstrual cycle patterns, presence of hot flashes, and other physical changes. The nature of the patient's symptoms is important because some physical symptoms of perimenopause such as sleep disturbances and sexual problems overlap with symptoms of major depression. A careful medical history is also necessary to rule out any organic etiology for mood changes, such as autoimmune or endocrine disorders. Finally, an inquiry into psychosocial stressors is essential, as major life changes such as the death of or separation from a loved one can contribute to a major depression in this population.

What Physical Examination and Laboratory Findings Are Helpful?

A patient who presents with menstrual irregularities along with mood symptoms should be referred for a gynecologic evaluation as she may be experiencing dysfunctional uterine bleeding rather than normal menopause. Important laboratory tests include an assessment of thyroid function, given the increased risk of thyroid disease in this age group, complete blood count, metabolic profile, and, if indicated, an evaluation of follicle-stimulating hormone and estradiol levels.

TREATMENT

What Are the Treatment Options for Depression in Peri/Postmenopausal Women?

The approach to treatment of depression associated with menopause is similar to that of any other major depression and includes psychotherapy or antidepressant medication, or both. Interestingly, studies of depression in menopause have shown that SSRIs and serotonergic noradrenergic reuptake inhibitors (SNRIs) such as venlafaxine are effective both for controlling depressive symptoms and for reducing hot flashes. Other options for treatment include individual psychotherapy and group therapy. A support group that focuses on issues unique to middle-aged women, such as loss of fertility, role transitions, or coping with medical problems, can be especially useful.

What about Hormone Replacement Therapy?

Hormone replacement therapy remains an issue of major controversy. Whereas short-term hormone therapy is effective for controlling the physical symptoms of menopause such as hot flashes and urogenital atrophy, long-term use is associated with an increased risk of breast cancer and cardiac disease. The efficacy of hormone replacement therapy for depression has not yet been established, although preliminary studies suggest that it may be a helpful short-term treatment for depressive symptoms associated with menopause.

KEY POINTS

- There are significant sex differences in prevalence, age of onset, symptom profile, and treatment responsiveness of most major psychiatric disorders.

- Women suffer from depressive disorders at twice the rate of men.

- Premenstrual dysphoric disorder is a real syndrome marked by premenstrual onset of depressive or anxiety symptoms, or both, that cause a marked impairment in functioning.

- Postpartum depression is usually severe and can be accompanied by psychotic symptoms. Common risk factors include a history of depression or previous postpartum depressive episodes, marital discord, and poor social supports.

- Perimenopause is associated with an increased vulnerability to depression.

Case 37-1

A 31-year-old woman with a history of major depression presents to your office 5 weeks after the birth of her first child with a chief complaint of "I don't deserve to be a mother." She reports that over the past 2 weeks she has experienced frequent crying episodes, low mood, insomnia, feelings of hopelessness, and excessive guilt. Upon further questioning, the patient admits that she has also been distressed by recurrent, intrusive thoughts about harming her baby. The patient has a psychiatric history significant for three previous depressive episodes that were responsive to sertraline; however, she discontinued the medication during the first month of her pregnancy.

    A. What is your initial diagnostic impression?
    B. What additional information do you need?
    C. What treatment do you recommend?

Case Answers

37-1 A. *Learning objective:* **Recognize the clinical features of a postpartum depression.** The hallmark of a postpartum depression is an onset within 4 weeks of delivery, with symptoms that persist for at least 2 weeks. This patient endorses at least five major depressive symptoms, along with intrusive thoughts of harming the infant, a phenomenon that is not uncommon among women with severe postpartum depression. The patient's history of recurrent major depression and the discontinuation of treatment during pregnancy are both significant risk factors in the development of a postpartum depression.

37-1 B.   *Learning objective:* **Appreciate the importance of asking about psychotic symptoms in women with postpartum depression.** Psychotic symptoms are present in approximately 10% of cases of postpartum depression. With this patient it is important to assess for psychotic symptoms and ask about any auditory hallucinations, paranoia, or delusions. It is particularly important to investigate her experience of obsessive thoughts about harming the baby. Is there a voice commanding her to harm the baby, or are the intrusive thoughts more typical of an OCD-like picture? Further, one must ask about any thoughts of self-harm or suicidality. The clinician should also consider other etiologies for her symptoms, including illicit drug use or an organic etiology.

37-1 C.   *Learning objective:* **Understand the approach to treatment of postpartum depression.** First, one must assess all of the patient's symptoms to determine medication management. The first-line medication for postpartum depression is generally an SSRI or atypical antidepressant, such as venlafaxine or bupropion. It is helpful to take a thorough psychiatric history so that you can select a medication that has been previously effective for that patient. In this case, we know that the patient has responded well to sertraline in the past, and it is a logical choice. Additional medications can be used to target other psychiatric symptoms, specifically an antipsychotic for psychotic symptoms or obsessionality, a benzodiazepine for anxiety, a sedative-hypnotic for insomnia. It is equally important to explore the patient's psychosocial supports and potential stressors; that is, does she have any help with child care? One might also explore the option of helping her to find a support group for new mothers. Finally, individual psychotherapy can be invaluable in helping the patient to cope with the major life transition of motherhood.

Practice Examination

MYRL R. S. MANLEY AND NATALIE GLUCK

The following 50 questions cover topics in clinical psychiatry including diagnosis, management, and treatment. They are written in the style and format of and with the approximate level of difficulty of questions on step 2 of the United States Medical Licensing Examination (USMLE) and the subject examination in psychiatry—often referred to as the "shelf" examination—prepared by the National Board of Medical Examiners. The psychiatry subject examination is commonly used as an end of clerkship examination. It consists of 100 questions, and students are allowed 2 hours and 10 minutes to complete it. Working through these questions will help you assess how prepared you are. If you are working at the pace necessary for completing the subject examination, you should be able to answer all 50 questions in under 1 hour and 5 minutes. It is helpful to keep the following points in mind:

1. The vocabulary, organization, and criteria of DMS-IV-TR are used throughout.
2. Only generic names of medications are used.
3. All signs and symptoms should be accepted as accurate. You need not, and should not, second-guess patients' self-report. (In real life, patients often say they are moderate drinkers when in fact they drink very heavily. In answering these questions, if a patient says he is a moderate drinker, that is what you should accept.)
4. Pay close attention to the chronological sequence of events; it may provide important diagnostic clues.
5. See Table 1 on page 426 for a list of normal laboratory values. You can refer to this as you are working through the examination.

1. A 19-year-old college student is brought to the college emergency department by his roommate because of bizarre behavior over the past 3 days. He has refused to come out of his room or answer the telephone or emails. He has not bathed for 3 days and appears distracted and frightened. Four months earlier he stopped attending classes and began to see friends less often, preferring to stay in his room by himself. Physical examination reveals a blood pressure of 125/75 and a heart rate of 65. Pupils are 2 mm and deep tendon reflexes are diffusely normal. Mental status examination reveals blunted emotional expression. He describes hearing several voices making threatening and derogatory comments. He believes that someone is stalking him and trying to kill him. He is oriented to

person, place, and time. He recalls three out of three objects after 5 minutes. Which of the following is the most likely diagnosis?

A. delusional disorder
B. paranoid personality disorder
C. psychotic disorder due to a general medical condition
D. schizophrenia
E. substance-induced psychotic disorder
F. schizophreniform disorder

2. A 56-year-old man comes to his internist for an annual medical examination. He describes increasing fatigue over the past month. He has been having trouble sleeping through the night, frequently waking at 4 or 5 in the morning and being unable to return to sleep. His appetite is low and he has lost 10 pounds over the last 4 weeks. He has continued to work as an insurance underwriter but is worried about doing a poor job because his concentration is poor. He denies feeling depressed but adds that he just doesn't seem to enjoy anything anymore. He drinks a glass of wine with most evening meals. He does not use other drugs or medications. Physical examination reveals no abnormalities. On mental status examination he appears tired and distracted. There are no visual or auditory hallucinations. He is oriented to person, place, and time. He has difficulty with serial 7 subtractions and remembers one out of three objects after 5 minutes. Which of the following is the most likely diagnosis?

A. breathing-related sleep disorder
B. chronic fatigue syndrome
C. dementia, Alzheimer's type
D. dysthymia
E. major depressive disorder
F. primary insomnia
G. substance-induced mood disorder

3. A 25-year-old woman is brought to an emergency department after she made several cuts into her thighs with a paring knife. The woman denies any intention to kill herself and says that cutting relieves anxiety. She and her boyfriend had been fighting after he told her he was going out of town for a week on a business trip. She shouted at him and began crying and then went into her bedroom, where she cut herself. She has been to the emergency department four times in the last year following similar episodes. Her boyfriend describes her as unpredictable and emotional, warm and affectionate at times but enraged at others. She smokes marijuana two or three times a week and drinks one or two glasses of wine with dinner. She has used cocaine on three occasions in the past but has had none for 6 months. Physical examination reveals four recent cuts 1/2 cm deep on each thigh. There are scars of old cuts on both legs and on her

left arm. Pupils are normal and reactive. Deep tendon reflexes are not increased. She appears angry and refuses to answer most questions. There are no visual or auditory hallucinations. She is alert and oriented to person, place, and time. Which of the following is the most appropriate long-term treatment recommendation?

A. cognitive therapy

B. diazepam therapy

C. dialectical behavioral therapy

D. disulfiram therapy

E. family therapy

F. quetiapine therapy

4. A 60-year-old man is brought to an emergency department by police from a bus station, where he was shouting and lunging at people. He is unable to give a coherent history. On physical examination, his blood pressure is 150/100, heart rate is 95 beats per minute, and respirations are 20 per minute. His temperature is 39°C. He is diaphoretic and tremulous. Deep tendon reflexes are increased. Pupils are dilated; his neck is supple. He is dysarthric. He acknowledges both auditory and visual hallucinations and he states that someone wants to kill him. He is oriented to person but not to place or time. He is unable to perform serial 7s or to remember three objects after 5 minutes. Laboratory studies show the following:

Sodium	140
Potassium	4.5
AST	50
GGTP	150
Urine toxicology	negative

Which of the following is the most appropriate next step in management?

A. amoxicillin therapy

B. chest radiograph

C. chlordiazepoxide therapy

D. haloperidol therapy

E. head CT scan

F. physical restraints

G. seclusion

5. A 17-year-old high school senior is referred by the school guidance counselor to his family physician after the boy fell asleep in class three times in 1 week. He tells his doctor that he has no trouble falling asleep at night. He wakes once to urinate and readily falls back to sleep. There has been no recent change in the usual duration of his total sleep time of 9 hours. He describes being suddenly overwhelmed by sleepiness during the day, whether during the week or on the weekend. Frequently he is unable to move any part of

his body for about 30 seconds when he wakes up in the morning. He typically sees colored shapes and figures as he is falling asleep at night. He does not drink alcohol and he uses no illicit drugs. His medical history is benign and he is not currently taking any medications. Physical examination reveals no abnormalities. He is 5 feet 9 inches tall and weighs 150 pounds. BMI is 22.1. There are no visual or auditory hallucinations. He is alert and oriented to person, place, and time. Concentration and memory are unimpaired. Which of the following investigations is the most likely to confirm the diagnosis?

A. electroencephalography (EEG)

B. head CT scan

C. Halstead-Reitan neuropsychological test battery

D. multiple sleep latency test

E. urine toxicology screen

6. A 35-year-old man comes to his family doctor for help with a sexual problem. During sexual intercourse he frequently experiences orgasm with intromission or very shortly after. He has experienced this difficulty off and on all of his adult life, but it has become more pronounced during the last 2 months coinciding with a new relationship. He does not have difficulty in delaying ejaculation when masturbating. The man has no significant medical history. He drinks one or two beers each evening and smokes a cigar once or twice a week. He does not use any illicit drugs. Physical examination is within normal limits. He is alert and oriented. Memory and concentration are unimpaired. Which of the following is the most appropriate medication recommendation?

A. atomoxetine

B. diazepam

C. diphenhydramine

D. paroxetine

E. oxcarbazepine

F. sildenafil

7. A 30-year-old woman comes to her family doctor for treatment of excessive daytime somnolence for the past month. She describes being tired all the time, frequently missing work, and sleeping 10 to 12 hours at night instead of her usual 7. She also reports a 5-pound weight gain, and she describes her mood as being very low with crying spells once or twice on most days. She has had thoughts of suicide, but she denies intent or plans. She experienced a similar episode 5 years ago. She received no treatment at the time, and all symptoms resolved after 4 months. She also describes several episodes over the years of increased energy and a need to sleep only 4 to 5 hours each night. During these periods her mind is particularly quick and she is able to accomplish a great deal. Her work and social

life have not been adversely affected during the periods of heightened energy, which typically last 4 to 6 weeks. Physical examination is within normal limits. She appears tired. She frequently becomes teary-eyed during the interview. There are no auditory or visual hallucinations. Which of the following is the most appropriate treatment recommendation?

A. clozapine therapy

B. cognitive-behavioral therapy

C. continuous positive airway pressure (CPAP) assistance

D. fluoxetine therapy

E. lamotrigine therapy

F. methylphenidate therapy

G. modafinil therapy

8. A 40-year-old man is referred to the company physician by his supervisor because of bizarre behavior over the past 3 months. For the past month he has been writing and rewriting reports four or five times. His productivity has decreased because of his checking and rechecking the results. In addition, when driving home he sometimes becomes worried that he may have struck a pedestrian despite the absence of any unusual sounds or movements. He will circle the block three times to look for evidence of an accident before driving on. His blood pressure is 135/85, heart rate 75, and temperature 37°C. He appears mildly anxious and distracted. He describes his mood as worried. His thoughts are organized and goal directed. He is oriented to person, place, and time. A medication affecting which of the following neurotransmitters is the most likely to be therapeutic?

A. acetylcholine

B. gamma-aminobutyric acid (GABA)

C. glutamate

D. norepinephrine

E. serotonin

9. A 25-year-old man is admitted to a hospital following a 2-day period of increasingly disorganized behavior, auditory hallucinations, and the belief that a microchip had been implanted in his brain to control his thoughts. He is treated with haloperidol. On the third day of medication he becomes withdrawn and uncommunicative. By the fourth day he is awake but nonresponsive. Over the course of the day he becomes obtunded. His body is diffusely rigid and it is difficult to flex or extend his arms and legs. His temperature is 40°C. His blood pressure is 150/95 and his heart rate is 90. Laboratory testing reveals the following:

leukocyte count	14,000
creatine kinase	1200
urinalysis	myoglobin

Which of the following is the most appropriate next step in management?

A. continue the haloperidol and add trihexyphenidyl

B. decrease the dose of haloperidol and add benztropine

C. discontinue the haloperidol and add dantrolene

D. discontinue the haloperidol and add quetiapine

E. discontinue the haloperidol and observe

F. increase the dose of haloperidol

10. A 45-year-old woman consults her internist because of increasing depression over the last 4 weeks. She had worked as a computer programmer for a nationally recognized company for 10 years. Two months ago she was informed that her job was being transferred overseas. She describes constant low mood, frequent crying spells, and preoccupation with her personal shortcomings. She has found it difficult to fall asleep and to stay asleep through the night. Over the past 3 weeks she has been drinking a half bottle of wine every night to help her get to sleep. She has very little appetite for food and describes a 10-pound weight loss over the last month. She acknowledges frequent thoughts of death but denies any plans or intention for suicide. She has no previous psychiatric history. She is 5 feet 7 inches tall and weighs 120 pounds. Her BMI is 18.8. She appears tired and is frequently tearful throughout the interview. She denies auditory or visual hallucinations. Her thinking is organized and goal directed. Which of the following is the most likely diagnosis?

A. adjustment disorder with depressed mood

B. bereavement

C. dysthymia

D. major depressive disorder

E. mood disorder due to a general medical condition

F. substance-induced mood disorder

11. A 45-year-old woman is referred to her employee health service because of increasingly bizarre behavior over the past 2 months. She has become more secretive, refusing to participate in meetings and refusing to let her supervisor review her work. She missed 5 days of work during the last month with no medical justification. This morning she was caught attempting to install a listening device on a coworker's telephone. The woman explains that the owner of the company, whom she has never met, is trying to get her fired. She believes this is because he is secretly in love with her and is afraid that her continued presence will jeopardize his marriage and his career. The woman's supervisor reports that the company is expanding and, far from laying people off, is actually planning to enlarge the work force. She denies any sleep or appetite changes. She does not take prescription medications or use any illicit drugs. On mental status examination she appears guarded. She denies auditory or visual

hallucinations. Her thinking is logical and goal directed. She is alert and oriented to person, place, and time. Which of the following is the most likely diagnosis?

A. bipolar disorder

B. borderline personality disorder

C. delusional disorder

D. narcissistic personality disorder

E. paranoid personality disorder

F. schizophrenia

12. A 22-year-old woman comes by herself to the emergency department complaining of flu-like symptoms for the past 12 hours. She complains of diffuse muscle aches and pains, arthralgias, and malaise. She appears restless and agitated. Her blood pressure is 140/95, heart rate is 95, and respirations are 20. Her pupils are dilated, and her eyes and nose are running. Muscle fasciculations are observed over both legs. She yawns frequently throughout the interview. She denies visual or auditory hallucinations. She is alert and oriented to person, place, and time. A urine toxicology screen is negative. Which of the following is the most likely diagnosis?

A. alcohol intoxication

B. alcohol withdrawal

C. amphetamine intoxication

D. amphetamine withdrawal

E. opiate intoxication

F. opiate withdrawal

G. phencyclidine intoxication

H. phencyclidine withdrawal

13. A 19-year-old college freshman comes to her family doctor asking for diet pills. For the past 6 months she reports difficulty controlling her appetite. Two to three times a week she eats much larger amounts than normal. Yesterday she ate an entire chocolate cake, a large bag of potato chips, a loaf of bread, and a pint of ice cream at one sitting. She says that sometimes when she starts eating she can't stop herself and finishes only when she runs out of food. Recently her grades have begun to suffer. She denies self-induced vomiting or use of laxatives. She periodically fasts in order to avoid weight gain. There has been no recent change in her menstrual cycle. She is 5 feet, 6 inches tall and weighs 130 pounds. Her BMI is 21. Her hair is thick and full. She denies suicidal plans but states that she is so disgusted with herself, it would serve her right to be struck by a truck. Which of the following is the most likely diagnosis?

A. anorexia nervosa

B. bipolar disorder

C. bulimia nervosa

D. dysthymia

E. morbid obesity

F. normal adolescence: no diagnosis

14. A 23-year-old man comes to his internist asking for something to help him stay awake. He has always been a heavy sleeper, typically sleeping 12 hours at night and occasionally napping an additional hour in the afternoon. He has no difficulty falling asleep, and if he wakes at night to urinate, he has no difficulty falling back to sleep. When he wakes in the morning he feels alert and refreshed. During high school and college he was able to work around his sleep schedule and still get good grades. One month ago he started law school, and he now finds he cannot keep up with the work unless he sleeps less. For the past 2 weeks he has been forcing himself to wake up after only 8 hours of sleep. He then feels tired, irritable, and has trouble concentrating. He has never noticed any difference in his sleep pattern on weekends or holidays. He is 6 feet tall and weighs 165 pounds. BMI is 22.4. He drinks one or two glasses of wine each week but does not use illicit drugs. Which of the following is the most appropriate treatment recommendation?

A. atomoxetine therapy

B. behavioral therapy

C. continuous positive airway pressure therapy

D. lorazepam therapy

E. modafinil therapy

F. psychodynamic psychotherapy

G. zolpidem therapy

15. A 45-year-old woman consults her family physician because of long-standing stage fright. The woman is a professional opera singer and has enjoyed a successful career singing mostly small roles in regional companies. A year ago she was hired to sing in a major, internationally famous opera house. Her performances are scheduled to begin in a week. She has always suffered stage fright and experiences sweaty palms and shortness of breath just before a performance begins. Once she starts singing, her anxiety subsides. She is worried that with the importance of the upcoming opera she will not be able to control her nervousness. She is concerned that her voice will crack and that her hands will shake so badly she will drop a prop. A medication targeting which of the following receptors is most appropriate?

A. α-adrenergic

B. β-adrenergic

C. D_2

D. 5-HT_2

E. muscarinic cholinergic

16. A 50-year-old man is brought to an emergency department by his wife after she found him attempting to hang himself in their garage.

He describes increasing despondency over the past 2 weeks, feeling that his life has been a failure. He has had difficulty sleeping through the night, often waking at 4 or 5 a.m. and not being able to fall back asleep. He has no appetite, and he feels so tired most days that he has not been able to go into work. He experiences frequent crying spells. One month ago he began hearing a voice commenting on his actions. He initially dismissed this as the result of overwork, but the voice continued and increased in frequency and loudness. He continued going to work, hoping to distract himself. Two weeks after the voice first occurred, his mood began to worsen. He has had two similar episodes in the past, each requiring hospitalization. He smokes a pack of cigarettes every day and drinks a glass of scotch most nights. His blood pressure is 150/90, heart rate 80, and respirations 15. On mental status examination he appears tearful and downcast. He states that he is disappointed that his suicide attempt was interrupted. He acknowledges hearing a voice talking about him, but he refuses to divulge the content. His thoughts are frequently disrupted and non–goal directed. He is alert and oriented to person, place, and time. Which of the following is the most likely diagnosis?

A. adjustment disorder with depressed mood

B. major depressive disorder

C. mood disorder due to a general medical condition

D. schizoaffective disorder

E. schizophrenia

F. substance-induced mood disorder

17. A 56-year-old woman comes to her doctor for a scheduled follow-up appointment to manage her depression. For the past 6 months she has experienced hopelessness, daily crying spells, fatigue, impaired concentration, and difficulty sleeping through the night. Her appetite is low and she has lost 15 pounds during this period. For the past month she has been taking bupropion without significant benefit and she now complains of worsening insomnia. She has had previous trials of fluoxetine, paroxetine, venlafaxine, and mirtazapine, but in each case the medication either was ineffective or caused intolerable side effects. She does not take any other prescription or illicit drugs. She does not use alcohol. She reports that for the last week she has heard the voice of her deceased father calling her to join him. She is 5 feet, 6 inches tall and weighs 115 pound; BMI is 18.6. Her blood pressure is 115/20, heart rate is 76. She appears tired and lethargic. She is tearful throughout the examination. She reports hearing the voice of her father. She denies suicidal plans but says that she is tired and can't continue living this way. She is oriented to person, place, and time. Laboratory testing is within normal limits. Which of the following is the most appropriate treatment recommendation?

A. continue bupropion therapy

B. cognitive-behavioral therapy

C. discontinue bupropion and begin olanzapine therapy

D. discontinue bupropion and begin sertraline therapy

E. electroconvulsive therapy (ECT)

F. psychodynamic psychotherapy

18. A 45-year-old woman consults her physician because of difficulty controlling her thoughts for the past 4 weeks. The woman is a criminal defense attorney working in a high-profile case of a corporate executive. She reports increasing difficulty concentrating, and she experiences frequent intrusive thoughts about shouting something obscene in the middle of court proceedings. She is embarrassed by such thoughts. She has discovered that she can control them to some extent by writing complex series of digits on the pad in front of her, but she feels the trial has reached a critical juncture and she can no longer afford to give less than full attention. She has had difficulty falling asleep but is generally able to stay asleep. There has been no change in sleep or appetite. She experienced similar symptoms during law school but didn't tell anyone, and they resolved on their own after several months. She drinks three to four glasses of wine each week. She is not taking any prescription medications. Physical examination is within normal limits. Her speech is loud and slightly pressured. She denies auditory or visual hallucinations. Thoughts are logical and goal directed. Which of the following is the most likely diagnosis?

A. adjustment disorder with anxiety

B. bipolar disorder

C. borderline personality disorder

D. obsessive-compulsive disorder

E. schizotypal personality disorder

F. substance-induced anxiety disorder

19. A 70-year-old woman is brought by police to an emergency department because of bizarre and uncooperative behavior. She was found living on an unused track in a train station. When questioned by police, she did not give any meaningful information. She carried no identification and was found with an empty wine bottle. On physical examination she is malodorous and unkempt. Blood pressure is 145/90 and heart rate is 72. Temperature is 37°C. Deep tendon reflexes are symmetrical and within normal limits. On mental status examination she appears cheerful and cooperative. She laughs occasionally. Her speech is articulate and moderate in volume. Her answers to questions are nonsensical and include multiple ideas, none of which is clearly related to another. She denies auditory or visual hallucinations. She can read a printed sentence accurately. She responds accurately to simple one-step commands. She recalls two out of three objects after 5 minutes. Laboratory testing reveals the following:

red blood cell count	4.5
leukocyte count	7000
AST	60
ALT	45
GGTP	65

Which of the following is the most likely diagnosis?

A. alcohol withdrawal delirium

B. dementia, Alzheimer's type

C. cardiovascular accident

D. schizophrenia

E. substance-induced amnestic disorder

F. substance-induced mood disorder

20. A 22-year-old woman is brought to an emergency department by her husband because of a sudden paralysis of her right hand 2 hours earlier. She had been chopping vegetables in the kitchen when her husband received a phone call. She was suspicious because he spoke on the phone in a low voice. She questioned him after he hung up, and he acknowledged that he was having an affair with one of the woman's friends. She screamed at him and started crying. Almost at once she noticed that she was unable to move her right hand. The woman has no prior medical or psychiatric history. She smokes marijuana once or twice a week and drinks a glass of wine with most evening meals. On physical examination, the muscle tone of her right hand appears normal. She does not feel or respond to light touch or pinprick from her wrist to the tips of all fingers on her right hand. On mental status examination she appears relaxed and cooperative. She is not tearful, but she does express contempt for her husband. Her speech is logical and goal directed. She denies auditory or visual hallucinations. Which of the following is the most likely diagnosis?

A. adjustment disorder with disturbance of conduct

B. brief psychotic episode

C. conversion disorder

D. hypochondriasis

E. somatization disorder

F. substance-induced mood disorder

21. A 25-year-old woman consults her internist because of not feeling right for the last 3 weeks. She reports a persistent sense of not being real and of observing herself from the outside as if in a movie. She finds these distorted perceptions unpleasant and distracting. She has not experienced similar feelings in the past. The woman works as a graphic designer and has been finding it increasingly difficult to concentrate at work. She reports no change in sleep and appetite.

She drinks one or two beers most evenings. She has smoked marijuana in the past but denies any use for the previous 6 months. There is no other significant psychiatric or medical history. Her physical examination is within normal limits. On mental status testing she appears mildly distracted and describes her mood as fair. Thoughts are logical and goal directed. She denies auditory or visual hallucinations. She is alert and oriented to person, place, and time. She performs serial 7 subtractions with difficulty. Which of the following is the most likely diagnosis?

A. avoidant personality disorder

B. depersonalization disorder

C. generalized anxiety disorder

D. major depressive disorder

E. paranoid personality disorder

F. post-traumatic stress disorder

G. schizoid personality disorder

H. schizophrenia

I. substance-induced anxiety disorder

22. A 7-year-old boy is referred by his school for a medical evaluation because he is disruptive in class. His teacher describes him as stubborn, defiant, quarrelsome, and having a short attention span. His mother states that at home he never keeps still for any length of time but is always running, jumping, rocking, or fiddling with something. He is extremely intrusive and disrupts any activity in which others are attempting to engage. During the evaluation the boy spends most of his time walking around the pediatrician's office or tilting a chair, leaning on its back, and rocking back and forth. He acknowledges having some trouble in school but feels it is because the other children pick on him. He is at the 40th percentile for height and weight. His vocabulary is appropriate for his age. Which of the following is the most likely diagnosis?

A. anxiety disorder of childhood

B. attention deficit/hyperactivity disorder

C. conduct disorder

D. mild mental retardation

E. oppositional defiant disorder

23. A 40-year-old woman with the diagnosis of chronic undifferentiated schizophrenia is hospitalized after a 2-week period of auditory hallucinations and disorganized behavior. She has been hospitalized 15 times in the past 20 years, usually for relapse of symptoms because of medication noncompliance. She is treated with olanzapine. Ten days later all symptoms have resolved. She is seen in the outpatient clinic for monthly follow-up visits. By the sixth month she has gained 40 pounds and is complaining of feeling overly sedated. Her vital signs are within normal limits. Mental status examination reveals logical and goal-directed

speech. There are no auditory or visual hallucinations. Laboratory tests reveal the following:

Glucose	165
Cholesterol	250
AST	35
ALT	50

Which of the following is the most appropriate next step in management?

A. continue olanzapine, add perphenazine

B. continue olanzapine, add topiramate

C. discontinue olanzapine, begin clozapine

D. discontinue olanzapine, begin perphenazine

E. discontinue olanzapine, observe off medication

F. increase the dose of olanzapine

24. A 35-year-old woman comes to her obstetrician for prenatal follow-up. She is 10 weeks pregnant after repeated attempts at in vitro fertilization. She has a history of bipolar disorder and has been hospitalized twice following serious suicide attempts. She had been taking lithium for several years but discontinued when she began fertility treatments. The woman now reports that she has not slept for the last three nights. Her speech is rapid and difficult to follow. She is experiencing auditory hallucinations, which she describes as God's instructions to her. She believes that the baby she is carrying was conceived through immaculate conception. She is alert, oriented, and does not appear tired. Which of the following is the most appropriate next step in treatment?

A. begin carbamazepine therapy

B. begin cognitive-behavioral therapy

C. begin diazepam therapy

D. begin electroconvulsive therapy (ECT)

E. begin lithium therapy

F. begin prenatal couple's counseling

G. begin valproic acid therapy

25. A 30-year-old woman consults her gynecologist for difficulty with sexual intercourse for the past 3 months. The woman is a lawyer who gave birth to her second child 6 months ago. Pregnancy, labor, and delivery were all uncomplicated. She returned to work 3 months after the baby was born. She now reports that although her desire for sex is normal, she is unable to have intercourse because the vaginal walls tighten to such an extent that penetration is not possible. She is able to achieve orgasm with manual stimulation. She has never before experienced similar difficulties. She denies pain or abnormal menstrual bleeding. Which of the following is the most likely diagnosis?

A. adjustment disorder

B. conversion disorder

C. dyspareunia

D. sexual arousal disorder

E. sexual orgasmic disorder

F. vaginismus

26. A 25-year-old man comes to an emergency department complaining of agitation for 24 hours. Two days ago he came to the emergency department with the complaint of auditory hallucinations for 4 days. The man was treated with haloperidol and was given a short supply with instructions to return to the crisis clinic the next morning. He did not keep the clinic appointment but continued to take the haloperidol as prescribed. He now describes feeling as if he is jumping out of his skin. He is unable to sit still for any length of time, but he has been able to sleep at night. On examination he is pacing back and forth in the room. When he sits in a chair, he jiggles his legs up and down. When asked, he can hold still only for several seconds before the urge to move overwhelms him. His gait is normal and he does not have a tremor. Deep tendon reflexes are diffusely normal. He appears distressed and states "I can't stand this." His thoughts are logical and goal directed. There are no auditory or visual hallucinations. A medication with which of the following actions is most appropriate?

A. block acetylcholine receptors

B. block β-adrenergic receptors

C. block dopamine D_2 receptors

D. block GABA receptors

E. block presynaptic norepinephrine reuptake

F. block presynaptic serotonin reuptake

G. block serotonin 5-HT_2 receptors

27. A 10-year-old boy is referred for evaluation on the advice of his teacher because of changes in his behavior over the past month. The boy has been getting into fights on the playground, teasing other children, and writing swear words on the blackboard. He had previously been a quiet, well-liked boy who was a good and attentive student. His parents report increasing arguments at home over bedtime and television privileges. Two months ago his mother accepted a new position that requires extensive travel. She is now away from home 3 to 4 days a week. The boy suffers from seasonal allergies and has mild asthma requiring the occasional use of a metaproterenol inhaler. He is in the 40th percentile for height and weight for boys his age. Physical examination is unremarkable. On mental status examination he describes feeling "OK." Speech is mostly monosyllabic. He appears restless and uncomfortable and avoids eye contact. He denies visual and auditory hallucinations. Which of the following is the most likely diagnosis?

A. adjustment disorder with disturbance of conduct

B. attention deficit/hyperactivity disorder

C. conduct disorder

D. dysthymia

E. mood disorder due to a general medical condition

F. oppositional defiant disorder

G. substance-induced mood disorder

28. A 69-year-old man is brought to an emergency department by emergency medical services after he was found unresponsive in the front seat of his car with the car engine running and the garage door locked. His home health aid had come by on her day off and found him. She reports that he was recently diagnosed with lung cancer. Although she has never seen him intoxicated, she suspects he is a heavy drinker because of the number of empty liquor bottles she finds. The man's wife died 2 years ago following a stroke. He has not had previous psychiatric counseling or treatment. He has never made a suicide attempt before. By the time he arrives in the emergency department he is fully awake and demands to be released. His blood pressure is 135/85, heart rate is 75, and temperature is 37.1°C. He describes his mood as excellent and insists that he was trying to repair his car engine and not take his life. He smiles frequently throughout the interview. He is alert and oriented to person, place, and time. Which of the following is the most appropriate next step in management?

A. admit to a locked psychiatric inpatient unit

B. admit to a medical intensive care unit

C. begin amitriptyline therapy

D. begin lithium therapy

E. begin quetiapine therapy

F. discharge to the care of the home health aid

G. schedule a follow-up appointment in the outpatient clinic

29. A 20-year-old man comes to his internist because of increasing anxiety and insomnia over the past 6 months. He experiences difficulty both in falling asleep and in maintaining sleep, and he has frequent nightmares that recall a private airplane accident 2 years earlier which he survived but in which two companions were killed. During the day he is tense, moody, and irritable. He is easily startled by loud noises, particularly by engines, which cause him to break out in a cold sweat. He has trouble concentrating, and he recently dropped out of college because of his inability to keep his mind on his studies. His physical examination is unremarkable. He describes his mood as "tired and frustrated." He can remember two out of three objects at 5 minutes. Which of the following is the most likely diagnosis?

A. acute stress disorder

B. dysthymia

C. generalized anxiety disorder

D. major depressive disorder

E. panic disorder

F. posttraumatic stress disorder

G. primary insomnia

30. A 3-year-old girl is brought by her father to the pediatrician on the recommendation of her day care teacher because of bizarre behavior since starting day care 2 months ago. The girl never plays with other children and seems oblivious to the presence of other people. Each day she follows a fixed routine, walking to a corner where she sits cross-legged playing with a toy bear. She moves the bear's eyelid up and down but has not been observed engaging in imaginative play. Her father reports that the girl never seemed to like being held when she was younger. She walked at 1 year of age and began to speak single words at 34 months of age. She now speaks simple two-word sentences, usually repeating what someone says to her. She does not initiate conversations or use words to ask for what she wants. She sleeps through the night. Which of the following is the most likely diagnosis?

A. Asperger's disorder

B. autistic disorder

C. Down syndrome

D. expressive language disorder

E. major depressive disorder

F. oppositional defiant disorder

G. schizophrenia

H. stereotypic movement disorder

31. A 15-year-old boy comes to his family physician asking if it is possible to have a face transplant. He has suffered mild facial acne since age 13, which has responded well to treatment. He believes that he will never be able to find a girlfriend and will not be accepted by any college because of his acne. He is receiving mostly B grades in classes; grades have been consistent over the last several years. He dated one girl for 2 months and then ended the relationship 6 months ago by mutual agreement. He has never been sexually active. He does not drink alcohol or use illicit drugs. He has no previous psychiatric history. There are small, scattered, mostly healed acne lesions on his forehead. The rest of the physical examination is within normal limits. He describes his mood as depressed. The range of affect is full and appropriate. He denies auditory or visual hallucinations. He is oriented to person, place, and time. Which of the following is the most likely diagnosis?

A. adjustment disorder with mixed features

B. body dysmorphic disorder

C. delusional disorder

D. hypochondriasis

E. major depressive disorder

F. social anxiety disorder

G. somatization disorder

32. A 45-year-old man comes to a physician for the first time for medical evaluation for insurance purposes. He denies any current physical or emotional symptoms. He has lived alone for the past 20 years and works the overnight shift at a data processing company. He has no friends and says that he enjoys his own company. He has never had romantic relationships or been sexually active. He sleeps 7 hours each night; his weight has been stable for 10 years. He enjoys reading and watching television in his spare time. He drinks one or two glasses of wine before going to bed. Two months ago his supervisor gave him a performance evaluation of only "fair." He states that he has no intention of changing the way he works and that he doesn't particularly care what anyone else thinks of him. He describes his mood as fine. His affect is variable and appropriate. His thoughts are logical and goal directed. He denies auditory or visual hallucinations. He is oriented to person, place, and time. Which of the following is the most likely diagnosis?

A. antisocial personality disorder

B. avoidant personality disorder

C. dysthymia

D. schizoid personality disorder

E. schizophrenia

F. social anxiety disorder

33. A 35-year-old man comes to his doctor for help with a sexual problem for the last 2 months. Six months ago the man was married to a woman he has known for 4 years. During the last 2 months he has ejaculated within seconds after intromission. Although this had happened occasionally in the past, it now occurs with every attempt with sexual intercourse. It does not happen with masturbation. He has no difficulty achieving an erection. He has no partners other than his wife. He states that his wife is understanding but that he is frustrated. He drinks one or two beers a week. He is taking no prescription medications. His sleep and appetite have not changed over the last 2 years. His blood pressure is 130/80, heart rate is 76. His physical examination is within normal limits. Blood tests for complete blood count and comprehensive metabolic studies reveal no abnormalities. Which of the following is the most appropriate treatment recommendation?

A. alprazolam therapy

B. cognitive-behavioral therapy

C. dialectical behavioral psychotherapy

D. psychodynamic psychotherapy

E. sildenafil therapy

F. supportive psychotherapy

G. testosterone therapy

34. A 40-year-old woman is admitted to an inpatient service for detoxification from methadone, which she has been buying on the street and abusing for 5 years. On the third day of admission she complains of diffuse muscle aches and pains. On physical examination her blood pressure is 150/95, heart rate 90, and temperature 37°C. Her eyes and nose are running and fasciculations are observed in both legs. She appears restless and she describes herself as being distressed and anxious. In addition to lorazepam, which of the following medications is most appropriate?

   A. amitriptyline
   B. clonidine
   C. fluoxetine
   D. phenelzine
   E. naltrexone
   F. risperidone
   G. venlafaxine

35. A 35-year-old man comes to his doctor for help in overcoming a life-long fear of dogs. If he encounters a dog on the sidewalk he feels anxious, short of breath, and lightheaded. Consequently, he goes out of his way to avoid chance encounters. He will not walk down blocks on which he has seen dogs in the past, and he will not shop in malls that house pet stores. He feels no anxiety or discomfort when he is away from dogs. His sleep and appetite are undisturbed. For the past 6 months his 8-year-old twin daughters have been asking for a puppy. Physical examination is unremarkable. On mental status examination he is friendly and affable. He describes his mood as good. There are no auditory or visual hallucinations, and he is oriented to person, place, and time. Which of the following is the most appropriate treatment recommendation?

   A. behavioral therapy
   B. buspirone therapy
   C. carbamazepine therapy
   D. group psychotherapy
   E. olanzapine therapy
   F. paroxetine therapy
   G. psychodynamic psychotherapy
   H. supportive psychotherapy

36. A 30-year-old man comes to his family doctor accompanied by his wife, who insisted that he be evaluated because of unusual behavior since their marriage 6 months ago. He is always on the go, never finishing one thing before beginning another. When they watch TV he controls the remote and will switch from channel to channel every 30 seconds or so. He has antagonized friends because he seems always to interrupt people in midsentence. When they have dinner, he is usually on his cell phone and often gets up from the

table to pace. The man says he has always been energetic and prides himself on being a quick thinker. He has received several tickets for driving too fast but has not otherwise been in trouble with the law. He denies any recent changes in appetite and says he sleeps 7 to 8 hours most nights. He drinks one to two glasses of wine with his evening meal and smokes marijuana once every 2 months. He has no previous psychiatric history. His medical history is significant for minor injuries sustained in several accidents over the past 5 years. Physical examination is unremarkable. He is friendly and outgoing. Speech is normal in rate and volume but he frequently interrupts the doctor. He describes his mood as good and appears euthymic. He has difficulty spelling "world" backward and in completing serial 7 subtractions. Laboratory studies show the following:

AST	20
ALT	35
GGTP	20
BUN	15
Creatinine	0.8
TSH	1.2

Which of the following is the most appropriate treatment recommendation?

A. alprazolam

B. atomoxetine

C. clonidine

D. disulfiram

E. lithium carbonate

F. risperidone

G. valproic acid

For each patient with sleep disturbance, select the most likely diagnosis.

A. bipolar disorder

B. circadian rhythm sleep disorder

C. generalized anxiety disorder

D. major depressive disorder

E. parasomnia

F. primary insomnia

G. sleep disorder due to a general medical condition

H. substance-induced sleep disorder

37. A 45-year-old man comes to his internist asking for medication to help him sleep. He reports irregular sleep over many years but increasing difficulty over the last 6 months. It takes 1 or 2 hours for him to fall asleep and he frequently wakes during the night. During the day he is irritable and fatigues easily. The man works as a real estate agent and has found it increasingly difficult to keep up with paper work. He describes constant worry that sales will slow and that

his income will decrease. He is concerned that he will not be able to maintain mortgage payments on his house and that he is not setting enough money aside for retirement and for his daughter's college education. The worries are with him most of the time and interfere with his ability to enjoy usual pastimes such as watching a movie. He drinks one or two glasses of wine with his evening meal but does not use illicit drugs or take prescription medications. Physical examination reveals a blood pressure of 145/90 and a heart rate of 80.

38. A 55-year-old woman comes to her company doctor for an annual insurance medical evaluation. She denies any recent change in her health but reports difficulty falling asleep over the past 2 years. She does not feel tired until late in the evening and finds it difficult to fall asleep before 1 or 2 a.m. She wakes at 6:30 a.m. in order to get to work on time but feels tired during the day. After her noon meal she finds it difficult to stay awake. She will nap for 45 minutes in the afternoon when her work schedule permits. One weekends and during vacations she usually sleeps from 3 a.m. to noon the next day and feels fully refreshed and energetic when she wakes up. She tried zolpidem to help her fall asleep earlier but found that it did not work or that she woke up after 2 hours and was unable to fall back asleep. She does not take any other medications or drink alcohol. Physical examination is within normal limits.

For each patient with pain, select the most likely diagnosis.

    A. body dysmorphic disorder
    B. delusional disorder
    C. generalized anxiety disorder
    D. hypochondriasis
    E. major depressive disorder
    F. opioid withdrawal
    G. phencyclidine intoxication
    H. primary insomnia
    I. somatization disorder
    J. somatoform pain disorder

39. A 60-year-old man comes to his doctor complaining of a 1-month period of diffuse aches and pains that vary in location and intensity. He has tried taking some old hydrocodone but he experienced inconsistent and short-lived benefit. He has not used any hydrocodone for 10 days. He describes difficulty falling asleep and staying asleep. His appetite has decreased and he has lost 10 pounds over the last month. One year ago his wife died of breast cancer. He lives alone; his grown son lives several hundred miles away. Although he is an avid golfer and tennis player he has not played golf or tennis for several weeks, and he stopped seeing his friends. Physical examination is unremarkable. On mental status examination he describes his mood as OK. He denies any suicidal thoughts or plans. He denies visual or auditory

hallucinations. He is oriented to person, place, and time. He has difficulty subtracting serial 7s from 100 and he is unable to spell "world" backward.

40. A 30 year-old-woman comes to her doctor with a complaint of stomach pain for 2 weeks. She experiences the pain in her lower abdomen and describes it as a dull ache that is always there. It is not affected by food or antacids. In addition, she describes being unable to reach orgasm with sexual intercourse for the past 4 weeks and occasional tingling in her fingers. She has experienced no change in sleep or appetite, and her weight is unchanged. She has been calling in sick from work because of the discomfort. She has a 5-year history of multiple physical problems including headache, cardiac palpitations, backache, nausea, fatigue, and dyspepsia. Her physical examination on previous office visits has always been within normal limits. Abdominal, chest, and spinal radiographs have not revealed any pathology. A CT scan of her head 2 years ago was read as normal. ECG on three occasions has been normal. She has been prescribed paroxetine and alprazolam in the past but discontinued each after a few days because of side effects. Her blood pressure is 125/85, heart rate is 72, and temperature 37°C. She is 5 feet 6 inches tall and weighs 135 pounds. BMI is 21.8. Physical examination is unremarkable. She describes her mood as upset but appears relaxed and cheerful. There are no auditory or visual hallucinations. She is oriented to person, place, and time.

For each patient with hallucinations, select the most likely diagnosis.

    A. alcohol withdrawal delirium

    B. bipolar I disorder

    C. major depressive disorder

    D. posttraumatic stress disorder

    E. psychotic disorder due to a general medial condition

    F. schizoaffective disorder

    G. schizophrenia

    H. substance-induced psychotic disorder

41. A 50-year-old man comes to his internist complaining of hearing voices making derogatory comments for the past 2 weeks. The voices are soft, intermittent, and present most days. The man is a corporate executive who 6 months earlier became implicated in a widely publicized insider trading scandal. He has experienced difficulty falling asleep and a 10-pound weight loss. He denies any change in libido. He has continued to work approximately 60 hours a week and to maintain social obligations. Ten years ago he took alprazolam for insomnia for a 5-week period. Since then he has taken no prescription medications. He drank three to four glasses of scotch every night for 20 years but has had no alcohol for 4 weeks on the recommendation of his doctor. Physical examination reveals a blood pressure of 135/85, heart rate 72, and

temperature 37°C. On mental status examination he describes his mood as "hanging in there." He exhibits normal range and intensity of affect. Thoughts are logical and goal directed. He is alert and oriented to person, place, and time.

42. A 17-year-old man is brought by his father to the family doctor because of bizarre behavior over the past 6 months. Although he was formerly a good student and active in sports, his is now failing all of his classes and no longer spends time with friends. Six months ago he broke up with his girlfriend. He now stays home from school 2 to 3 days a week and spends hours on his computer. He keeps the shades down and curtains closed in his bedroom because he is afraid someone is watching him. He describes seeing devils in the corners of his room and asked his parents if they also see them. He has not experienced any change in appetite or sleep. He has smoked marijuana four times in the past year. His blood pressure is 115/70, heart rate is 60, and temperature 37°C. His physical examination is within normal limits. He describes his mood as good but appears emotionally blunted. His speech is frequently disrupted by long pauses; he sometimes forgets what he was saying. He denies auditory hallucinations. He is alert and oriented to person, place, and time.

For each patient with memory loss, select the most likely diagnosis.

   A. Alzheimer's disease
   B. amnestic disorder due to a general medical condition
   C. dissociative fugue disorder
   D. factitious disorder
   E. major depressive disorder
   F. schizophrenia
   G. social anxiety disorder
   H. substance-induced amnestic disorder

43. A 65-year-old woman comes with her husband to their family doctor for evaluation of memory problems over the last 3 months. She has been increasingly forgetful around the house and on numerous occasions has not been able to find her keys, her purse, or her checkbook. Her husband reports that she frequently does not remember events of the previous few days. Twice she has left stove burners turned on when she went to bed. She has been sleeping 10 hours per day for the last month. She complains of extreme lethargy and often complains of feeling cold. The woman has a history of bipolar disorder well managed with lithium for the past 20 years. She takes no other medications and she does not drink alcohol or use illicit drugs. Her blood pressure is 110/70, heart rate is 60. She is 5 feet 5 inches tall and weighs 175 pounds. BMI is 29.1. Pupils are 2 mm and reactive. Her hair is thin and dry. Deep tendon reflexes are diffusely decreased. She remembers one out of three objects after 5 minutes. She is

unable to do serial 7 subtractions. Laboratory studies show the following:

Lithium level	0.9
WBC	11,000
BUN	16
Creatinine	1.0
TSH	20

44. A 35-year-old woman is brought to an emergency department by police because of bizarre statements she made after she was arrested for shoplifting. After trying on expensive designer scarves in a department store, the woman walked out wearing one without paying for it. When questioned by police, she gave her name as Antoinette DuPlessis. The police confirmed that a woman by that name was living in the rooming house she gave as her address for the past 3 months. However, in her purse, the police found a driver's license with her photo giving her name as Madge Midley with an address in a city 500 miles away. The woman did not recognize the driver's license and couldn't remember ever being in that city. When they called the phone number listed for that address, a man answered who identified himself as the husband of Madge Midley. She had been missing for 3 months after leaving their home to buy groceries. An intense search had failed to turn up her whereabouts. The woman appears pleasant, personable, and forthcoming. She describes her mood as good. Her thoughts are logical and goal directed. She denies auditory or visual hallucinations. She is oriented to place and time and gives her name as Miss DuPlessis. She remembers three out of three objects after 5 minutes. She spells "world" forward and backward. She cannot remember where she was or what she was doing 4 months ago. She is uncertain of where she grew up or where she went to school.

For each patient with mood symptoms, select the most likely diagnosis.

A. adjustment disorder with depressed mood
B. bipolar disorder
C. dysthymia
D. major depressive disorder
E. mood disorder due to a general medical condition
F. schizoaffective disorder
G. substance-induced mood disorder

45. A 65-year-old man comes to an emergency department with his wife after she found him in their garage with a rope around his neck preparing to hang himself. She reports that he has not been himself for the last 2 months. He eats very little and frequently does not sleep through the night. About a month ago he stopped seeing friends and going to social events. Most of his time is spent sitting in a chair in his study. He often appears tearful and had recently been telling her he didn't think he could go on. Last week he reported for the first time hearing voices making derogatory and threatening comments. Six months ago he retired from his job with an accounting office where he had worked for 40 years. He has no previous psychiatric history. He has been treated for moderate hypertension for the past 6 years with stable doses of atenolol. He is 6 feet tall and weighs 155 pounds. BMI is 21. His blood pressure is 140/80, heart rate 64. The remainder of his physical examination is within normal limits. He is quietly crying through most of the interview and expresses regret that he did not succeed in killing himself. He states that his life is worthless and he sees no hope for the future. He acknowledges hearing a voice telling him to kill himself.

46. A 40-year-old woman comes to her doctor for a scheduled follow-up examination. Three years ago she was diagnosed with hepatitis C, and she has been treated with interferon alpha for the past 2 months. She now describes extreme fatigue, disinterest in all normal activities, and a constant low mood with frequent crying spells for the past month. She experiences multiple myalgias and arthralgias. The woman does not drink alcohol and has never used illicit drugs. She received a blood transfusion following the birth of her son 15 years ago. She has been divorced for 2 years after her husband revealed that he had been having an affair. She has worked as a freelance graphic artist, but she has not been able to do any work for the last month. On mental status examination she appears tired and withdrawn. She describes her mood as very blue and is teary-eyed during the interview. Her speech is slow and soft but articulate. She denies auditory or visual hallucinations. She is alert and oriented to person, place, and time. Laboratory studies reveal the following:

AST	65
ALT	75
Total bilirubin	0.5
GGTP	120
Leukocyte count	9.0
Hematocrit	39

For each patient with anxiety, select the most likely diagnosis.

    A. anxiety disorder due to a general medical condition

    B. delusional disorder

    C. generalized anxiety disorder

    D. major depressive disorder

    E. panic disorder

    F. schizophrenia

    G. separation anxiety disorder

    H. social anxiety disorder

    I. substance-induced anxiety disorder

47. A 45-year-old woman consults her doctor because of anxiety and insomnia over the past 2 weeks. She feels edgy, short of breath, and has a growing sense of dread and discomfort. These feelings are always present. She has difficulty falling asleep and she wakes several times during the night. Her appetite has decreased but she has not lost weight. For the past week she has left her job as a projects manager for a real estate developer shortly after noon because she could not concentrate. She has type 2 diabetes that has been well controlled with a stable dose of tolbutamide for the past 10 years. Five years ago she began taking clonazepam at night following the death of her father. She continued the medication until 1 month ago, when she discontinued because she thought it no longer necessary. On physical examination her blood pressure is 160/90, heart rate is 96. She is tremulous; deep tendon reflexes are diffusely increased. Pupils are 2 mm and reactive to light. She appears restless and describes her mood as anxious. She denies auditory or visual hallucinations. She is oriented to person, place, and time.

48. A 10-year-old girl is brought by her parents to a pediatrician because of difficulty in school attendance since the start of school 1 month ago. She frequently complains of stomach aches or headaches and insists that she stay home. When her parents let her stay home, she seems to be in normal health and in a good mood. When they have insisted on her going to school she resists, sometimes crying and saying she is too sick. Her teacher says she appears worried and distracted. The girl often asks to call home to make sure her mother is OK. Last summer the mother underwent surgery for breast cancer, followed by radiation therapy. The cancer is now in remission. The girl has been taking diphenhydramine for a month to help her sleep at night. Physical examination is unremarkable. On mental status examination she avoids eye contact. Her answers are mostly one or two words. She describes her mood as OK. She denies auditory or visual hallucinations.

For each person with suicidal thoughts, choose the most likely diagnosis.

- **A.** adjustment disorder with depressed mood
- **B.** antisocial personality disorder
- **C.** bipolar disorder
- **D.** borderline personality disorder
- **E.** delusional disorder
- **F.** dependent personality disorder
- **G.** major depressive disorder
- **H.** mood disorder due to a general medical condition
- **I.** panic disorder
- **J.** schizophrenia
- **K.** somatoform pain disorder
- **L.** substance-induced mood disorder

49. A 30-year-old G1 P1 woman brings her 1-month-old baby to her family medicine doctor for a scheduled well baby examination. When he tells her the baby is well and thriving, she says she doesn't know how that could be. He asks her how she has been feeling, and she acknowledges feeling very low for the past 2 weeks. She has trouble falling asleep and staying asleep. She has very little appetite and has lost 10 pounds since giving birth. She feels sorry for the baby because she knows she will be a terrible mother. The woman has a history of serious headaches occurring about once a month, for which she takes hydrocodone. The last headache was the month before giving birth. The doctor performs a physical examination on the mother and the results are unremarkable. She is tearful. For the past week she has heard a voice telling her she should take her life in order to spare the baby. She acknowledges thinking about suicide but denies any plans.

50. A 15-year-old boy is brought by his mother to an emergency department after she found him trying to hang himself from a light fixture in his bedroom. She describes changes in his behavior since the start of the school year 6 months ago. He has spent much more time by himself, and his schoolwork has deteriorated. Four months ago she found a bag of marijuana in his jacket pocket, but he denied knowing how it got there. For the past 2 weeks he has complained of hearing voices of people talking about him. He believes that someone is trying to control his thoughts through his computer. Physical examination reveals a blood pressure of 110/75, heart rate 60. Pupils are 2 mm and reactive, sclerae are white, and conjunctivae are clear. Retinal examination reveals no hemorrhages. There are abrasions around his neck. He states that he feels "empty," and he has a blank expression. His speech is disrupted by many pauses, and he frequently forgets what he was about to say. He acknowledges auditory hallucinations.

Table 1

Laboratory Values

Test	Reference Range
Blood, Plasma, Serum	
Alanine aminotransferase (ALT)	8–20 U/L
Amylase	25–125 U/L
Aspartate aminotransferase (AST)	8–20 U/L
Bilirubin, total	0.1–1.0 mg/dL
Calcium	8.4–10.2 mg/dL
Cholesterol	200 mg/dL
Creatine kinase: Female	10–70 U/L
Male	25–90 U/L
Creatinine	0.6–1.2 mg/dL

(continued)

Table 1	
Laboratory Values (Continued)	
Test	**Reference Range**
Electrolytes	
Sodium	136–145 mEq/L
Chloride	95–105 mEq/L
Potassium	3.5–5.0 mEq/L
Bicarbonate	22–28 mEq/L
Gamma-glutamyl transpeptidase (GGTP)	0–50 U/L
Glucose (fasting)	70–110 mg/dL
Lactate dehydrogenase (LDH)	45–90 U/L
Thyroid-stimulating hormone (TSH)	0.5–5.0 µU/mL
Thyroxine (T₄)	5–12 µg/dL
Blood urea nitrogen (BUN)	7–18 mg/dL
Hematologic erythrocyte count (RBC)	
Male	4.3–5.9 million/mm
Female	3.5–5.5 million/mm
Hematocrit	
Male	41%–53%
Female	36%–46%
Leukocyte count (WBC)	4500–11,000/mm
Platelet count	150,000–400,000/mm
Body Mass Index (BMI)	
Underweight	18.5
Normal weight	18.5–24.9
Overweight	25–29.9
Obesity	30

Answers and Explanations

1. **The answer is F: Schizophreniform disorder.** Although the emotional blunting, social withdrawal, and auditory hallucinations are characteristic of schizophrenia, the symptoms have not been present for at least 6 months, as is required for a diagnosis of schizophrenia. Consequently, the diagnosis must be (at least for now) schizophreniform disorder. Prominent auditory hallucinations are inconsistent with a diagnosis of delusional disorder and paranoid personality disorder. The negative physical findings, intact orientation, and unimpaired memory make medical or drug-related disorders less likely.

2. **The answer is E: Major depressive disorder.** The man meets diagnostic criteria for an episode of major depression, which require either a depressed mood or anhedonia: "...he doesn't seem to enjoy anything

anymore." His fatigue, sleep disturbance, concentration, and memory problems can all be explained by depression and it is not necessary to invoke another diagnosis such as chronic fatigue, primary insomnia, breathing-related sleep disorder, or Alzheimer's disease—any one of which would be inadequate to explain the full complement of symptoms he is experiencing. Dysthymia requires the presence of symptoms for 2 years. A glass of wine with most evening meals is unlikely to result in a clinical picture that suggests a major mood disorder.

3. **The answer is C: Dialectic behavioral therapy.** The impulsivity, self-destructive behavior, emotional lability, drug use, and the stormy romantic relationship all suggest borderline personality disorder. Dialectical behavioral therapy was developed specifically as a treatment for borderline personality disorder, and there is considerable empirical support for its efficacy. Her extreme emotionality would make cognitive therapy alone difficult, and there is little in the case to suggest benefit from family therapy. Diazepam therapy is not a good choice in someone already abusing drugs. Moreover, the disinhibition resulting from benzodiazepine intoxication could worsen the emotional lability and impulsive behavior. Disulfiram therapy will help only motivated drinkers to abstain. Quetiapine therapy may prove to be a useful adjunct, but there are no data to suggest that it is effective in the long term as the sole treatment of borderline personality disorder.

4. **The answer is C: Chlordiazepoxide therapy.** The altered level of consciousness, perceptual abnormalities, and disorientation describe a delirium. Given the laboratory data and physical findings, delirium tremens is a leading consideration. Because DTs are a medical emergency and potentially fatal, it is urgent to treat presumptively, even while continuing his work-up. The benzodiazepine chlordiazepoxide is cross-tolerant with alcohol and will stop the progression of symptoms. There is nothing in the history to suggest that physical restraints are necessary (he seems to be cooperating enough for blood to have been drawn and a physical examination performed.) Seclusion is contraindicated in someone with a rapidly evolving medical condition.

5. **The answer is D: Multiple sleep latency test.** Sudden attacks of sleep accompanied by sleep paralysis and hypnagogic hallucinations (hallucinations that occur while falling asleep) in a medically healthy person who is not abusing drugs are very likely narcolepsy. Of all the tests listed, only the multiple sleep latency test will help diagnose narcolepsy. An EEG performed at the time of his falling asleep would also be helpful (sleep-onset REM is diagnostic of narcolepsy), but the response as given does not make it clear that the test would be more than a standard waking EEG.

6. **The answer is D: Paroxetine.** A side effect of SSRIs such as paroxetine is prolonging the time to reach orgasm. This side effect is sometimes exploited in treating premature ejaculation, the condition described by this man. None of the other medications have similar

actions. (Sildenafil helps in achieving and maintaining an erection, but that does not seem to be the concern in this case.)

7. **The answer is E: Lamotrigine therapy.** The woman's daytime somnolence seems to be due to her psychiatric condition. Consequently, it is necessary to establish the diagnosis before recommending treatment. She describes periods of depression with physical symptoms and suicidal thoughts and periods of increased energy, decreased need for sleep, and increased productivity. Because the latter do not interfere with her functioning and do not include psychotic symptoms, they are hypomanic (not manic) episodes. The combination of major depressive and hypomanic episodes in a chronic relapsing clinical course indicates a bipolar II disorder. The treatment of choice for bipolar II depression is lamotrigine.

8. **The answer is E: Serotonin.** The checking behaviors that are interfering with the man's productivity and causing distress are compulsions. Obsessive-compulsive disorder is the presence of obsessions or compulsions or both. The appropriate medication therapy for OCD is an SSRI, a drug blocking presynaptic reuptake of serotonin. (Note that compulsions seem to respond to medication therapy better than obsessions, particularly when combined with cognitive-behavioral therapy.)

9. **The answer is C: Discontinue the haloperidol and add dantrolene.** Rigidity, obtundation, and high fever in the context of starting a typical antipsychotic represent neuroleptic malignant syndrome, a diagnosis supported by the elevated leukocyte count and creatine kinase. NMS is a medical emergency. All medications must be stopped, especially the offending antipsychotic. Dantrolene is a powerful peripheral muscle relaxant that will help to reverse the rigidity and decrease the creatine kinase and any myoglobinuria, thereby decreasing the likelihood of renal damage. Anticholinergic medication is ineffective in treating NMS. Switching from haloperidol to an atypical such as quetiapine may be useful but not until the NMS is under control. (All atypicals have the potential to cause NMS.)

10. **The answer is D: Major depressive disorder.** The woman meets criteria for a diagnosis of a major depressive episode. Although the history suggests that her depression is in response to the major change at work, a diagnosis of adjustment disorder is not made if the individual qualifies for another Axis I diagnosis such as major depressive disorder. Similarly, a diagnosis of bereavement is superseded by a diagnosis of major depression when symptoms become severe enough to qualify for the latter diagnosis. The weight loss appears to be caused by her depression and not a sign of an underlying medical illness. Her drinking a half bottle of wine at night began after the onset of mood symptoms, making a diagnosis of substance-induced mood disorder unlikely.

11. **The answer is C: Delusional disorder.** The single, prominent feature in this case is a delusion, which is clearly interfering with the woman's ability to function well. None of the personality disorders present

with elaborated delusions lasting 2 months. (Paranoid personality disorder describes an individual with pathologic levels of suspiciousness but not delusions.) A diagnosis of schizophrenia cannot be made without additional symptoms such as hallucinations, disorganized speech, or negative symptoms. Although bipolar disorder can certainly include paranoid delusions, there are no mood symptoms to justify that diagnosis. This woman's delusional belief is "nonbizarre," that is, something that could happen in real life, however unlikely. (A person with "bizarre" delusions cannot be diagnosed with delusional disorder.)

12. **The answer is F: Opiate withdrawal.** This woman presents with the signs and symptoms classically associated with opiate withdrawal: myalgias and arthralgias, dilated pupils, rhinorrhea, lacrimation, and muscle fasciculations with no perceptual disturbances and with a clear sensorium. There really is no other substance-related condition that this could be. A negative toxicology screen is expected in withdrawal states.

13. **The answer is C: Bulimia nervosa.** This young woman is suffering from an eating disorder that is affecting her grades and her self-image. The key to the diagnosis of bulimia nervosa is that the patient has discrete periods of overeating during which she experiences a feeling of lost control. Self-induced vomiting is not necessary for a diagnosis of bulimia, which has two subtypes—purging and nonpurging. Despite her heavy binge eating, she is able to maintain a normal weight through food restriction between binges. Consequently, she cannot be given a diagnosis of either anorexia nervosa or morbid obesity, both of which require abnormal weight. There are not sufficient mood symptoms present to warrant a diagnosis of either bipolar disorder or dysthymia.

14. **The answer is E: Modafinil therapy.** The only sleep abnormality this man experiences appears to be the amount of sleep he needs to feel rested—12 hours. He has no trouble falling asleep or staying asleep, and he does not feel excessive daytime drowsiness when he is able to sleep 12 or 13 hours per day. Because there is no information given suggesting that his need for sleep is caused by an underlying medical, psychiatric, or drug-related condition, the most likely diagnosis is primary hypersomnia. Of the treatments listed, only the antinarcolepsy drug modafinil will promote wakefulness. The drug atomoxetine is used to increase concentration and focus in ADHD, but it is not a stimulant and will not help keep a sleepy person awake. Continuous positive airway pressure is of no use in someone who does not have a breathing-related sleep disorder such as sleep apnea. A breathing-related sleep disorder would leave him feeling tired all the time no matter how many hours he slept. There are no data to suggest that psychotherapy alone can be helpful in primary hypersomnia.

15. **The answer is B: β-adrenergic.** β-Blockers such as propranolol are quite effective in controlling the peripheral manifestations of anxiety in situations such as stage fright, a form of social phobia. (CBT can also be useful, but this is not listed as a choice and it

would not be effective as quickly as needed here.) An advantage of β-blockers is that they do not cause sedation or impair performers' concentration, unlike benzodiazepines. (Benzodiazepines are GABA agonists; GABA is not listed as a possible choice.) Antipsychotics and antihistaminic drugs (D_2 and $5-HT_2$) might at best be somewhat sedating and are both poor choices. Anticholinergic drugs help control abnormal movements caused by antipsychotics, but that is not the issue in this case.

16. **The answer is D: Schizoaffective disorder.** Schizoaffective disorder, unlike schizophrenia, includes prominent mood symptoms. Unlike major depressive disorder with psychotic symptoms, schizoaffective disorder includes a period of at least 2 weeks during a given episode during which there are psychotic symptoms without mood symptoms. Nothing in the history, physical findings, or mental status examination suggests a substance-related disorder or a condition due to a general medical condition. The diagnosis of an adjustment disorder is not made if the patient meets criteria for another Axis I disorder.

17. **The answer is E: Electroconvulsive therapy (ECT).** There is no evidence of benefit from bupropion after 4 weeks. It is possible that continuing bupropion will eventually help, but the benefit is by no means certain and the clinical situation is dire. Switching to olanzapine should diminish the psychotic symptoms but is unlikely to help her depression. Switching to sertraline might help, but she has not benefited from two previous trials of an SSRI, and there might be several weeks' delay before any improvement would be seen. The woman is seriously depressed and at considerable risk for self-harm. Cognitive-behavioral therapy and psychodynamic psychotherapy are not indicated for patients with psychotic symptoms. Moreover, both therapies take some time to be helpful, even in a nonpsychotic patient. (CBT is most helpful with mild to moderate depression.) ECT is safe and relatively quick. It is indicated for major depression with psychotic symptoms.

18. **The answer is D: Obsessive-compulsive disorder.** The woman is experiencing both obsessions and compulsions. She had an episode of similar symptoms several years ago. The features of a personality disorder are nonepisodic, and a personality disorder is unlikely to explain her presenting symptoms. Her speech is loud and pressured, but there is nothing else to suggest bipolar disorder. The diagnosis of an adjustment disorder is not made if the person meets criteria for another Axis I disorder, as is the case here.

19. **The answer is D: Schizophrenia.** Although the woman was found with a wine bottle and although she has mildly elevated liver function tests, the diagnosis of a psychiatric condition is based solely on the signs, symptoms, and clinical course. (The duration of symptoms is unknown for this woman, but they appear to be long-standing given her living circumstances and personal hygiene.) The main consideration in the differential is between a thought disorder and a cognitive disorder such as delirium or dementia. An altered level of consciousness and disorientation are not described, making a delirium much less

likely. She recalls only two out of three objects at 5 minutes, but this is a fairly mild deficit compared with the degree of functional impairment. Her ability to read accurately, to hear and follow one-step commands, and her articulate speech all speak against a neurologic disorder. Her inability to make sense is most likely the result of a thought disorder. Disorganized speech and impaired ability to function in the absence of medical or neurologic impairment are evidence of schizophrenia, most likely of the disorganized subtype. (It is possible to diagnose schizophrenia in the absence of hallucinations.)

20. **The answer is C: Conversion disorder.** In conversion disorder, the patient presents with symptoms that suggest a neurologic or medical etiology, such as paralysis. The diagnosis is made when the physician has sufficient evidence that there is no physical explanation for the symptoms and that the patient is not voluntarily producing them. Conversion symptoms appear acutely and often follow an upsetting or stressful event, as was the case for this patient. A brief psychotic episode would involve bizarre delusions, hallucinations, or disordered thinking, which are not evident here. Somatization disorder is characterized by multiple neurologic, sexual, gastrointestinal, and pain symptoms. Hypochondriasis involves a preoccupation with or fear of illness and has a duration of at least 6 months. Although the patient's marijuana and alcohol use may be exacerbating an underlying mood disturbance, her use would not explain the current symptoms.

21. **The answer is B: Depersonalization disorder.** Depersonalization disorder is characterized by a sense of "unrealness" or being outside oneself. It often occurs in the context of stress, as in this patient, or as part of a primary psychotic or mood disorder. The patient does not have any of the core symptoms of either major depression or schizophrenia, making these diagnoses unlikely. Her presenting problems are acute rather than long-standing, which is inconsistent with a personality disorder. Her substance use does not explain the depersonalization phenomenon.

22. **The answer is B: Attention deficit/hyperactivity disorder.** This patient has symptoms consistent with the core features of ADHD, which are inattentiveness and hyperactivity. The symptoms of ADHD are usually evident by the age of 7 and occur in multiple settings, as with this patient. Both oppositional defiant disorder and conduct disorder can coexist with ADHD, sometimes making the diagnosis difficult. However, oppositional defiant disorder is diagnosed when there is a clear pattern of disruptive behaviors, rule breaking, and disregard for authority. Conduct disorder, a more extreme version of behavioral disturbance, always involves violation of the rights of others. (Children with conduct disorder are at high risk for future violent or criminal behavior.)

23. **The answer is D: Discontinue olanzapine, begin perphenazine.** The olanzapine should be discontinued because this patient is showing signs of metabolic syndrome, which puts her at significant risk for developing cardiovascular disease and diabetes. Signs of metabolic syndrome include central obesity, high glucose levels, elevated

triglyceride levels, and hypertension. The majority of atypical antipsychotics can cause metabolic syndrome; however, olanzapine and clozapine pose the greatest risk.. Perphenazine, a midpotency typical antipsychotic, is a good choice for this patient because it is less likely to cause weight gain or other metabolic changes. Topiramate is an anticonvulsant believed to have some mood-stabilizing properties and is associated with weight loss. It will not reverse a metabolic syndrome caused by olanzapine.

24. **The answer is D: Begin electroconvulsive therapy (ECT).** Although lithium appears to have worked well in the past in controlling bipolar disorder in this woman, there are two reasons why it is not the treatment of choice now. Lithium is teratogenic and poses a risk to the baby of heart and great vessel abnormalities when taken by the mother during the first trimester. (The risk is actually rather small—about one in a thousand—and the risk of treating must be weighed against the risk of not treating.) In addition, lithium will not be immediately effective; it might be necessary for her to take it for several weeks before the manic symptoms subside. ECT is both safer and faster. Carbamazepine, diazepam, and valproic acid all pose greater teratogenic risks than lithium. Cognitive-behavioral therapy will not improve psychotic symptoms. Prenatal counseling may be desirable, but it will do nothing for the woman's urgent psychiatric condition.

25. **The answer is F: Vaginismus.** Vaginismus is a condition in which the muscles of the vaginal wall involuntarily contract upon penetration, preventing sexual intercourse. It is often associated with a history of sexual abuse or trauma, but may be related to stresses associated with sexual intercourse. Dyspareunia simply refers to pain on intercourse. As this patient is able to achieve orgasm with manual stimulation, her symptoms cannot be considered an orgasmic disorder or a problem with arousal. In conversion disorder, the symptoms or deficits affect voluntary muscle or sensory deficits; in vaginismus the vaginal contractions are involuntary. The diagnosis of an adjustment disorder is not made when a patient meets criteria for another Axis I disorder.

26. **The answer is: B. Block β-adrenergic receptors.** The patient's description of feeling as if he is jumping out of his skin is called akathisia, a common EPS side effect of the high-potency typical antipsychotics. Akathisia is characterized by a subjective sense of restlessness and is usually experienced within days of starting an antipsychotic. The treatment of choice for akathisia is a β-blocker. Benzodiazepines, which bind to but do not block GABA receptors, can also be used to relieve the symptoms of akathisia. Anticholinergic medications are used to treat other EPSs caused by antipsychotics, but they are less effective in akathisia.

27. **The answer is A: Adjustment disorder with disturbance of conduct.** The sudden change in the boy's behavior began shortly after the change in his mother's schedule, suggesting that the change is in

response to her increasing absence. There is no evidence that this boy has problems with inattentiveness or impulsivity as seen in ADHD or that he shows a consistent pattern of rule breaking or violent behavior, which is more characteristic of ODD and conduct disorder. Dysthymia, when diagnosed in children, requires at least 1 year of depressed or irritable mood.

28. **The answer is A: Admit to a locked psychiatric inpatient unit.** Suicidality is a psychiatric emergency that often requires hospitalization. The psychiatric and medical seriousness of this attempt is in favor of hospitalization despite the man's attempt to minimize its significance. Furthermore, this patient has significant risk factors for suicide: a previous attempt, his increased age, widowhood, active alcohol use, and recent diagnosis of a serious illness. Amitriptyline or lithium therapy can be considered when the patient has been hospitalized. A home health aid worker who lacks professional training and does not have the backup resources of an inpatient unit should not be given responsibility for a seriously suicidal patient.

29. **The answer is F: Posttraumatic stress disorder.** Posttraumatic stress disorder occurs when a patient has experienced or witnessed an event that involved actual or threatened death or serious injury. This patient is describing symptoms that are characteristic of PTSD, including reexperiencing of the trauma (nightmares) and hyperarousal, demonstrated by his exaggerated startle response. PTSD can also be associated with irritability, impaired concentration, and moodiness, as this patient reports. Acute stress disorder is also associated with a traumatic event, but the symptoms are transient and experienced within 1 month of the trauma. Dysthymia and generalized anxiety disorder describe some of his symptoms but not the full symptom complex. Primary insomnia is not diagnosed when another psychiatric disorder is believed to be the cause of sleep disturbance.

30. **The answer is B: Autistic disorder.** The main distinction between autistic disorder and Asperger's disorder is the preservation of normal language in the latter. This girl's language is not normal for a 34-month-old child. She speaks only two-word sentences, repeats phrases said by others (echolalia), and does not initiate conversation. Her seeming indifference to other people is not typical of Down syndrome or expressive language disorder. The social and language deficits would not be seen in stereotypical movement disorder. Mood, thinking, and behavioral abnormalities that would justify a diagnosis of major depression, oppositional defiant disorder, or schizophrenia are not present. Schizophrenia in children, as with adults, requires the presence of psychotic symptoms at some point in the clinical course.

31. **The answer is B: Body dysmorphic disorder.** He seems to be doing pretty well in school and his social adjustment seems age appropriate. The only symptom is an exaggerated concern about a perceived physical deficit and a distorted sense of its impact on his life. He is not delusional because his belief is based on reality, although the conclusions he draws are grossly disproportionate. He does not have the

conviction of serious, undetected illness that would be seen in hypochondriasis or the multiple, changing, physical complaints over time seen in somatization disorder. The breakup with his girlfriend—"by mutual consent"—does not appear to have been particularly traumatic. He is not experiencing vegetative symptoms that would raise suspicion of major depression. The request for a "face transplant" is odd but not psychotic in a 15-year-old boy who is concerned about his physical appearance.

32. **The answer is D: Schizoid personality disorder.** The diagnosis of schizoid personality disorder describes people with few if any friends or social acquaintances, no desire to be with other people, and an indifference to the opinions of others. A person with avoidant personality disorder desires the company of others but avoids social situations out of fear of rejection or embarrassment. An individual with a social anxiety disorder also desires the company of others but feels overwhelming anxiety in social situations. Antisocial personality disorder describes people who violate the rights of others. There is no evidence that this man is unhappy in a way that would justify the diagnosis of dysthymia, and the absence of psychotic symptoms rules out the possibility of schizophrenia. It should be noted that the diagnosis of any personality disorder—as is true for all psychiatric disorders—requires the presence of distress or disability. In this case, his indifference is getting in the way of good work performance and evaluations. If he were happy and with no work difficulties, he could be diagnosed only with schizoid "traits."

33. **The answer is B: Cognitive behavioral therapy.** The treatment of choice for premature ejaculation is cognitive-behavioral therapy. It is one of the most easily treated of all sexual dysfunctions. He does not have difficulty with libido or in achieving erections. Accordingly, sildenafil or testosterone would not be indicated. Alprazolam therapy might make him more relaxed but would not provide consistent or predictable help with his sexual problem. Dialectical behavioral therapy is specifically indicated for borderline personality disorder. There are no data showing psychodynamic psychotherapy effective for premature ejaculation.

34. **The answer is B: Clonidine.** Clonidine, an α_2-agonist, is the only medication among those listed that reduces the signs and symptoms of opiate withdrawal. Naltrexone, an opiate antagonist that blocks the euphoric effects of opioid drugs, would not help and might make symptoms worse.

35. **The answer is A: Behavioral therapy.** Simple phobias such as a fear of dogs are among the most treatable of all psychiatric conditions. The treatment of choice is behavioral therapy, which neutralizes anxiety through exposure to the phobic stimulus. Treatments used in other anxiety disorders (buspirone for generalized anxiety disorder, group therapy for PTSD, paroxetine therapy for generalized social anxiety disorder) are not by themselves effective treatments for phobias. Psychodynamic psychotherapy and supportive psycho-

therapy may both be effective in reducing symptomatic anxiety in general but not in curing a simple phobia.

36. **The answer is B: Atomoxetine.** Treatment is predicated on diagnosis. His symptoms and mental status findings are most consistent with a diagnosis of attention deficit disorder. His good mood, normal sleep, and appetite make a mood disorder very unlikely. Moderate alcohol use does not cause the kinds of behaviors described here, and his occasional marijuana use does not correlate with the onset of symptoms. (Remember to accept as accurate reports of how much a person drinks or uses drugs when you are taking the shelf examination or step 2 of the boards.) No psychotic symptoms are described that would justify use of an antipsychotic such as risperidone. Atomoxetine is a nonstimulant drug used to treat ADHD. It is potentially hepatotoxic and is contraindicated in people with preexisting liver disease. This man's liver function tests are within normal limits.

37. **The answer is C: Generalized anxiety disorder.** Depression and anxiety can both interfere with sleep, and the distinction between major depressive disorder and generalized anxiety disorder may be difficult in clinical practice. In this case, criteria for generalized anxiety disorder are met, those for depression are not. (Keep in mind that major depression can be diagnosed in the absence of a significant mood component if there is anhedonia.) The manic phase of bipolar disorder typically results in a decreased need for sleep in which there is no fatigue. There is no suggestion that the man's sleep would be restful and restorative if he altered his sleep hours, as would be true in circadian rhythm sleep disturbance. "Parasomnia" refers to abnormal phenomena such as sleep walking or bruxism that occur in the context of otherwise normal sleep. Alcohol can cause rebound insomnia, but it is unlikely that one or two glasses of wine with the evening meal would be enough to cause this level of disturbance. Primary insomnia is diagnosed only when there is no evidence of a psychiatric or medical condition causing the sleep disturbance.

38. **The answer is B: Circadian rhythm sleep disturbance.** Unlike the man in case 37, this woman does get good sleep when she is able to alter her sleep hours (getting up at noon rather than 6:30 A.M.). There is no evidence of a medical, drug-related, or psychiatric problem contributing to her sleep difficulties. Her experience with zolpidem is typical of people with circadian rhythm problems. At best the medication may help the person fall asleep, but it is usually not enough to keep the individual asleep for the entire night.

39. **The answer is E: Major depressive disorder.** This man's aches and pains are part of a larger symptom complex (including insomnia, fatigue, decreased appetite with weight loss, and social withdrawal) most characteristic of major depression. Somatization disorder and somatoform pain disorder present with physical symptoms but without the associated symptoms seen here. The pain is not caused by opioid withdrawal because it began before he started taking hydrocodone. He does not express a preoccupation with having serious illness

that would be required in hypochondriasis. "Mood disorder due to a general medical condition" is not included among the possible answers, but good clinical practice would mandate ruling out an underlying physical illness in this case.

40. **The answer is I: Somatization disorder.** Multiple, changing physical complaints over a long period of time for which no physical basis can be found are best described by the diagnosis of somatization disorder. In somatoform pain disorder, the only complaint would be pain. A patient with body dysmorphic disorder would be preoccupied by an imaginary or exaggerated physical defect but would not come in repeatedly with different physical complaints. Hypochondriasis describes worry about having a serious medical illness, not having multiple physical symptoms to which no particular meaning is ascribed.

41. **The answer is H: Substance-induced psychotic disorder.** Alcohol withdrawal results in two syndromes with psychotic symptoms. The major withdrawal syndrome—delirium tremens—typically occurs several days after the last drink; it always includes alterations in the level of consciousness along with other mental status abnormalities such as disorientation and evidence of autonomic instability on physical examination: elevated temperature, blood pressure, and heart rate; diaphoresis; increased deep tendon reflexes; and tremulousness. Alternatively, some chronically heavy drinkers experience auditory hallucinations days to weeks after the last drink, occurring in a clear sensorium without other ancillary physical or mental status findings. This is sometimes referred to as "alcohol hallucinosis" and is classified in DSM-IV-TR as a substance-induced psychotic disorder. This man's continuing productivity (60-hour work weeks) and the absence of mood symptoms make major depression unlikely. He does not seem to reexperience the traumatic event through nightmares or daytime flashbacks, and he has no symptoms of hyperarousal as would be seen in posttraumatic stress disorder.

42. **The answer is G: Schizophrenia.** A diagnosis of schizophrenia is high on the differential of a 17-year-old man who experiences hallucinations, emotional blunting, and disorganized speech after a 6-month period of social withdrawal and declining school performance. A drug-related or general medical condition would have to be investigated, but no information to support either of those diagnoses is presented here. (Marijuana can cause psychotic symptoms but typically with very heavy use and not simply four times in the past year.) The 6-month clinical course rules out a brief psychotic episode (maximum duration of symptoms is 1 month), and the absence of pronounced mood symptoms makes major depression and schizoaffective disorder very unlikely.

43. **The answer is B: Amnestic disorder due to a general medical condition.** Not all memory impairment in elderly people is Alzheimer's. This woman is suffering from hypothyroidism, as made clear by the elevated TSH and supported by the findings on her physical examination (thin,

dry hair and decreased deep tendon reflexes). The dementia caused by hypothyroidism is usually reversible with the administration of thyroid hormone. (Her long-standing treatment for bipolar disorder raises the suspicion of thyroid damage caused by lithium.)

44. **The answer is C: Dissociative fugue disorder.** The mental status examination reveals no current memory deficits. What this woman has lost is all memory pertaining to her personal life before a particular date. In addition, she suddenly and unexpectedly left home, justifying a diagnosis of dissociative fugue. Although the assumption of a new identify (as here) is possible, it is in fact not common in dissociative fugue. A diagnosis of factitious disorder requires evidence of purposeful fabrication of signs or symptoms, which is not present here. Social anxiety disorder describes fearfulness of some social situations but not a broad loss of memory.

45. **The answer is D: Major depressive disorder.** A 2-month history of vegetative symptoms, serious mood symptoms, suicidality, and the recent onset of auditory hallucinations is best explained by a diagnosis of major depressive disorder. In schizoaffective disorder, the hallucinations would have to be present for at least a 2-week period during which there were no mood symptoms. A diagnosis of dysthymia requires symptoms to be present for at least 2 years. Atenolol can cause depression (although usually not this severe), but his dose has been unchanged for 6 years, making a substance-related depression extremely unlikely. The normal findings on physical examination do not support a diagnosis of depression due to a general medical condition. As before, however, a thorough assessment must include evaluation of possibly undetected physical disease.

46. **The answer is G: Substance-induced mood disorder.** One of the serious potential side effects of the antiviral medication interferon is depression, sometimes serious enough to cause suicidality. Depression accompanied by fatigue, myalgias, and arthralgias in the context of starting interferon therapy is most likely due to the drug. Hepatitis can cause depression, but she was first diagnosed 3 years ago, and the mood symptoms began abruptly 1 month ago just after she started interferon. The diagnosis of an adjustment disorder is not made if the person meets diagnostic criteria for another Axis I disorder, as is the case here.

47. **The answer is I: Substance-induced anxiety disorder.** Psychiatric symptoms accompanied by pronounced physical signs should always lead to the suspicion of an underlying medical or drug-related cause. The only information we are given about her medical status is that she has type 2 diabetes that has been well controlled for many years, an unlikely cause of her current anxiety and insomnia. On the other hand, she was taking the benzodiazepine clonazepam for 5 years before stopping a month ago. Clonazepam has a long half-life—up to 4 days. It is common for symptoms of withdrawal from clonazepam to appear several days after stopping the drug. Her blood pressure, heart rate, increased deep tendon reflexes, and

tremulousness are all consistent with benzodiazepine withdrawal, although more severe than is usually seen.

48. **The answer is G: Separation anxiety disorder.** The refusal to go to school is a common form of separation anxiety disorder in school-age children. Her physical complaints, her worry about her mother's well-being when the girl is at school, and her normal health and good mood when she does stay home are all consistent with that diagnosis. The diagnosis of social anxiety disorder in children requires the presence of symptoms for 6 months (not 1 month as here). More important, the anxiety in social anxiety disorder is focused on scrutiny by others, not on concern about the safety of parents. Generalized anxiety disorder would result in excessive worry in all situations, not just school.

49. **The answer is G: Major depressive disorder.** DSM-IV-TR classifies post-partum depression as major depressive disorder with postpartum onset; even if there have not been previous episodes of depression. Childbirth is not considered a general medical condition. An adjustment disorder is not diagnosed if criteria for another Axis I disorder are met. Hydrocodone last taken 2 months ago would not be sufficient to account for her current state. The woman is experiencing auditory hallucinations. Psychotic symptoms are compatible with a diagnosis of major depression, and schizophrenia is not diagnosed when psychotic symptoms occur only during an episode of major mood symptoms.

50. **The answer is J: Schizophrenia.** The onset of psychotic symptoms in a previously healthy 15-year-old boy will always raise the suspicion of substance use or an underlying medical condition. Although his mother found marijuana in his jacket 4 months ago, he does not have signs of intoxication on his physical examination, and it is unlikely that marijuana alone would account for his overall 6-month clinical course. Similarly, there are no symptoms or physical findings that would make a medical condition the leading diagnosis. Although suicidality cannot be used in making the diagnosis, it is worth remembering that the risk of suicide in people with schizophrenia is 15 times greater than that in the general population.

A Table of Medications Used in Psychiatry

DILLON EULER

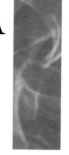

Antipsychotic Medications

Drug Class/Pharmacology	Agents	Indications/ Contraindications	Adverse Effects and Toxicities
Typical Antipsychotics Mechanism of action: Antagonism at dopamine D2 receptors Therapeutic efficacy against *positive symptoms* (delusions, hallucinations) is believed due to D2 blockade in **mesolimbic** dopamine pathway. D2 blockade in other dopamine tracts causes "typical" side effect profile: • **Nigrostriatal** blockade yields EPSs • **Tuberoinfundibular** blockade causes hyperprolactinemia • **Mesocortical** blockade worsens *negative symptoms* (alogia, avolition) and *cognitive symptoms* (poor attention and vigilance)	**High Potency** *haloperidol (Haldol)* PO, IM, and depot IM (decanoate) forms available *fluphenazine (Prolixin)* PO, IM, and depot IM (decanoate) forms available *pimozide (Orap)* *thiothixene (Navane)* *trifluoperazine (Stelazine)* **Midpotency** *perphenazine (Trilafon)* PO, IM forms available *molindone (Moban)* *loxapine (Loxitane)*	√ Psychotic disorders, including: • Schizophrenia • Schizoaffective disorder • Brief psychotic disorder • Substance- and medication-induced psychosis √ Psychotic symptoms in mood disorders: • Major depression with psychotic features • Acute manic, depressed, and mixed manic states of bipolar disorder √ Tourette's disorder √ Huntington's disorder	**Adverse Effects:** Extrapyramidal symptoms (EPSs), including: • Akathisia, intense restlessness and anxiety, which can be treated with anticholinergics, β-blockers, or benzodiazepines • Dystonic reactions, painful muscle spasms usually involving extremities, neck, and ocular muscles, which can be treated with PO or IM anticholinergic agents • *Parkinsonism,* including tremor, bradykinesia, masked facies, festinating gait, and cogwheeling rigidity, which can also be treated with anticholinergics, dopaminergic agents (amantadine), or β-blockers Hyperprolactinemia, with associated gynecomastia and impotence in males, amenorrhea in females Sedation Weight gain Anticholinergic side effects, including dry mouth, constipation, blurry vision, urinary retention, confusion, ECG changes Orthostatic hypotension Decreased seizure threshold (more in low-potency agents) Sexual dysfunction Dermatologic effects, including dermatitis and photosensitivity

Typical antipsychotics also block muscarinic, α-adrenergic, and histamine-1 receptors.

All agents are equal in efficacy and are grouped by potency, which predicts their side effect profiles:

High-potency agents cause worse EPSs

Low-potency agents cause more anticholinergic, antihistaminergic, and antiadrenergic side effects

Midpotency agents have a balanced profile

Atypical Antipsychotics
Mechanism of action: antagonism at dopamine D2 receptors and serotonin 2A receptors

Low Potency
chlorpromazine (Thorazine)
Highly sedating
Significant hypotension and anticholinergic effects, but low EPSs

mesoridazine (Serentil)

thioridazine (Mellaril)
Least EPSs of all typicals
Significant QT prolongation; at doses >800 mg/day, retinitis pigmentosa

clozapine (Clozaril)
Wide antagonism at 5HT2A, D1, D2, D4, H1, muscarinic, and α1 receptors
Most efficacious

√ Typical antipsychotic indications
√ Treatment-refractory schizophrenia
√ Schizophrenia concurrent with tardive dyskinesia

Serious Adverse Effects:
Tardive dyskinesia, involuntary choreoathetoid movements of face, neck, trunk, and extremities, which is often permanent and can be grossly debilitating.

Neuroleptic malignant syndrome, life-threatening condition of hyperpyrexia, autonomic instability, muscle rigidity, and delirium. Although uncommon, it can occur with all antipsychotics.

Sedation
Anticholinergic side effects, including dry mouth, constipation, blurry vision, urinary retention, confusion
ECG changes
Orthostatic hypotension
Weight gain, which can be substantial

(continued)
√ = indications (Includes FDA approved indications and common evidence-based off-label uses)
X = contradications (Includes both absolute and relative contraindications)

Antipsychotic Medications *(continued)*

Drug Class/Pharmacology	Agents	Indications/ Contraindications	Adverse Effects and Toxicities
Therapeutic efficacy against *positive symptoms* (delusions, hallucinations) is due to D2 blockade in **mesolimbic** dopamine pathway.	antipsychotic	X Granulocytopenia X Diabetes/hyperlipidemias	Hypersalivation Seizures, especially with high doses or fast titrations Metabolic problems, including diabetes and hyperlipidemias **Serious Adverse Effects** Agranulocytosis, necessitating frequent WBC monitoring
Dopamine transmission is normally *suppressed* by serotonin transmission in the mesocortical, nigrostriatal, and tuberoinfundibular dopamine tracts. Thus, serotonin 2A blockade enhances dopamine transmission, mitigating "typical" side effects.	*risperidone (Risperdal/ Consta/M-tabs)* Antagonist at 5HT2A, D2, and α1 receptors PO, dissolvable tab, and depot IM forms available	√ Typical antipsychotic indications √ Acute mania	Orthostatic hypotension, reflex tachycardia, and dizziness Insomnia Agitation Weight gain Hyperprolactinemia At higher dosages (above 6 mg daily), EPSs may develop Metabolic problems

Atypical antipsychotics also block muscarinic, α-adrenergic, and histamine-1 receptors to varying degrees.

Compared with typicals, atypicals cause higher rates of metabolic problems—hyperglycemia, type II diabetes, and hyperlipidemias—but have a lower incidence of tardive dyskinesia, neuroleptic malignant syndrome, and EPSs, with the exception of risperidone. Risk of metabolic syndrome appears greatest for olanzapine and clozapine.

Drug	Indications / Contraindications	Side effects
olanzapine (Zyprexa, Zydis) Like clozapine, wide antagonism at 5HT2A, D1, D2, D4, H1, muscarinic, and α1 receptors PO and dissolvable tab forms available Among atypicals, may have efficacy second only to clozapine	√ Typical antipsychotic indications √ Acute mania √ Bipolar maintenance X Diabetes/hyperlipidemias	Anticholinergic side effects, including dry mouth, constipation, blurry vision, urinary retention, confusion, ECG changes Orthostatic hypotension and dizziness Sedation Weight gain, which can be substantial Hyperglycemia, type 2 diabetes, diabetic ketoacidosis Hyperlipidemias
quetiapine (Seroquel) Antagonist at 5HT2A, D2, α1 and 2, and H1 receptors	√ Typical antipsychotic indications √ Acute mania	Orthostatic hypotension and dizziness Sedation Weight gain Metabolic problems

(continued)

√ = indications (Includes FDA approved indications and common evidence-based off-label uses)

X = contradications (Includes both absolute and relative contraindications)

Antipsychotic Medications (continued)

Drug Class/Pharmacology	Agents	Indications/ Contraindications	Adverse Effects and Toxicities
All atypicals (with the exception of clozapine) have recently won indications for acute mania; olanzapine and aripiprazole are indicated for prophylaxis of recurrent mania, or *bipolar maintenance.*	*ziprasidone (Geodon)* Antagonist at 5HT1A and 2A, D2, D3 receptors, and monoamine (NE, 5HT, DA) reuptake pumps PO and fast-acting IM forms available	√ Typical antipsychotic indications √ Acute mania	Sedation Weight gain, to lesser extent than clozapine, olanzapine, and risperidone Metabolic problems, including diabetes and hyperlipidemias, probably at a lower rate than olanzapine and clozapine Possible increased risk for prolongation of QT interval
	aripiprazole (Abilify) Antagonist at 5HT2A, partial agonist at D2 and 5HT1A	√ Typical antipsychotic indications √ Acute mania √ Bipolar maintenance	Sedation Weight gain, to lesser extent than clozapine, olanzapine, and risperidone Metabolic problems

Antidepressant Medications

Drug Class/Pharmacology	Agents	Indications/ Contraindications	Adverse Effects and Toxicities
Tricyclic Antidepressants (TCAs) Proposed mechanism of action: antagonism at dopamine (DA), serotonin (5HT), and norepinephrine (NE) presynaptic reuptake pumps. Mechanism is not precisely understood. It has been postulated to involve receptor and downstream second messenger and gene transcription changes. Tricyclic antidepressants also block muscarinic, α-adrenergic, and histamine-1 receptors.	**Tertiary Amines** *amitriptyline (Elavil)* Wide use for pain, headache and insomnia *clomipramine (Anafranil)* Highly serotonergic, indicated for OCD *doxepin (Sinequan)* Used for pain, insomnia, and anxiety *trimipramine (Surmontil)*	√ Major depressive disorder √ Bipolar depression √ Dysthymia √ Panic disorder √ Generalized social phobia √ Generalized anxiety disorder √ Obsessive-compulsive disorder (OCD) (clomipramine) √ Pain disorders (migraines/ neuralgias) X Cardiac conduction delays X Arrhythmias	**Adverse Effects** Anticholinergic side effects, including dry mouth, constipation, blurry vision, urinary retention, confusion, ECG changes Sedation Weight gain Orthostatic hypotension Sexual dysfunction—erectile dysfunction and delayed ejaculation in men, anorgasmia in women Mania in bipolar patients Seizures (rare) **Serious Adverse Effects** *Cardiotoxicity:* TCAs slow cardiac conduction, potentially causing ECG changes, arrhythmias, and A√ block *Neurotoxicity:* tremor and ataxia; in overdose, agitation, delirium, coma, and death.

(continued)

√ = indications (Includes FDA approved indications and common evidence-based off-label uses)

X = contraindications (Includes both absolute and relative contraindications)

Antidepressant Medications *(continued)*

Drug Class/Pharmacology	Agents	Indications/Contraindications	Adverse Effects and Toxicities
Therapeutic effect begins only after 3–4 weeks of administration. Variable in efficacy for several mood and anxiety disorders, tricyclic antidepressants are grouped by amine configuration, which predicts side effect profile: • *Tertiary amines* have greater α, histamine-1, and muscarinic blockade • Newer, *secondary amines,* have fewer side effects, are less sedating, and are safer in overdose	*imipramine (Tofranil)* Useful for panic, enuresis **Secondary amines** *desipramine (Norpramin)* Demethylated imipramine Least anticholinergic *nortriptyline (Pamelor)* Demethylated amitriptyline Least orthostasis		

Tricyclic antidepressants can be *lethal in overdose* and carry substantial adverse effects. Therapeutic blood monitoring is commonly performed.

protriptyline (Vivactil)

Monoamine Oxidase Inhibitors (MAOIs)

Proposed mechanism of action: these drugs are irreversible MAOIs. MAO metabolizes monoamines (5HT, DA, NE) in the presynaptic neuron; MAO inhibition, then, disables monoamine degradation.

All available MAOIs block both MAO_A and MAO_B, though only MAO_A blockade is necessary for the antidepressant effect.

MAOIs also block alpha-1

phenelzine (Nardil)

tranylcypromine (Parnate)

√ Major depressive disorder
√ Atypical depression
√ Panic disorder
√ Social phobia
√ OCD

X Coadministration with:
    Demerol
    Another antidepressant,
        (especially SSRIs)
    Sympathomimetic drugs
    Dietary tyramine

Orthostatic hypotension may be severe and may require support stockings, hydration, and increased salt intake.
Weight gain
Sexual dysfunction
Insomnia
Myoclonus, muscle pains, and paresthesias
Mania

Serious Adverse Effects

Tyramine-induced hypertensive crisis
Patients taking MAOIs must be put on low-tyramine diet. Common sources of tyramine are aged cheese, fava beans, and liver. Tyramine is normally broken down in the GI tract by MAO_A. In MAOI patients, it gets into the blood stream undigested and acts as a false transmitter in adrenergic

(continued)

√ = indications (Includes FDA approved indications and common evidence-based off-label uses)
X = contraindications (Includes both absolute and relative contraindications)

Antidepressant Medications (continued)

Drug Class/Pharmacology	Agents	Indications/ Contraindications	Adverse Effects and Toxicities
			pathways. It can precipitate a sudden, catastrophic rise in blood pressure. Many cold medications and pain killers can precipitate a similar crisis.
			Note, minimal to no anticholinergic side effects
Selective Serotonin Reuptake Inhibitors (SSRIs) Proposed mechanism of action: selective antagonism at serotonin (5HT) presynaptic reuptake pumps. Site of action thought to be frontal serotonin projection. As with TCAs, therapeutic effect begins only after 3–4 weeks of administration.	*fluoxetine (Prozac, Sarafem, Prozac Weekly)* Longest half-life Efficacy in bulimia *paroxetine (Paxil, Paxil CR)* More sedating than fluoxetine and sertraline	√ Major depressive disorder √ Premenstrual dysphoric disorder (PMDD) √ PTSD √ Bulimia √ Panic disorder √ Social phobia √ OCD X Coadministration with MAOIs	**Serotonergic side effects,** due to overstimulation of various 5HT receptors widely distributed through the body. By receptor, • $5HT_3$—GI system; overstimulation leads to *diarrhea, nausea, and vomiting* • $5HT_{2C}$—central nervous system (CNS); overstimulation leads to *anxiety* and *mental agitation* • $5HT_{2A}$—CNS, spinal cord; overstimulation leads to *anxiety and mental agitation, akathisia, insomnia, myoclonus,* and *sexual dysfunction* Weight gain Mania *Serotonin discontinuation syndrome,* consisting of headache, dizziness, irritability, and fatigue upon abrupt discontinuation

Safe, well tolerated, and widely indicated, SSRIs heralded a new era in pharmacologic treatment of mood and anxiety disorders.

fluvoxamine (Luvox)
Indicated for OCD

citalopram (Celexa)

escitalopram (Lexapro)

Serious Adverse Effects

Serotonin syndrome, associated with hyperthermia, myoclonus, autonomic instability, rigidity, coma, and death, possible with coadministration of SSRI and MAOI. MAOI washout of 2 weeks necessary prior to initiation of SSRI treatment.

Serotonin and Norepinephrine Reuptake Inhibitors (SNRIs)
Proposed mechanism of action: selective antagonism at norepinephrine (NE) and serotonin (5HT) presynaptic reuptake pumps.

No α, histamine-1, or muscarinic blockade, thus avoiding many side effects typical of TCAs.

venlafaxine (Effexor)
Suggested to have superior efficacy for depression among all new antidepressants

duloxetine (Cymbalta)
Nausea common
Also approved for diabetic neuropathy

√ Major depressive disorder
√ Generalized anxiety disorder
√ Panic disorder
√ Generalized social phobia

X Coadministration with MAOIs

Tremor
Agitation
Tachycardia
Hypertension
Diarrhea, nausea, and vomiting
Anxiety and mental agitation
Akathisia
Insomnia
Myoclonus
Sexual dysfunction
Seizures (rare)
Mania

(continued)
√ = indications (Includes FDA approved indications and common evidence-based off-label uses)
X = contraindications (Includes both absolute and relative contraindications)

Antidepressant Medications (*continued*)

Drug Class/Pharmacology	Agents	Indications/ Contraindications	Adverse Effects and Toxicities
Has additional dopamine reuptake inhibition at higher dosages, yielding a curvilinear dose response.			Discontinuation syndrome, consisting of headache, dizziness, irritability, and fatigue upon abrupt discontinuation
Noradrenergic and Specific Serotonergic Antidepressants (NaSSAs) Proposed dual mechanism of action: 1. Antagonism at central α2 autoreceptors (and subsequent disinhibition of NE and 5HT release) 2. Stimulation of α1 somatodendritic receptors on serotonin neurons, boosting 5HT release	*mirtazapine (Remeron)* Also blocks 5HT2A, 2C, 3 and H1 receptor	√ Major depressive disorder X Coadministration with MAOIs	**Adverse Effects** Sedation (significant, often used as sleep aid) Increased appetite and weight gain **Serious Adverse Effects** Agranulocytosis and other blood dyscrasias

Serotonin Antagonists and Reuptake Inhibitors (SARIs)
Proposed mechanism of action: selective antagonism at serotonin (5HT) presynaptic reuptake pumps with simultaneous 5HT2A blockade.

trazodone (Desyrel)

nefazodone (Serzone)

√ Major depressive disorder
√ Dysthymia

X Coadministration with MAOIs

Sedation
Nausea
Dizziness
Mania

Serious Adverse Effects:
Trazodone: priapism (rare)
Nefazodone: liver toxicity (black box warning)

*Note, due to 5HT2A blockade, sexual dysfunction is avoided

Noradrenergic and Dopamine Reuptake Inhibitors
Proposed mechanism of action: antagonism of presynaptic norepinephrine and dopamine reuptake pumps.

bupropion (Wellbutrin, Zyban)

√ Major depressive disorder
√ Dysthymia
√ Bipolar depression
√ ADHD
√ Smoking cessation

X Coadministration with MAOIs
X Anorexia nervosa
X Bulimia nervosa
X Seizure disorder

Activation
Insomnia
Nausea
Tremor

Serious Adverse Effects:
Seizures at higher doses

(continued)

√ = indications (Includes FDA approved indications and common evidence-based off-label uses)
X = contradications (Includes both absolute and relative contraindications)

Sedative-Hypnotic Medications

Drug Class/Pharmacology	Agents	Indications/ Contraindications	Adverse Effects and Toxicities
Benzodiazepines Mechanism of action: full agonism at benzodiazepine binding site on GABA$_A$ receptor. Binding potentiates GABA by causing increased frequency of chloride channel openings. Grouped in terms of: 1. *Potency* (the higher the more efficacious and addictive), and 2. *Half-life* (the shorter the more rapid in onset and addictive) Benzodiazepines are *cross tolerant* with alcohol and barbiturates, allowing their use in detoxification in sedative and alcohol addiction.	**Short half-life (in order of decreasing potency)** *alprazolam (Xanax),* Highly addictive, but very effective for panic *lorazepam (Ativan)* Available in PO, IM, and IV forms Widely used *oxazepam (Serax)* *temazepam (Restoril)* Effective short-term sleep aid	√ Generalized anxiety disorder √ Situational anxiety/phobias √ Panic disorder √ Epilepsy √ Muscle spasms √ Akathisia √ Alcohol withdrawal √ Agitation √ Anxiety associated with other psychiatric disorders X Substance dependence	Drowsiness Dizziness and ataxia Cognitive impairments and/or amnesia Tolerance Dependence Withdrawal symptoms that are common include anxiety, insomnia, restlessness, agitation, irritability, and muscle tension. As with alcohol, benzodiazepine withdrawal can be potentially life threatening. Dose-related sedation can progress to hypnosis and coma. Owing to their high therapeutic index, benzodiazepines are generally not lethal in overdose but can be in cases of preexistent cardiopulmonary compromise or when mixed with other sedatives or alcohol. Benzodiazepine overdose can be counteracted with flumazenil, a benzodiazepine antagonist.

Mainstay of treatment for a variety of anxiety disorders since the 1960s due to increased safety profile, better tolerability, and less addictive potential than previous sedatives.

*Note lorazepam, oxazepam, and temazepam are not metabolized in the liver, but are glucuronidated throughout the body, making them safe to use in liver disease

Long half-life (in order of decreasing potency)

clonazepam (Klonopin)

diazepam (Valium)
Fast onset but with active metabolite

chlordiazepoxide (Librium)
Alcohol detoxification

Nonbenzodiazepine Sedatives
Of various forms and mechanisms, generally are nonaddictive.

Prototypical agent of choice for agents listed.

buspirone (BuSpar)
5HT1A agonist, effective in anxiety via unclear mechanism

Onset of action at least 2 weeks

√ Generalized anxiety disorder
√ Adjunctive use in major depressive disorder

Dizziness
Headache
Fatigue
GI distress

*Note, does not have sedation or addictive potential of benzodiazepines

(continued)

√ = indications (Includes FDA approved indications and common evidence-based off-label uses)
X = contradications (Includes both absolute and relative contraindications)

Sedative-Hypnotic Medications (continued)

Drug Class/Pharmacology	Agents	Indications/Contraindications	Adverse Effects and Toxicities
	hydroxyzine (Atarax, Vistaril) Sedating antihistamine	√ Situational anxiety	Sedation and weight gain Anticholinergic side effects
Nonbenzodiazepine Hypnotics Although not benzodiazepines, all but diphenhydramine and ramelteon are GABAergic. Zolpidem and zaleplon yield progressive tolerance and dependence.	zolpidem (Ambien) GABAergic	√ Insomnia	Dizziness Nausea Vomiting GI distress
	zaleplon (Sonata) GABAergic Short-acting, can dose in middle of night	√ Insomnia	Dizziness Dyspepsia
Primary insomnia is less common than secondary insomnia. Treatment of insomnia should address possible underlying medical or psychiatric etiologies and employ sleep hygiene techniques.	eszopiclone (Lunesta) GABAergic Suggested not to yield tolerance	√ Insomnia	Headache

diphenhydramine (Benadryl) Sedating antihistamine	√ Insomnia		Sedation Weight gain Anticholinergic side effects
ramelteon (Rozarem) Agonist at melatonin MT-1 and MT-2 receptors, thought to normalize circadian rhythms	√ Insomnia		Dizziness Fatigue
Propranolol (Inderal) β-Adrenergic blocker	√ Performance anxiety	X Asthma	Dizziness Fatigue Bradycardia and hypotension

(continued)

√ = indications (Includes FDA approved indications and common evidence-based off-label uses)

X = contraindications (Includes both absolute and relative contraindications)

Mood-Stabilizing Medications

Drug Class/Pharmacology	Agents	Indications/Contraindications	Adverse Effects and Toxicities
Mood Stabilizers—Lithium Mechanism of action: unknown; theories posit that its effect is in modulation of second messenger systems, leading to changes in signal transduction, downstream enzymes, or gene expression. Lithium is not metabolized in the liver but is cleared almost entirely by the kidney.	*lithium (Eskalith, Lithobid)*	√ Bipolar I disorder, especially euphoric mania √ Bipolar II disorder √ Bipolar maintenance √ Intermittent explosive disorder √ Adjunct to antidepressants ✗ Pregnant women—can cause Ebstein's anomaly, abnormality of the great vessels ✗ Caution with thiazide diuretics, ACE inhibitors, and NSAIDs, all of which can raise lithium levels	**Adverse Effects** GI irritation Polyuria, polydipsia, nephrogenic diabetes insipidus Tremor, subtle incoordination, cognitive blunting Benign leukocytosis Weight gain **Serious Adverse Effects** *Lithium toxicity,* a serious concern given lithium's low therapeutic index, causes nausea, diarrhea, vomiting, oliguria, ataxia, coarse tremor, increased DTRs, obtundation, seizure, and death Thyrotoxicity Long-term nephrotoxicity Cardiac arrhythmias and T-wave flattening Lithium's toxicity profile necessitates periodic therapeutic blood monitoring and thyroid and kidney function testing.

Mood Stabilizers—Anticonvulsants

Mechanism of action: unknown; theoretical mechanisms vary by agent.

Of all anticonvulsants, carbamazepine and valproic acid have the most established evidence in treating mania.

Lately, many other anticonvulsants have been tried off-label in mania with varying degrees of success.

Carbamazepine (Tegretol)
Has effects at Na/K channels, possibly enhances GABA

√ Bipolar I disorder, especially mixed mania and rapid cycling
√ Bipolar II disorder
√ Epilepsy and neuralgias
√ Alcohol withdrawal

X Pregnant women—can cause craniofacial abnormalities such as cleft lip and palate, neural tube defects, and learning disorders

Adverse Effects
Nausea, vomiting, diarrhea
Sedation, lightheadedness, tremor
Cognitive blunting
Electrolyte abnormalities, including hyponatremia
Anticholinergic side effects
Rash, which may progress to Stevens-Johnson syndrome
Weight gain

Serious Adverse Effects
Blood dyscrasias (aplastic anemia, agranulocytosis, thrombocytopenia)
Hepatotoxicity

Overdose can lead to coarse tremor, coma, and death.

Carbamazepine's toxicity profile necessitates periodic therapeutic blood
monitoring and blood count, liver, and metabolic function testing.

Valproic acid (Depakene/Depakote)
Inhibits Na/Ca channels, thereby

√ Bipolar I disorder, especially mixed mania and rapid cycling
√ Bipolar II disorder
√ Epilepsy and neuralgias

Adverse Effects
Nausea, vomiting, diarrhea
Sedation, lightheadedness, tremor
Cognitive blunting

(continued)

√ = indications (Includes FDA approved indications and common evidence-based off-label uses)
X = contraindications (Includes both absolute and relative contraindications)

Mood-Stabilizing Medications *(continued)*

Drug Class/Pharmacology	Agents	Indications/ Contraindications	Adverse Effects and Toxicities
	boosting GABA and decreasing glutamate (It is not known whether this is the mechanism that provides mood-stabilizing properties.) Can be rapidly loaded for quicker therapeutic effect	√ Alcohol withdrawal X Pregnant women—can cause neural tube defects, to a greater degree than carbamazepine X Childbearing age women—can cause polycystic ovaries	Weight gain Hair loss **Serious Adverse Effects** Thrombocytopenia Hemorrhagic pancreatitis Hepatotoxicity Polycystic ovaries Overdose can lead to coarse tremor, coma, and death. Valproic acid's toxicity profile necessitates periodic therapeutic blood monitoring and blood count, liver and pancreatic function testing.
	oxcarbazepine (Trileptal) Has effects at Na/K/Ca channels, possibly enhances GABA Structurally related to carbamazepine	√ Bipolar I disorder, adjunctive treatment √ Epilepsy and neuralgias	Nausea, vomiting, diarrhea Sedation, lightheadedness, tremor Cognitive blunting Rash Compared with carbamazepine, oxcarbazepine has much less potential for hematologic, dermatologic, and hepatotoxicity. Therapeutic blood monitoring is not necessary.

lamotrigine (Lamictal)
Has effects at Na channels, possibly inhibits glutamate
Unique efficacy in bipolar depression

√ Bipolar depression
√ Bipolar maintenance
√ Epilepsy and neuralgias
X Caution when administered with valproic acid (due to boosted blood levels)

Nausea, vomiting, diarrhea
Sedation, lightheadedness, tremor
Cognitive blunting
Weight gain

Serious Adverse Effects
Rash (common), may progress to Stevens-Johnson syndrome

gabapentin (Neurontin)
GABAergic, excreted renally
Ineffective as monotherapy for mania
Also off-label use in GAD and social anxiety

√ Bipolar I disorder, adjunctive treatment
√ Epilepsy and neuralgias
X Caution in renal disease

Sedation, lightheadedness, tremor
Nausea, vomiting, diarrhea

topiramate (Topamax)
Ineffective as monotherapy for mania

√ Bipolar I disorder, adjunctive treatment
√ Epilepsy and neuralgias

Sedation, lightheadedness, cognitive dulling
Nausea
Nephrolithiasis
Anorexia and weight loss

(continued)
√ = indications (Includes FDA approved indications and common evidence-based off-label uses)
X = contraindications (Includes both absolute and relative contraindications)

Drugs Used to Promote Attention and Wakefulness

Drug Class/Pharmacology	Agents	Indications/ Contraindications	Adverse Effects and Toxicities
Central Nervous System Stimulants Mechanism of action: stimulation of α- and β-adrenergic receptors triggering release of dopamine and norepinephrine from presynaptic terminals	*methylphenidate (Ritalin)*; both regular and sustained release	√ Attention deficit disorder √ Narcolepsy	**Adverse Effects** Anxiety Insomnia Anorexia Tachycardia
	methylphenidate extended release (Concerta, Metadate CD, Metadate ER)	X Coadministration with MAOIs X Narrow angle glaucoma	
	dexmethylphenidate (Focalin); both regular and extended-release		**Serious Adverse Effects** Drug dependence Hypertension Cardiac arrhythmias Cardiovascular collapse (rare)
	dextroamphetamine (Dexedrine)		
	amphetamine/dextro-amphetamine (Adderall) Both regular and extended release		
	pemoline (Cylert)		

Novel CNS Stimulants
Mechanism of action is
unclear; not adrenergic
agonists

modafinil (Provigil)

√ Narcolepsy
√ Attention deficit disorder
√ Primary and secondary
  hypersomnia

X Coadministration with MAOIs

Headache
Nausea
Rhinitis
Anxiety
Insomnia

Mechanism of action is
unclear. May be related to
selective inhibition of
presynaptic reuptake of
norepinephrine

atomoxetine (Strattera)

√ Attention deficit disorder
X Coadministration with MAOIs
X Narrow angle glaucoma

Adverse Effects
Dyspepsia
Nausea, vomiting
Anorexia
Dizziness
Insomnia
Sexual dysfunctions

Serious Adverse Effects
Suicidal ideation (black box warning)
Severe liver injury

√ = indications (Includes FDA approved indications and common evidence-based off-label uses)
X = contradictions (Includes both absolute and relative contraindications)

463

Scale for the Assessment of Negative Symptoms (SANS) *

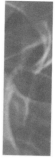

0 = None 1 = Questionable 2 = Mild 3 = Moderate 4 = Marked
5 = Severe

Affective Flattening or Blunting

1. *Unchanging Facial Expression*   0 1 2 3 4 5
   The patient's face appears wooden, changes less than expected as emotional content of discourse changes.

2. *Decreased Spontaneous Movements*   0 1 2 3 4 5
   The patient shows few or no spontaneous movements, does not shift position, move extremities, etc.

3. *Paucity of Expressive Gestures*   0 1 2 3 4 5
   The patient does not use hand gestures, body position, etc., as an aid to expressing his ideas.

4. *Poor Eye Contact*   0 1 2 3 4 5
   The patient avoids eye contact or "stares through" interviewer even when speaking.

5. *Affective Nonresponsivity*   0 1 2 3 4 5
   The patient fails to smile or laugh when prompted.

6. *Lack of Vocal Inflections*   0 1 2 3 4 5
   The patient fails to show normal vocal emphasis patterns, is often monotonic.

7. *Global Rating of Affective Flattening*   0 1 2 3 4 5
   This rating should focus on overall severity of symptoms, especially unresponsiveness, eye contact, facial expression, and vocal inflections.

Alogia

8. *Poverty of Speech*   0 1 2 3 4 5
   The patient's replies to questions are restricted in amount and tend to be brief, concrete, and unelaborated.

---

*Available from Nancy C. Andreasen, MD, PhD, Department of Psychiatry, College of Medicine, The University of Iowa, Iowa City, IA 52242. Copyright 1984 Nancy C. Andreasen. Reprinted with permission.

9. *Poverty of Content of Speech*   0 1 2 3 4 5
   The patient's replies are adequate in amount but tend to be
   vague, overconcrete, or overgeneralized and convey little
   information.

10. *Blocking*   0 1 2 3 4 5
    The patient indicates, either spontaneously or with prompting,
    that his train of thought was interrupted.

11. *Increased Latency of Response*   0 1 2 3 4 5
    The patient takes a long time to reply to questions; prompting
    indicates the patient is aware of the question.

12. *Global Rating of Alogia*   0 1 2 3 4 5
    The core features of alogia are poverty of speech and poverty of
    content.

Avolition-Apathy

13. *Grooming and Hygiene*   0 1 2 3 4 5
    The patient's clothes may be sloppy or soiled, and he may have
    greasy hair, body odor, etc.

14. *Impersistence at Work or School*   0 1 2 3 4 5
    The patient has difficulty seeking or maintaining employment,
    completing school work, keeping house, etc. If an inpatient,
    cannot persist at ward activities, such as occupational therapy and
    playing cards.

15. *Physical Anergia*   0 1 2 3 4 5
    The patient tends to be physically inert. He may sit for hours and
    does not initiate spontaneous activity.

16. *Global Rating of Avolition-Apathy*   0 1 2 3 4 5
    Strong weight may be given to one or two prominent symptoms if
    particularly striking.

Anhedonia-Asociality

17. *Recreational Interests and Activities*   0 1 2 3 4 5
    The patient may have few or no interests. Both the quality and
    quantity of interests should be taken into account.

18. *Sexual Activity*   0 1 2 3 4 5
    The patient may show a decrease in sexual interest and activity or
    in enjoyment when active.

19. *Ability to Feel Intimacy and Closeness*   0 1 2 3 4 5
    The patient may display an inability to form close or intimate
    relationships, especially with the opposite sex and family.

20. *Relationships with Friends and Peers*   0 1 2 3 4 5
    The patient may have few or no friends and may prefer to spend
    all of his time isolated.

21. *Global Rating of Anhedonia-Asociality*   0 1 2 3 4 5
    This rating should reflect overall severity, taking into account the
    patient's age, family status, etc.

Attention

22. *Social Inattentiveness*   0 1 2 3 4 5
    The patient appears uninvolved or unengaged. He may seem
    spacey.

23. *Inattentiveness during Mental Status Testing*   0 1 2 3 4 5
     Tests of "serial 7s" (at least five subtractions) and spelling
     "world."
     backward: Score: 2 = one error; 3 = two errors; 4 = three errors.
24. *Global Rating of Attention*   0 1 2 3 4 5
     This rating should assess the patient's overall concentration,
     clinically and on tests.

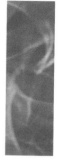

Scale for the Assessment of Positive Symptoms (SAPS)*

0 = None 1 = Questionable 2 = Mild 3 = Moderate 4 = Marked 5 = Severe

Hallucinations

1. *Auditory Hallucinations*   0 1 2 3 4 5
   The patient reports voices, noises, or other sounds that no one else hears.

2. *Voices Commenting*   0 1 2 3 4 5
   The patient reports a voice which makes a running commentary on his behavior or thoughts.

3. *Voices Conversing*   0 1 2 3 4 5
   The patient reports hearing two or more voices conversing.

4. *Somatic or Tactile Hallucinations*   0 1 2 3 4 5
   The patient reports experiencing peculiar physical sensations in the body.

5. *Olfactory Hallucinations*   0 1 2 3 4 5
   The patient reports experiencing unusual smells which no one else notices.

6. *Visual Hallucinations*   0 1 2 3 4 5
   The patient sees shapes or people that are not actually present.

7. *Global Rating of Hallucinations*   0 1 2 3 4 5
   This rating should be based on the duration and severity of the hallucinations and their effects on the patient's life.

Delusions

8. *Persecutory Delusions*   0 1 2 3 4 5
   The patient believes he is being conspired against or persecuted in some way.

---

*Available from Nancy C. Andreasen, MD, PhD, Department of Psychiatry, College of Medicine, The University of Iowa, Iowa City, IA 52242. Copyright 1984 Nancy C. Andreasen. Reprinted with permission.

9. *Delusions of Jealousy*   0 1 2 3 4 5
The patient believes his spouse is having an affair with someone.

10. *Delusions of Guilt or Sin*   0 1 2 3 4 5
The patient believes that he has committed some terrible sin or done something unforgivable.

11. *Grandiose Delusions*   0 1 2 3 4 5
The patient believes he has special powers or abilities.

12. *Religious Delusions*   0 1 2 3 4 5
The patient is preoccupied with false beliefs of a religious nature.

13. *Somatic Delusions*   0 1 2 3 4 5
The patient believes that somehow his body is diseased, abnormal, or changed.

14. *Delusions of Reference*   0 1 2 3 4 5
The patient believes that insignificant remarks or events refer to him or have some special meaning.

15. *Delusions of Being Controlled*   0 1 2 3 4 5
The patient feels that his feelings or actions are controlled by some outside force.

16. *Delusions of Mind Reading*   0 1 2 3 4 5
The patient feels that people can read his mind or know his thoughts.

17. *Thought Broadcasting*   0 1 2 3 4 5
The patient believes that his thoughts are broadcast so that he himself or others can hear them.

18. *Thought Insertion*   0 1 2 3 4 5
The patient believes that thoughts that are not his own have been inserted into his mind.

19. *Thought Withdrawal*   0 1 2 3 4 5
The patient believes that thoughts have been taken away from his mind.

20. *Global Rating of Delusions*   0 1 2 3 4 5
This rating should be based on the duration and persistence of the delusions and their effect on the patient's life.

Bizarre Behavior

21. *Clothing and Appearance*   0 1 2 3 4 5
The patient dresses in an unusual manner or does other strange things to alter his appearance.

22. *Social and Sexual Behavior*   0 1 2 3 4 5
The patient may do things considered inappropriate according to usual social norms (e.g., masturbating in public).

23. *Aggressive and Agitated Behavior*   0 1 2 3 4 5
The patient may behave in an aggressive, agitated manner, often unpredictably.

24. *Repetitive or Stereotyped Behavior*   0 1 2 3 4 5
The patient develops a set of repetitive actions or rituals that he must perform over and over.

25. *Global Rating of Bizarre Behavior*   0 1 2 3 4 5
This rating should reflect the type of behavior and the extent to which it deviates from social norms.

Positive Formal Thought Disorder

26. *Derailment*   0 1 2 3 4 5
A pattern of speech in which ideas slip off track onto ideas obliquely related or unrelated.

27. *Tangentiality*   0 1 2 3 4 5
Replying to a question in an oblique or irrelevant manner.

28. *Incoherence*   0 1 2 3 4 5
A pattern of speech which is essentially incomprehensible at times.

29. *Illogicality*   0 1 2 3 4 5
A pattern of speech in which conclusions are reached which do not follow logically.

30. *Circumstantiality*   0 1 2 3 4 5
A pattern of speech which is very indirect and delayed in reaching its goal idea.

31. *Pressure of Speech*   0 1 2 3 4 5
The patient's speech is rapid and difficult to interrupt; the amount of speech produced is greater than that considered normal.

32. *Distractible Speech*   0 1 2 3 4 5
The patient is distracted by nearby stimuli which interrupt his flow of speech.

33. *Clanging*   0 1 2 3 4 5
A pattern of speech in which sounds rather than meaningful relationships govern word choice.

34. *Global Rating of Positive Formal Thought Disorder*   0 1 2 3 4 5
This rating should reflect the frequency of abnormality and degree to which it affects the patient's ability to communicate.

Inappropriate Affect

35. *Inappropriate Affect*   0 1 2 3 4 5
The patient's affect is inappropriate or incongruous, not simply flat or blunted.

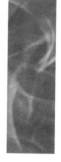

Hamilton Rating Scale for Depression*

For each item select the "cue" which best characterizes the patient.

1: Depressed Mood (Sadness, hopelessness, helplessness, worthlessness)
- 0   Absent
- 1   These feeling states indicated only on questioning
- 2   These feeling states spontaneously reported verbally
- 3   Communicates feeling states nonverbally—e.g., through facial expression, posture, voice, and tendency to weep
- 4   Patient reports VIRTUALLY ONLY these feeling states in his spontaneous verbal and nonverbal communication

2: Feelings of Guilt
- 0   Absent
- 1   Self-reproach, feels he has let people down
- 2   Ideas of guilt or rumination over past errors or sinful deeds
- 3   Present illness is a punishment; delusions of guilt
- 4   Hears accusatory or denunciatory voices and/or experiences threatening visual hallucinations

3: Suicide
- 0   Absent
- 1   Feels life is not worth living
- 2   Wishes he were dead or any thoughts of possible death to self
- 3   Suicide ideas or gesture
- 4   Attempts at suicide (any serious attempt rates 4)

4: Insomnia (Early)
- 0   No difficulty falling asleep
- 1   Complains of occasional difficulty falling asleep—i.e., more than 1/4 hour
- 2   Complains of difficulty falling asleep every night

*Reprinted with permission from Hamilton M. A rating scale for depression. J Neurol Neurosurg Psychiatry 1960;23:56–62.

5: Insomnia (Middle)
  0   No difficulty
  1   Patient complains of being restless and disturbed during the night
  2   Waking during the night—any getting out of bed (except for purpose of voiding) rates 2

6: Insomnia (Late)
  0   No difficulty
  1   Waking in early hours of the morning but goes back to sleep
  2   Unable to fall asleep again if gets out of bed

7: Work and Activities
  0   No difficulty
  1   Thoughts and feelings of incapacity, fatigue, or weakness related to activities, work, or hobbies
  2   Loss of interest in activity, hobbies, or work—either directly reported by patient, or indirect in listlessness, indecision, and vacillation (feels he has to push self to work or activities)
  3   Decrease in actual time spent in activities or decrease in productivity. In hospital, rate 3 if patient does not spend at least 3 hours a day in activities (hospital job or hobbies) exclusive of ward chores
  4   Stopped working because of present illness. In hospital, rate 4 if patient engages in no activities except ward chores, or if patient fails to perform ward chores unassisted

8: Retardation (Slowness of thought and speech; impaired ability to concentrate; decreased motor activity)
  0   Normal speech and thought
  1   Slight retardation at interview
  2   Obvious retardation at interview
  3   Interview difficult
  4   Complete stupor

9: Agitation
  0   None
  1   "Playing with" hands, hair, etc.
  2   Hand wringing, nail biting, hair pulling, biting of lips

10: Anxiety (Psychic)
  0   No difficulty
  1   Subjective tension and irritability
  2   Worrying about minor matters
  3   Apprehensive attitude apparent in face or speech
  4   Fears expressed without questioning

Hamilton Rating Scale

11: Anxiety (Somatic) (Physiologic concomitants of anxiety*)

0	Absent	*Gastrointestinal—dry mouth, wind, indigestion, diarrhea, cramps, belching
1	Mild	Cardiovascular—palpitations, headaches
2	Moderate	Respiratory—hyperventilation, sighing
3	Severe	Urinary frequency
4	Sweating	Incapacitating

12: Somatic Symptoms—Gastrointestinal

0   None
1   Loss of appetite but eating without staff encouragement; heavy feelings in abdomen
2   Difficulty eating without staff urging; requests or requires laxatives or medication for bowels or medication for GI symptoms

13: Somatic Symptoms—General

0   None
1   Heaviness in limbs, back, or head; backaches, headache, muscle aches
2   Loss of energy and fatigability
3   Any clear-cut symptom rates 2

14: Genital Symptoms (Such as loss of libido, menstrual disturbances)

0   Absent
1   Mild
2   Severe

15: Hypochondriasis

0   Not present
1   Self-absorption (bodily)
2   Preoccupation with health
3   Frequent complaints, requests for help, etc.
4   Hypochondriacal delusions

16: Loss of Weight

A: WHEN RATING BY HISTORY
    0   No weight loss
    1   Probable weight loss associated with present illness
    2   Definite (according to patient) weight loss
B: ON WEEKLY RATINGS BY WARD PSYCHIATRIST, WHEN ACTUAL WEIGHT CHANGES ARE MEASURED
    0   Less than 1 lb weight loss in 1 week
    1   Greater than 1 lb weight loss in 1 week
    2   Greater than 2 lb weight loss in 1 week

Hamilton Rating Scale

17: Insight
   0   Acknowledges being depressed and ill
   1   Acknowledges illness but attributes cause to bad food, climate, overwork, virus, need for rest, etc.
   2   Denies being ill at all

18: Diurnal Variation*

AM	PM		
0	0	Absent	*If symptoms are worse in the
1	1	Mild	morning or evening, note which
2	2	Severe	it is and rate severity of variation

19: Depersonalization and Derealization (Such as feelings of unreality, nihilistic ideas)
   0   Absent
   1   Mild
   2   Moderate
   3   Severe
   4   Incapacitating

20: Paranoid Symptoms
   0   None
   1   Suspiciousness
   2   Ideas of reference
   3   Delusions of reference and persecution

21: Obsessional and Compulsive Symptoms
   0   Absent
   1   Mild
   2   Severe

22: Helplessness
   0   Not present
   1   Subjective feelings which are elicited only by inquiry
   2   Patient volunteers his helpless feelings
   3   Requires urging, guidance, and reassurance to accomplish ward chores or personal hygiene
   4   Requires physical assistance for dress, grooming, eating, bedside tasks, or personal hygiene

23: Hopelessness
   0   Not present
   1   Intermittently doubts that "things will improve" but can be reassured
   2   Consistently feels "hopeless" but accepts reassurance
   3   Expresses feelings of discouragement, despair, pessimism about future, which cannot be dispelled
   4   Spontaneously and inappropriately perseverates "I'll never get well" or its equivalent

Hamilton Rating Scale

24: Worthlessness (Ranges from mild loss of esteem, feelings of inferiority, self-depreciation to delusional notions of worthlessness)
- 0 Not present
- 1 Indicates feelings of worthlessness (loss of self-esteem) only on questioning
- 2 Spontaneously indicates feelings of worthlessness (loss of self-esteem)
- 3 Different from 2 by degree. Patient volunteers that he is "no good," "inferior," etc.
- 4 Delusional notions of worthlessness—e.g., "I am a heap of garbage" or its equivalent

Index

Note: Page numbers followed by the letter b refer to boxed material. Page numbers followed by the letter f refer to figures, and those followed by t refer to tables.

Domestic violence, outpatient triage for, 28, 31
Donepezil (Aricept), for Alzheimer's disease, 277, 278t, 278–280
Dopamine
depression and, 182
in ADHD, 355
in medication-induced movement disorders, 383
Dopamine agonist/reuptake inhibitors, 452–453
for neuroleptic malignant syndrome, 387
Double depression, 185–186
Down syndrome
diagnostic timing of, 373
mental retardation versus, 373
typical physical features of, 373, 375f
Doxepin (Sinequan), 447
Drug addiction
as matter of control, 250
description of, 249
in somatoform disorders, 346
Drug dependence, 249
on sedative-hypnotics, 149
treatment of, 260, 261
Drug-induced hallucinations, 87, 88t, 89
toxicology screens for, 90
treatment of, 92
Drug-induced mood disturbances, 107, 108t
evaluation of, 110
Drug rehabilitation, detoxification versus, 258
Drug-related diagnoses
DSM-IV-TR coding of, 66
Drug tolerance
of benzodiazepines, 307
of sedative-hypnotics, 149
Drug toxicity
in ADHD, 356
of carbamazepine, 214
of lithium, 213, 214t
prevention of, 213
of valproate, 213
Drug withdrawal, 249
case studies, 263
delirium associated with, 266, 267t
evaluation of, 267
hallucinations caused by, 88t, 90–91
treatment of, 92
patient assessment for, 253
signs and symptoms of, 253f, 254f, 255t
treatment of, 258, 259, 260
Dual agency, in forensic psychiatry, 59
Dual diagnosis, in substance use disorders, 262
Duloxetine (Cymbalta), 451
for depression, 188, 189t
Dyspareunia, 318t, 320
medical work-up for, 320t

Dysthymia
depression associated with, 185–186
treatment of, 198
in children and adolescents, 363
Dystonia, medication-induced, 381, 382t
classic arising of, 381
tardive, 381, 382–383
treatment of, 385–386

E

Eating disorders
amenorrhea in, 298
anorexic, 295
body weight changes in, 161, 298
bulimic, 295
case studies, 303–304
definitions of, 295
etiology of, 296t
evaluation of, 162, 296
factitious, 161
laboratory abnormalities in, 299, 300t
medical or drug-related conditions in, 301
obesity as, 296
personality type in, 296t, 298
physical findings in, 298, 299f, 300t
prevalence of, 295, 296
prognosis for, 303
psychiatric conditions in, 297
self-induced vomiting in, 307
sex differences in, 295, 296
symptoms of, 296–297
treatment of, 301
clinical settings for, 301, 302t
drugs for, 302
goals of, 301
psychotherapy for, 302
Education
for caregivers, of Alzheimer's patients, 280
in group therapy, 8t
Egosyntonic symptoms, in personality disorders, 284
Elderly patients
cognitive decline in, 126–127, 128
depression in, 181
SSRIs for, 193
Electrocardiogram (ECG)
baseline, for lithium therapy, 212
for dissociative fugue, 334
for severe weight loss, 162
Electroconvulsive therapy (ECT), 194
dangers of, 195
depression indications, 194, 194–195t
electrode placement for, 195, 196f, 197f
for appetite changes, 162–163
for bipolar disorders, 218
for pregnant patient, 393
postpartum indications, 396
for psychiatric disorders, 19–20